# Case Studies in Hypertension

# Case Studies in Hypertension

Editor: Ayla Rose

AMERICAN
MEDICAL PUBLISHERS
www.americanmedicalpublishers.com

AMERICAN
MEDICAL PUBLISHERS
www.americanmedicalpublishers.com

**Cataloging-in-Publication Data**

Case studies in hypertension / edited by Ayla Rose.
p. cm.
Includes bibliographical references and index.
ISBN 979-8-88740-604-6
1. Hypertension. 2. Hypertension--Treatment. I. Rose, Ayla.
RC685.H8 H96 2023
616.132--dc23



American Medical Publishers,
41 Flatbush Avenue,
1st Floor, New York,
NY 11217, USA

ISBN 979-8-88740-604-6 (Hardback)

# Contents

# Preface

Hypertension refers to a long-term medical condition wherein the blood pressure (BP) of an individual is higher than normal. Informally, it is known as high blood pressure. It usually has no symptoms but it can increase the risk of serious health conditions such as heart disease and stroke. Blood pressure is a vital body parameter. The overall blood pressure is measured with the help of two components, namely systolic and diastolic pressure. The pressure in blood vessels when the heart contracts is known as systolic, whereas pressure in blood vessels when the heart is at rest is called diastolic. The normal BP is 120/80 and BP less than 130/80 with or without comorbidities is medically recommended. A BP that lies in the range of 130-139/80-89, is called as stage 1 hypertension. It can be used to make diagnostic and treatment decisions based on multiple high quality BP measurements. The case studies included in this book will serve as an excellent guide to develop a comprehensive understanding about hypertension and to help develop a better understanding of the latest advances in its diagnosis and management. It will provide comprehensive knowledge to the readers.

This book unites the global concepts and researches in an organized manner for a comprehensive understanding of the subject. It is a ripe text for all researchers, students, scientists or anyone else who is interested in acquiring a better knowledge of this dynamic field.

I extend my sincere thanks to the contributors for such eloquent research chapters. Finally, I thank my family for being a source of support and help.

**Editor**

# 1

# Management of Pulmonary Artery Aneurysms in Pulmonary Hypertension: A Single-Center Review of 3 Cases

**Talha Ahmed,[1] Gautam V. Ramani,[2] Mehrdad Ghoreishi,[3] Ayesha Safdar,[4] and Bartley P. Griffith[3]**

[1]*Department of Medicine, University of Maryland Midtown Campus, USA*
[2]*Department of Medicine, University of Maryland, USA*
[3]*Department of Surgery, University of Maryland, USA*
[4]*Army Medical College, Pakistan*

Correspondence should be addressed to Talha Ahmed; atalha858@yahoo.com

Academic Editor: Ertugrul Ercan

Pulmonary artery aneurysms (PAAs) are defined as having pulmonary artery diameter of greater than 40 mm. PAAs are rare and can occur in various pulmonary diseases. There are no clear-cut guidelines regarding the management of PAAs, and recommendations for management are made based on expert consensus opinion, case reports, and institutional experience. This series highlights three patients with pulmonary hypertension (PH) and PAA. The clinical course and diagnostic findings and the decision-making involved in the treatment are reviewed. An overview of three distinct management strategies including medical management, heart/lung transplant, and surgical aneurysm repair is presented.

## 1. Case 1

A 51-year-old female with long-standing pulmonary hypertension (PH) on sildenafil, suspected to be pulmonary arterial hypertension (PAH) with known prior history of pulmonary artery aneurysm (PAA) but was lost to follow-up, presented to the hospital with hemoptysis. She suffered from profound anxiety and often missed appointments due to fear of leaving the home. Computerized tomography (CT) scan of the chest showed an aneurysm of the main pulmonary artery (PA) measuring 85 mm in diameter with an intimal flap concerning for pulmonary artery dissection (Figure 1(a)). Transthoracic echocardiogram (TTE) revealed a hypertrophied, moderately dilated, and dysfunctional right ventricle (RV) with an estimated right ventricular systolic pressure (RVSP) of 78 mmHg and severe dilation of main PA compatible with severe PH (Figures 1(b) and 1(c)). Due to the massive size of the PAA with suspected dissection, PA catheterization was deferred. She was evaluated for lung and lung/heart transplant but was not deemed a suitable candidate due to her significant psychiatric history. Her risks of surgical or percutaneous repair were felt to be prohibitive due to the degree of PH and RV dysfunction. A decision was made to manage her medically, and she was started on intravenous treprostinil which was rapidly uptitrated. This was done as a palliative measure for symptomatic improvement of her PH which was suspected to be most likely idiopathic as well as the fact that the case posed limited diagnostic and therapeutic evaluation. Her functional status improved after a few months of parenteral treprostinil from WHO Functional Class (FC) III to FC II. Routine follow-up studies including 6-minute walk test (6MWT), pulmonary function tests (PFTs), and repeat TTE were not performed primarily due to patient anxiety. She was found deceased on the ground three years after the hospital admission most likely as a complication of PAA rupture, though no autopsy was performed.

## 2. Case 2

A 57-year-old female with a long-standing history of fibrocystic sarcoidosis developed PH 18 years following her initial diagnosis. A CT scan of the chest revealed findings

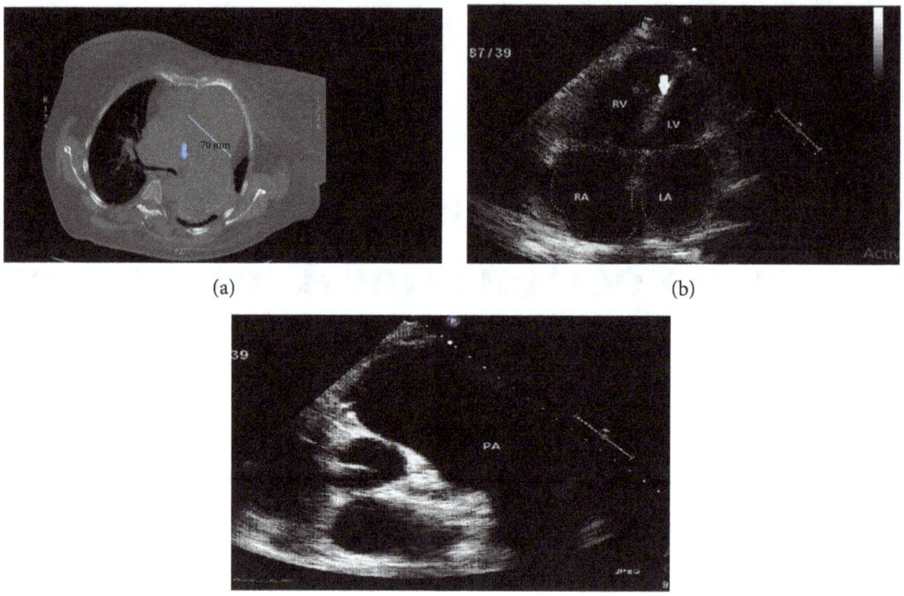


(a) (b)

(c)

Figure 1: (a) Noncontrast chest CT showing main pulmonary artery aneurysm measuring 70 mm with blue arrow pointing the possible intimal flap. Rapid tapering of pulmonary vessels can be appreciated on the right lung zones. (b) Transthoracic echocardiogram apical four-chamber view showing severely dilated right ventricle and septal flattening (white arrow). (c) Transthoracic echocardiogram parasternal short axis view at the level of aortic valve showing severe dilation of pulmonary artery.

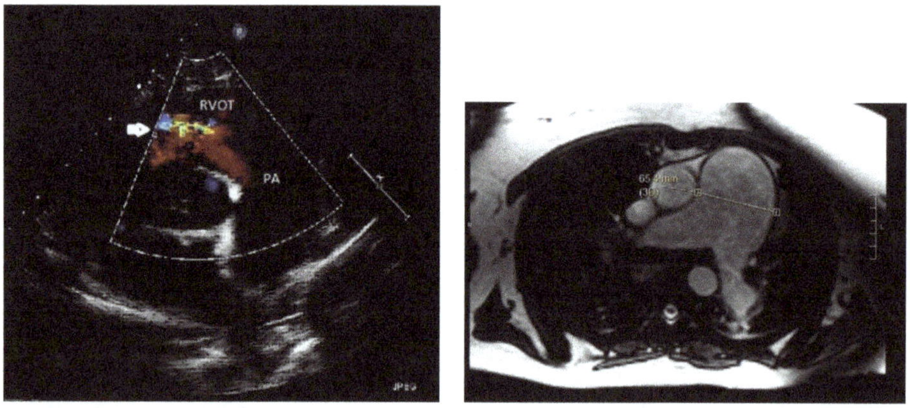


(a) (b)

Figure 2: (a) Transthoracic echocardiogram parasternal short axis color Doppler showing severe pulmonic regurgitation (white arrow) and dilated pulmonary artery. (b) Cardiac MRI showing marked aneurysmal enlargement of the main PA.

compatible with advanced pulmonary sarcoidosis with primarily apical involvement, bilateral hilar lymphadenopathy, and PH with aneurysmal dilation of main PA to 65 mm. Right heart catheterization (RHC) showed elevated right-sided filling pressures with a mean PA pressure (mPAP) of 46 mm Hg, normal pulmonary capillary wedge pressure (PCWP) of 12 mmHg, and pulmonary vascular resistance (PVR) of 7.1 Wood units. TTE revealed severe dilation with dysfunction of the RV and severe pulmonary valvular regurgitation (PVR) (Figure 2(a)). Despite the etiology of WHO Group 5 PH, she was started on sildenafil and macitentan given the severity of her symptoms. Inhaled treprostinil was added later due to persistent dyspnea. Her symptoms and supplemental oxygen requirement did not improve, and she was admitted for clinical worsening. A cardiac MRI was performed. The study did not reveal findings of cardiac sarcoidosis; however, it did reveal PAA and severe pulmonic regurgitation (Figure 2(b)). PFTs showed severe restrictive lung disease (FEV1 of 55%, FVC of 44% with FEV1/FVC of 126%). Preoperative ventilation/perfusion (V/Q) scan showed heterogeneous ventilation as well as perfusion activity in both lungs but with no V/Q mismatch. She was considered for bilateral lung transplant due to severe and progressive pulmonary sarcoidosis refractory to medical management (steroids) as well as severe and progressive PH. However, due to coexisting PAA and severe PVR, it was decided to proceed with heart-lung transplantation. Surgery was performed under venoarterial extracorporeal

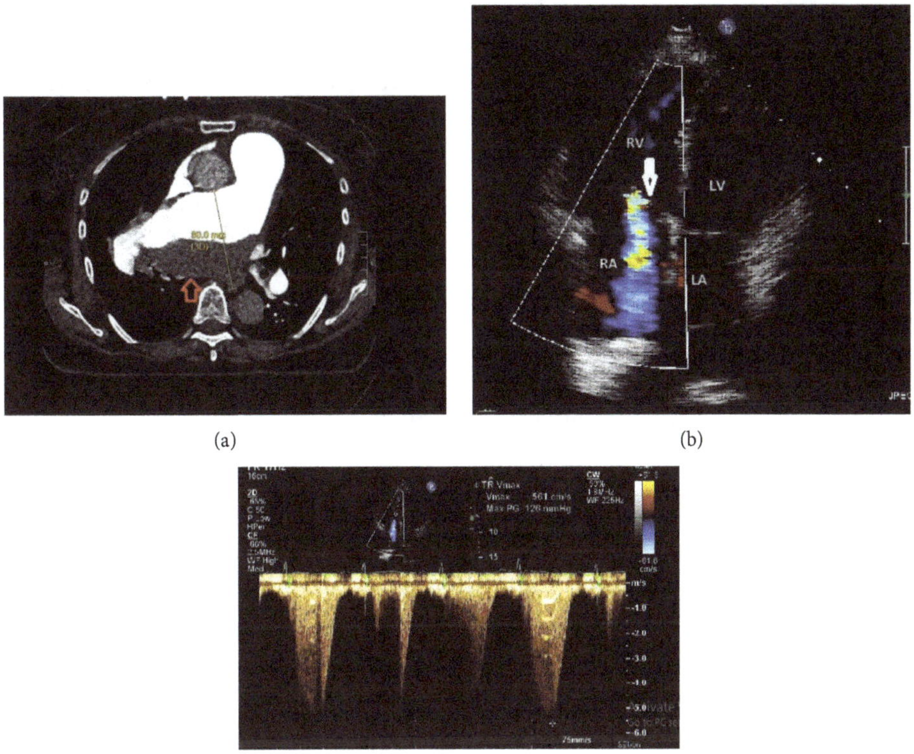


(a) (b) (c)

Figure 3: (a) CTA chest showing right pulmonary artery aneurysm measuring 80 mm in the greatest dimension with laminated thrombus in the aneurysmal sac (red arrow). (b) Transthoracic echocardiogram apical four-chamber view showing dilated RV, severe TR (white arrow), and systolic septal flattening consistent with RV pressure overload. (c) Extremely elevated estimated PA systolic pressure measurements to 134 mmHg indicating severe PH.

membrane oxygenation (VA-ECMO) support. A 7 cm proximal PA aneurysm was found. After achieving hemostasis by clamping the aorta, the heart was removed followed by the removal of PA intrapericardially till the bifurcation, and then, the anterior segments of the right and left PA were resected leaving the posterior segment behind followed by intrapericardial stapling of pulmonary veins. This was followed by lung removal and successful placement of the heart and lung into the pericardial and pleural space, respectively, with anastomosis to the pulmonary vessels. She was successfully decannulated from VA-ECMO and had an unremarkable postoperative course. At 2-year follow-up, the patient had marked improvement of symptoms, was walking 3 miles a day on treadmill, and had a normal surveillance TTE and PFTs (FEV1 of 86%, FVC of 89% with FEV1/FVC of 102%).

## 3. Case 3

A 73-year-old female was referred from an outside hospital with worsening edema, dyspnea, and concern for acute pulmonary embolism (PE). On presentation to the outside hospital, she was hypoxic with asymmetric lower extremity swelling. The lower extremity venous Doppler did not reveal any evidence of deep venous thrombosis (DVT).

Computerized tomography angiography (CTA) of the chest revealed a right PAA measuring 80 mm in diameter with laminated clot burden and compression of the right bronchus (Figure 3(a)). There was a question of acute PE vs. chronic thromboembolic pulmonary disease (CTED) vs. in situ thrombus within the aneurysm sac. She was started on intravenous heparin. A careful review of the images, however, did not reveal classic findings of CTED, and there was a suspicion for PAH and associated PAA with clot formation in the aneurysmal sac. A V/Q scan showed low probability for pulmonary embolism. TTE showed right ventricular dysfunction with elevated RVSP of 134 mmHg and severe tricuspid regurgitation (TR) (Figures 3(b) and 3(c)). RHC was deferred due to the presence of the aneurysm. PFTs revealed a restrictive pattern with FEV1 of 32%, FVC of 28%, and FEV1/FVC of 115%. Owing to significant bronchial compression by the massive aneurysm and profound PA dilatation, a decision was made to proceed with surgical repair. During surgery, a large deeply hidden aneurysm situated just at the bifurcation of the main pulmonary trunk was opened and found full of clotted blood. There was evidence of dissection of aneurysm involving both right and left PAs. She underwent aneurysmectomy and homograft repair, and her postoperative course was unremarkable. On subsequent outpatient visits, patient's symptoms improved from WHO FC III at the time of presentation to WHO FC II, but RV dilatation/dysfunction persisted on TTE. An outpatient RHC was completed which revealed mPAP of 45 mmHg and increased PVR to 10 Wood units compatible with PAH. She was subsequently started on tadalafil and ambrisentan with plan for lifelong anticoagulation. At 9-month follow-up, the patient had improvement in her symptoms and could walk up and down a 1-2 flight of stairs (WHO FC II) and walked 425 m (98% of predicted) during 6MWT on room air with improvement of RV size and function on TTE.

## 4. Discussion

PAAs are not routinely encountered in clinical practice and can occur in a spectrum of pulmonary and systemic diseases. The true incidence of PAAs remains unclear in the general population, but in 1947, Deterling and Clagett reported eight cases in a series of more than 100,000 autopsies (0.00008%) [1]. Risk factors for PAA include increasing age, male sex, elevated mPAP, duration of PH, vasculitis, and connective tissue diseases [2]. In patients with PH, regardless of etiology, the incidence is significantly higher (1.25%) [2].

The normal diameter of the PA on CT ranges 25 mm ± 3 mm with 29 being the upper limit of normal. For the left and right PAs, the upper range of normal is 20 mm. Most of the studies have defined a PAA as a main PA > 40 mm.

The course of patients with isolated PAA is clinically less severe than the patients with an underlying cardiopulmonary disease including PH, congenital heart disease, and infections such at tuberculosis and syphilis (which are rare in the western world). Some of the high-risk features of PAA include PA diameter exceeding 75 mm, rapid pulmonary artery diameter growth (>2 mm/year), and high mean PA pressures on RHC (exceeding 50 mmHg) [3]. Common complications of PAAs include in situ thrombosis, pulmonary embolism, compression of adjacent structures including left main coronary artery as well as adjacent bronchi, and dissection of the pulmonary artery [4]. PAAs can progress to rupture, and one-third of all the reported cases of PAA died of complications resulting from rupture including lethal hemoptysis, asphyxiation, exsanguination, and sudden death. There are no established guidelines for the management of PAAs, and treatment usually is individualized. Surgical repair is usually recommended for large (>60 mm) PAAs due to the risk of rupture or dissection. These criteria are however based on case studies [5, 6]. Other potential indications include development of symptoms related to bronchial compression, thrombus formation in the aneurysm sac, and evidence of valvular pathology such as severe pulmonic regurgitation. In case of pulmonary valve insufficiency, timing of surgical intervention is determined by changes in RV size and function [7]. Results from previous case reports have also demonstrated improvements in lung function and PH after surgical repair [8]. Data from case reports and series in the past also suggest that treating PH with vasodilators does not affect the growth rate of PAAs. Lung transplant is an option when significant parenchymal or progressive pulmonary vascular disease is present [9].

Various surgical management options have been described in the literature. Aneurysmectomy with homograft repair is being increasingly utilized, especially when the aneurysm is compressing adjacent structures, and PA pressures are manageable [10]. The third patient in our series did well after surgical repair indicating that despite the presence of PAH, with an experienced team, good surgical outcomes are feasible. Angioplasty with plication, reconstruction of the main pulmonary artery with autologous or prosthetic tissue has been reported in the literature in the absence of underlying PH [11]. Endovascular coiling and embolization of peripheral PAA have also been reported in some cases in the past [12].

In this case series, we highlight three distinct approaches to PAA management in PH. These include medical management alone with pulmonary arterial vasodilators, transplant including lung or heart/lung transplant, and surgical resection (aneurysmectomy). Each of these options has its strength and weakness, and case-based management is usually considered based on individual patient profile.

## References

[1] R. A. Deterling Jr. and O. T. Clagett, "Aneurysm of the pulmonary artery: Review of the literature and report of a case," *American Heart Journal*, vol. 34, no. 4, pp. 471–499, 1947.

[2] A. L. Duijnhouwer, E. P. Navarese, A. P. J. Van Dijk, B. Loeys, J. W. Roos-Hesselink, and M. J. De Boer, "Aneurysm of the Pulmonary Artery, a Systematic Review and Critical Analysis of Current Literature," *Congenital Heart Disease*, vol. 11, no. 2, pp. 102–109, 2016.

[3] P. Wood, "The Eisenmenger syndrome or pulmonary hypertension with revised cardiac shunt," *British Medical Journal*, vol. 2, no. 5099, pp. 755–762, 1958.

[4] F. Butto, R. V. Lucas Jr., and J. E. Edwards, "Pulmonary Arterial Aneurysm," *Chest*, vol. 91, no. 2, pp. 237–241, 1987.

[5] S. J. Deb, K. J. Zehr, and R. C. Shields, "Idiopathic Pulmonary Artery Aneurysm," *The Annals of Thoracic Surgery*, vol. 80, no. 4, pp. 1500–1502, 2005.

[6] M. Sakuma, J. Demachi, J. Suzuki, J. Nawata, T. Takahashi, and K. Shirato, "Proximal pulmonary artery aneurysms in patients with pulmonary artery hypertension: complicated cases," *Internal Medicine*, vol. 46, no. 21, pp. 1789–1793, 2007.

[7] M. Kreibich, M. Siepe, J. Kroll, R. Hohn, J. Grohmann, and F. Beyersdorf, "Aneurysms of the pulmonary artery," *Circulation*, vol. 131, no. 3, pp. 310–316, 2015.

[8] S. Akagi, K. Ejiri, S. Kasahara, K. Nakamura, and H. Ito, "Improvement of lung function and pulmonary hypertension after pulmonary aneurysm repair: case series," *Pulmonary Circulation*, vol. 9, no. 1, p. 204589401983121, 2019.

[9] Ö. Senbaklavaci, Y. Kaneko, A. Bartunek et al., "Rupture and dissection in pulmonary artery aneurysms: Incidence, cause, and treatment—Review and case report," *The Journal of Thoracic and Cardiovascular Surgery*, vol. 121, no. 5, pp. 1006–1008, 2001.

[10] O. Ucar, D. Sahin, M. Vural, and S. Aydogdu, "Thrombosed giant proximal pulmonary artery aneurysm," *Archives of the Turkish Society of Cardiology*, vol. 37, no. 7, pp. 493–496, 2009.

[11] B. Boerrigter, G. J. Mauritz, J. T. Marcus et al., "Progressive Dilatation of the Main Pulmonary Artery Is a Characteristic of Pulmonary Arterial Hypertension and Is Not Related to Changes in Pressure," *Chest*, vol. 138, no. 6, pp. 1395–1401, 2010.

[12] H. J. Shin and Y. J. Suh, "Novel pulmonary artery reduction plasty for pulmonary artery aneurysm with pulmonary arterial hypertension," *World Journal for Pediatric and Congenital Heart Surgery*, vol. 7, no. 1, pp. 96–99, 2016.

2

# Pulmonary Artery Dissection: A Fatal Complication of Pulmonary Hypertension

**Chuanchen Zhang,[1] Xiaoyong Huang,[2] Shuhua Li,[1] Hengchen Yao,[3] and Bin Zhang[4]**

[1]*Department of Radiology, Liaocheng People's Hospital, Shandong University, 67 Dongchang West Road, Liaocheng District, Shandong 252000, China*
[2]*Department of Radiology, Anzhen Hospital, Capital Medical University, 2 Anzhen Road, Chaoyang District, Beijing 100029, China*
[3]*Department of Cardiology, Liaocheng People's Hospital, Shandong University, 67 Dongchang West Road, Liaocheng District, Shandong 252000, China*
[4]*Department of Surgery, Liaocheng People's Hospital, Shandong University, 67 Dongchang West Road, Liaocheng District, Shandong 252000, China*

Correspondence should be addressed to Bin Zhang; zhangbin252000@163.com

Academic Editor: Michael S. Firstenberg

Pulmonary artery dissection is extremely rare but it is a really life-threatening condition when it happens. Most patients die suddenly from major bleeding or tamponade caused by direct rupture into mediastinum or retrograde into the pericardial sac. What we are reporting is a rare case of a 46-year-old female patient whose pulmonary artery dissection involves both the pulmonary valve and right pulmonary artery. The patient had acute chest pain and severe dyspnea, and the diagnosis of pulmonary artery dissection was confirmed by ultrasonography and CT angiography. Moreover, its etiology, clinical manifestations, and management are also discussed in this article.

## 1. Introduction

Pulmonary artery dissection is an exceptionally rare and deadly condition, usually paired with pulmonary hypertension [1, 2]. Unlike aortic dissection, pulmonary artery dissection progresses rapidly and typically ruptures rather than developing a reentry site, which causes cardiogenic shock or sudden death [2–4]. It is thus mainly involved in the pulmonary artery trunk, without involvement of its branches or pulmonary valve [4, 5]. Furthermore, pulmonary artery dissection involving both the pulmonary valve and right pulmonary artery has never been reported.

In this article, there is presentation of the first pulmonary artery dissection case including both the pulmonary valve and right pulmonary artery with a patent ductus arteriosus (PDA). We discuss specific ultrasound and multidetector computed tomography (CT) angiography findings and briefly review the etiology, clinical manifestations, and management.

## 2. Case Report

With chest pain and shortness of breath, a 46-year-old woman was admitted to the emergency department. One day before her admission, her symptoms developed into acute chest pain and severe dyspnea during physical exertion. Her symptoms were described as severe, substernal pressure radiating into the shoulder associated with shortness of breath and nausea. At the age of forty one, the patient suffered dyspnea and edema in the lower limbs (New York Heart Association Functional Class IV). She was admitted to a regional hospital center and was diagnosed with severe pulmonary hypertension secondary to a patent ductus arteriosus (PDA). Because of high mortality of anesthesia, surgical intervention was not suggested. Thereafter, the patient was treated with a long-term medical regimen of diuretics and digoxin.

Generic approval was given by the Ethics Committee at our institution for retrospective analysis of clinical and

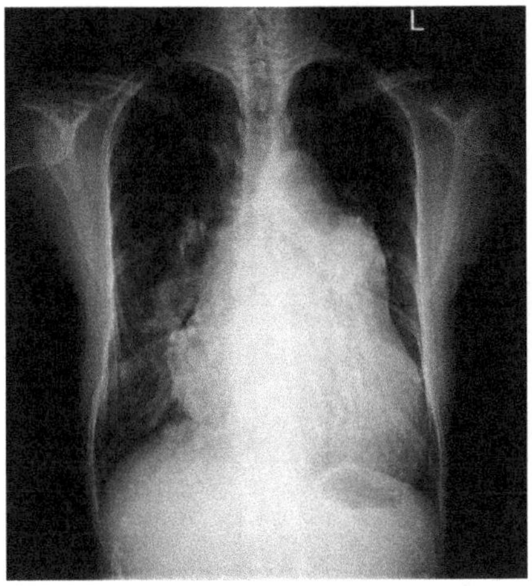


FIGURE 1: Plain radiographic features of pulmonary artery dissection. Posteroanterior chest radiograph showing cardiac enlargement and pulmonary arterial overcirculation. Pulmonary arterial overcirculation is indicated by prominent pulmonary arterial segments and greatly dilated hilar vessels.

imaging data (the chairperson of the ethics committee: Guozhang Liu, the protocol number: 2014110802, and the date of approval: Nov 8, 2014). The patient's husband provided permission to publish these features of this case.

A physical examination revealed a regular heart rate of 90 beats $min^{-1}$, a respiratory rate of 25 breaths $min^{-1}$, and blood pressure of 95/60 mmHg. She was afebrile, with elevated jugular venous pressure. Cardiac auscultation revealed a continuous murmur located at the upper left sternal border and a loud pulmonary component sound from the second heart sound, heard loudest over the left sternal edge.

The laboratory analyses revealed mild anemia (hemoglobin 98 g/L), hyponatremia (serum sodium 122 mmol/L), and elevated blood urea nitrogen (10.97 mmol/L). Her ECG showed sinus rhythm, right atrial enlargement, biventricular hypertrophy, and right axis deviation. A chest radiograph revealed moderate cardiomegaly and enormous dilatation of the pulmonary artery and its branches. The lungs and pleura were normal (Figure 1).

Echocardiography showed enlarged right heart chambers, a greatly dilated main pulmonary trunk 64 mm in diameter with severe pulmonary regurgitation, as well as a PDA measured at 16 mm. We noted a dissection flap within the main pulmonary trunk (Figure 2) and performed an ECG-gated pulmonary CT angiography for further evaluation with a 64-slice CT scanner. CT axial images demonstrated marked dilation of the main pulmonary trunk (62.4 mm in diameter) and its central branches (Figure 3(a)). The intimal flap in the main and right pulmonary arteries was depicted as a dark line separating the true and false lumen (Figures 3(a) and 3(b)). Multiplanar reconstruction (MPR) clearly showed that the flap extended retrograde to the pulmonary valve from the inciting intimal tear in the proximal main pulmonary trunk (Figure 3(c)). Three-dimensional volume rendered (VR) images more validly demonstrated the relationship between the pulmonary valve and intimal flap (Figure 3(d)).

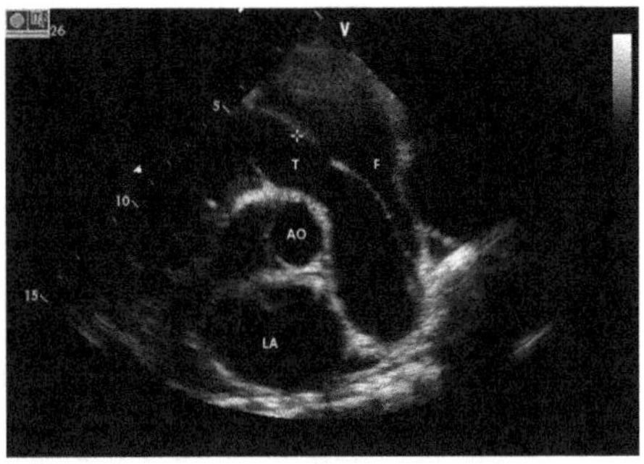


FIGURE 2: Echocardiogram. Two-dimensional transthoracic echocardiography in short-axis view of the heart base showing a greatly dilated pulmonary trunk with the dissection membrane (+). AO, aorta; LA, left atrium; T, true lumen; F, false lumen.

Combined lung and heart transplantations were proposed for this patient. Unfortunately, she suddenly collapsed and died 8 days after the onset of acute chest pain, before surgical intervention was possible. Her family declined an autopsy as the patient's diagnosis was clearly known.

## 3. Discussion

The diagnosis of pulmonary artery dissection is usually made in postmortem studies because it progresses rapidly and tends to rupture, causing cardiogenic shock or sudden death. Only 26 cases were documented in living patients so far since it was first described by Helmbrechtr in 1842 [4–8]. A review by Inayama et al. [5] indicated that the main pulmonary trunk is the dissection site in 72% of cases, followed by the intrapulmonary arteries (10%), the trunk and right main artery (6%), the left main artery (6%), the right main artery (4%), and the trunk plus both main arteries (2%).

The initiating event of artery dissection is known to be a tear through the intima into the mid or deep media, causing propagation of the dissection along intramedia planes. Pressurized blood in the media dissects the media longitudinally between concentric layers of elastin sheets, forming the false lumen. Even in aorta which is notable for thick media dominated by layers of elastin sheets, the dissection propagates more anterogradely than retrogradely with poorly understood reasons. The media of pulmonary artery are much thinner compared with that of aorta due to lower resistance to flow in the lung. Therefore, in pulmonary dissection, the false lumen tends to rupture rather than to develop a reentry site, as is usual in aortic dissection [6]. Interestingly, despite the dissection extents to the distal right pulmonary artery, her proximal pulmonary valve was also involved.

Pulmonary artery dissection occurs in both sexes with a slight female predominance (male : female 1 : 1.2). Patient ages ranged from 26 days to 85 years with incidence peaks occurring in the third and sixth decades [5, 6]. The etiology of pulmonary artery dissection remains unclear because few cases have been reported so far. Postmortem findings indicated the majority of pulmonary artery dissections occur in the presence of medial degeneration with fragmentation

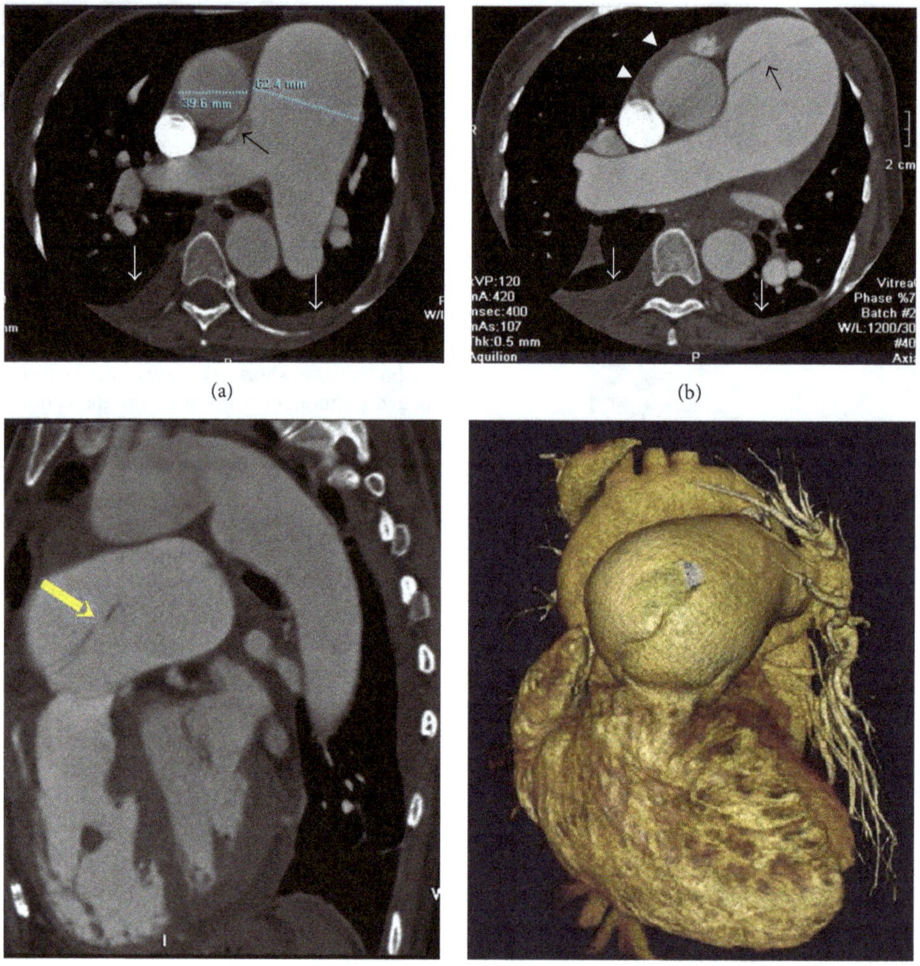


(a) (b) (c) (d)

Figure 3: Intimal flap features determined on CT angiography. Transverse sections of CT pulmonary angiography (a, b) showing dilated central pulmonary arteries with an intimal flap (black arrow) in the main pulmonary trunk and right pulmonary artery. Pericardial effusion (white arrowheads) and bilateral pleural effusion (white arrows) are also noted. Sagittal MPR reconstruction (c) revealed the primary entry tear (arrow) in the proximal main pulmonary trunk and retrograde extension of the intimal flap to the pulmonary valve. Volume rendered images (d) vividly demonstrated the relationship between the intimal flap and pulmonary artery root.

of elastic fibres and generalized dilatation of the pulmonary arterial tree. Pulmonary artery dissections are normally caused by chronic pulmonary hypertension and secondary to congenital cardiovascular anomalies, acquired valvular diseases, altered perfusion ventilation in COPD, or primary pulmonary hypertension [7–10], while minority of pulmonary artery dissections occur in aneurysm which associated with congenital lesions, infection, trauma, atherosclerosis or connective tissue disorders [11, 12].

Pulmonary artery dissection symptoms are nonspecific, and 82% of patients have exertional dyspnea, 67% have retrosternal chest pain, and 52% have central cyanosis [6, 12]. Pulmonary artery dissection is suspected in the face of sudden hemodynamic decomposition in an otherwise previously stable patient with known presentation of pulmonary hypertension or pulmonary artery aneurysm [13]. The condition progresses rapidly, so prompt diagnosis permits surgical treatment, which improves prognosis [14, 15]. Fortunately, several imaging modalities, such as chest radiograph, echocardiography, CT angiography, MRI, and cardiac catheterization, have been available for the evaluation of pulmonary artery dissection.

Chest radiograph is a commonly used imaging method to evaluate chest pain patients. Unfortunately, chest radiographs are abnormal in almost all pulmonary artery dissection cases but nonspecific. Common radiographic abnormalities include cardiomegaly, central pulmonary artery dilatation, and pleural effusion [16]. Chest radiographic findings may indicate if echocardiography or CT angiography should be the next evaluation method.

Khattar et al. [10] suggested ultrasonography should be performed first due to its ready accessibility, ease of use, and low cost and the fact that it is very sensitive at detecting main pulmonary artery dissection. However, for the left and right main pulmonary arteries or peripheral artery dissection, intimal flaps might not be readily identified by ultrasonography. Pulmonary CT angiography can show pulmonary artery dissection directly, as does pulmonary angiography. It is also noninvasive, cheaper, and widely available [17]. The segmented and subsegmented vessels are better demonstrated and findings are easier to interpret. CT scanning is the only test that can provide significant additional information related to alternate diagnoses such as pulmonary embolism (PE), which is important in an acute setting. Also, abundant postprocessing CT techniques make pulmonary artery dissection diagnosis more accurate and convenient.

Although investigators have reported the feasibility of MRI and conventional angiography at evaluating pulmonary artery dissection, MRIs are mostly limited to the evaluation of patients who have renal dysfunction or other contraindications for the use of iodinated contrast material, and conventional angiography is limited to patients in whom other results are nondiagnostic (clinical suspicion is high) [13, 18].

Several factors determine the best modality for the initial evaluation and postoperative follow-up of pulmonary artery dissection. These factors include the patient's condition stability, renal function, suspected postoperative complication, and each imaging modality's availability. Although the intimal flap can be detected by echocardiography, CT, MRI, and catheter angiography, we believe that echocardiography should be the first choice to evaluate the cause of chest pain or shortness of breath which is not only to look for pulmonary artery dissection but also to exclude other causes of chest pain, assess the valves, measure the PA pressure, and further assess underlying cardiovascular pathophysiology and haemodynamics. In the emergency setting, echocardiography will also be the most readily available test and the easiest way to apply in a bedside manner. Nevertheless, CT or MR pulmonary angiography could provide additional or confirmatory information. There is no definite guideline as the optimal treatment for pulmonary artery dissection. Surgical intervention may be necessary for most patients but it is usually followed by fatal consequences [12, 14]. Unfortunately, this patient suddenly died before surgical intervention.

In summary, although pulmonary artery dissection is an extremely rare condition, it should be suspected in patients with chronic pulmonary arterial hypertension presenting with chest pain, worsening dyspnea, or hemodynamic instability. Physicians should familiarize themselves with clinical features and imaging modalities of this condition so that a definitive diagnosis can be made and a proper treatment can be carried out.

## Acknowledgments

The authors are grateful to the patient's husband, who consented to publishing this case report and the figures. This article is funded by the Natural Science Foundation of Shandong Province (ZR2013HL017).

## References

[1] M. A. Navas Lobato, R. Martín Reyes, P. Lurueña Lobo et al., "Pulmonary artery dissection and conservative medical management," *International Journal of Cardiology*, vol. 119, no. 1, pp. e25–e26, 2007.

[2] R. D. A. Corrêa, L. C. D. S. Silva, C. J. Rezende, R. C. Bernardes, T. A. Prata, and H. L. Silva, "Pulmonary hypertension and pulmonary artery dissection," *Jornal Brasileiro de Pneumologia*, vol. 39, no. 2, pp. 238–241, 2013.

[3] H.-H. Hsu, C. Tzao, C.-S. Tsai, G.-H. Sun, and C.-Y. Chen, "Acute concomitant pulmonary artery and aortic dissection with rupture," *International Journal of Cardiovascular Imaging*, vol. 23, no. 3, pp. 411–414, 2007.

[4] K. B. Shilkin, L. P. Low, and B. T. Chen, "Dissecting aneurysm of the pulmonary artery," *The Journal of Pathology*, vol. 98, no. 1, pp. 25–29, 1969.

[5] Y. Inayama, Y. Nakatani, and H. Kitamura, "Pulmonary artery dissection in patients without underlying pulmonary hypertension," *Histopathology*, vol. 38, no. 5, pp. 435–442, 2001.

[6] Ö. Senbaklavaci, Y. Kaneko, A. Bartunek et al., "Rupture and dissection in pulmonary artery aneurysms: incidence, cause, and treatment—review and case report," *Journal of Thoracic and Cardiovascular Surgery*, vol. 121, no. 5, pp. 1006–1008, 2001.

[7] N. Tøonder, L. Køber, and C. Hassager, "Pulmonary artery dissection in a patient with Eisenmenger syndrome treated with heart and lung transplantation," *European Journal of Echocardiography*, vol. 5, no. 3, pp. 228–230, 2004.

[8] W. A. Wuyts, P. Herijgers, W. Budts, W. De Wever, and M. Delcroix, "Extensive dissection of the pulmonary artery treated with combined heart-lung transplantation," *Journal of Thoracic and Cardiovascular Surgery*, vol. 132, no. 1, pp. 205–206.e1, 2006.

[9] M. A. N. Lobato, R. Martín Reyes, P. Lurueña Lobo et al., "Pulmonary artery dissection and conservative medical management," *International Journal of Cardiology*, vol. 119, no. 1, pp. e25–e26, 2007.

[10] R. S. Khattar, D. J. Fox, J. E. Alty, and A. Arora, "Pulmonary artery dissection: an emerging cardiovascular complication in surviving patients with chronic pulmonary hypertension," *Heart*, vol. 91, no. 2, pp. 142–145, 2005.

[11] B. Degano, G. Prevot, L. Têtu, O. Sitbon, G. Simonneau, and M. Humbert, "Fatal dissection of the pulmonary artery in pulmonary arterial hypertension," *European Respiratory Review*, vol. 18, no. 113, pp. 181–185, 2009.

[12] S. Westaby, B. J. Evans, and O. Ormerod, "Pulmonary-artery dissection in patients with Eisenmenger's syndrome," *The New England Journal of Medicine*, vol. 356, no. 20, pp. 2110–2112, 2007.

[13] A. Smalcelj, V. Brida, M. Samarzija, A. Matana, E. Margetic, and N. Drinkovic, "Giant, dissecting, high-pressure pulmonary artery aneurysm: case report of a 1-year natural course," *Texas Heart Institute Journal*, vol. 32, no. 4, pp. 589–594, 2005.

[14] Q. Li, A. Wang, D. Li et al., "Dissecting aneurysm of the main pulmonary artery: a rare complication of pulmonary balloon valvuloplasty diagnosed 1 month after the procedure," *Circulation*, vol. 119, no. 5, pp. 761–763, 2009.

[15] Y. Sakamaki, M. Minami, M. Ohta et al., "Pulmonary artery dissection complicating lung transplantation for primary pulmonary hypertension," *Annals of Thoracic Surgery*, vol. 81, no. 1, pp. 360–362, 2006.

[16] S. L. Hoye, C. P. Gale, D. J. M. Tolan, and C. B. Pepperl, "An unusual presentation of pulmonary artery dissection," *Thorax*, vol. 64, no. 4, article 368, 2009.

[17] M. A. Neimatallah, W. Hassan, M. Moursi, and Y. Al Kadhi, "CT findings of pulmonary artery dissection," *The British Journal of Radiology*, vol. 80, no. 951, pp. e61–e63, 2007.

[18] E. J. Stern, C. Graham, G. Gamsu, J. A. Golden, and C. B. Higgins, "Pulmonary artery dissection: MR findings," *Journal of Computer Assisted Tomography*, vol. 16, no. 3, pp. 481–483, 1992.

3

# Pulmonary Hypertension and Hypocholesterolemia Secondary to Thyrotoxicosis

**Narangoda Liyanage Ajantha Shyamali**[1] **and Chandrike Ponnamperuma**[2]

[1]*University of Sri Jayewardenepura, Gangodawila, Nugegoda, Sri Lanka*
[2]*National Hospital of Sri Lanka, Colombo 10, Sri Lanka*

Correspondence should be addressed to Narangoda Liyanage Ajantha Shyamali; ajaliyanage@yahoo.com

Academic Editor: Lucy Mastrandrea

*Background.* Thyroid disorders commonly affect the cardiovascular system. Thyrotoxicosis leading to pulmonary hypertension has been increasingly reported during recent years. Thyroid dysfunction affects the lipid metabolism, and thyrotoxicosis can be associated with low lipid levels. Thyrotoxicosis presenting with right ventricular dysfunction is rare, and only few cases had been reported. *Case Presentation.* A 53-year-old woman presented with progressive shortness of breath and swelling of body for four months. Examination showed generalized oedema and a systolic murmur over the left sternal border. Transthoracic echocardiography confirmed pulmonary hypertension with tricuspid regurgitation. Investigations revealed thyrotoxicosis and very low cholesterol levels. Diagnosis of Graves' disease was confirmed with detection of thyrotropin receptor antibodies. Pulmonary pressure was normalized six months after antithyroid therapy. *Conclusion.* Thyrotoxicosis is a recognized cause of reversible pulmonary hypertension and acquired hypocholesterolemia. However, most clinicians are not aware of these associations. This case illustrates the importance of assessing thyroid function in patients presenting with pulmonary hypertension.

## 1. Introduction

Thyrotoxicosis is well known to associate with left ventricular dysfunction due to long-standing effects of thyroid hormones. However, the association of hyperthyroidism with right ventricular dysfunction secondary to pulmonary hypertension has been reported in the literature since 1980 [1]. The exact mechanism of pulmonary hypertension in thyrotoxicosis is ill-defined [2, 3]. Several studies have reported the resolution of pulmonary hypertension secondary to thyrotoxicosis with antithyroid therapy [4]. The association of hypothyroidism with hyperlipidemia has been well known for a long period. However, low cholesterol level secondary to thyrotoxicosis is not widely appreciated. Only few cases of Graves' thyrotoxicosis with pulmonary hypertension and hyperlipidemia have been reported in the literature.

## 2. Case Presentation

A 53-year-old previously healthy woman presented with fever for 3 days associated with a four-month history of progressive shortness of breath and generalized body swelling. She has also noted increased sweating which she considered as a perimenopausal symptom. On examination, she was febrile with a heart rate of 101/min and oxygen saturation of 98% on room air. She had bilateral ankle oedema and extensive abdominal wall oedema. Jugular venous pressure was elevated, and there was a pansystolic murmur over the left sternal border. Respiratory system examination was clinically normal.

Her basic blood investigations of full blood count, erythrocyte sedimentation rate, C-reactive protein levels, renal function tests, and liver function tests were normal. She was found to have low cholesterol levels with total

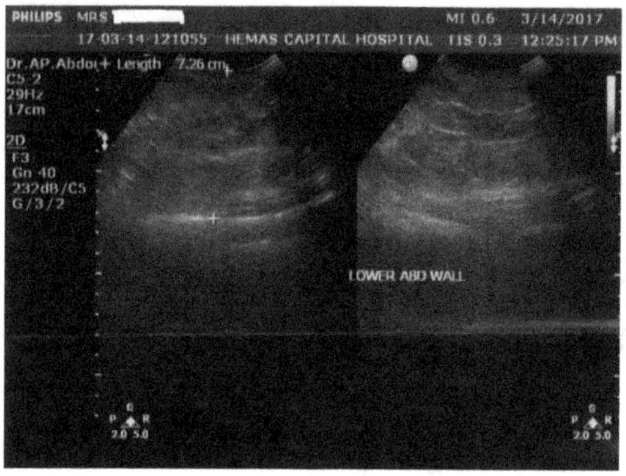


Figure 1: Ultrasound scan of the abdomen showing extensive abdominal wall oedema.

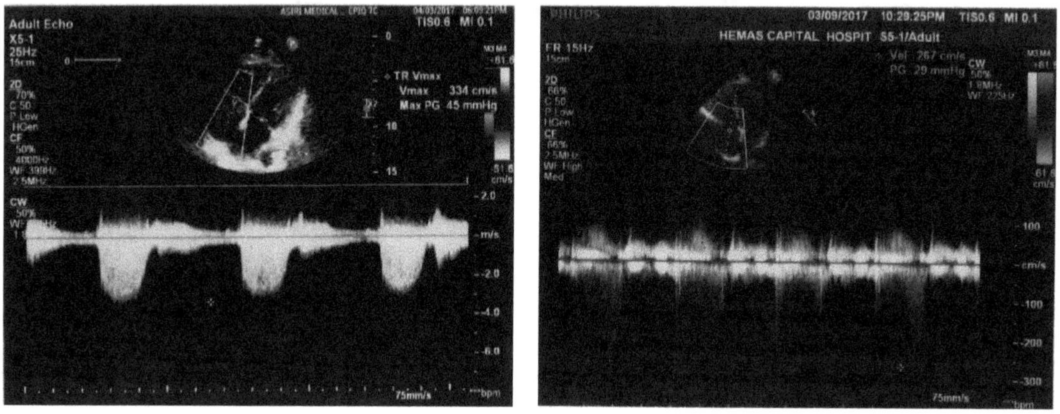


(a) (b)

Figure 2: Transthoracic echocardiography demonstrating pulmonary artery pressures before (a) and after (b) the treatment of thyrotoxicosis.

cholesterol of 61 mg/dl (normal range: 140–239), low-density lipoprotein cholesterol (LDLC) of 26 mg/dl (normal range: 75–159), and high-density lipoprotein cholesterol (HDLC) of 20 mg/dl (normal range: 35–85). Thyroid-stimulating hormone (TSH) level was 0.004 $\mu$IU/ml (normal range: 0.4–4.0) with free thyroxin (FT4) 5.48 ng/dl (normal range: 0.89–1.76) and free triiodothyronine (FT3) 11.48 pg/dl (normal range: 1.5–4.1). TSH receptor antibodies were positive with 4.39 IU/L (normal < 2 IU/L). Ultrasound of the thyroid showed diffusely enlarged glands with increased vascularity, and ultrasound scan of the abdomen revealed marked lower abdominal wall oedema without organomegaly (Figure 1). Transthoracic echocardiography showed right ventricular enlargement with tricuspid regurgitation. The systolic pulmonary artery pressure gradient was 45 mmHg (normal < 25 mmHg) (Figure 2(a)).

Graves' thyrotoxicosis was diagnosed, and she was started on antithyroid medication. She underwent computed tomographic pulmonary angiography (CT-PA) ten days after starting thyrostatic drugs which did not show evidence of chronic thromboembolic pulmonary hypertension or abnormalities of lung parenchyma. After six months of treatment, her symptoms improved. The systolic pulmonary artery pressure gradient was reduced to 29 mmHg in repeated transthoracic echocardiography (Figure 2(b)). TSH level increased to 0.48 μIU/ml with normalization of thyroid hormone levels. Her serum lipid levels returned to normal with total cholesterol of 185 mg/dl, LDLC of 109 mg/dl, and HDLC of 61 mg/dl.

## 3. Discussion

The association of thyrotoxicosis with right ventricular dysfunction was first reported in the literature in 1973 [5]. Thyrotoxicosis as a cause for pulmonary hypertension and reduction of pulmonary artery pressure with treatment of antithyroid medication have been clearly established recently [6, 7]. Therefore, most clinicians are not aware of this important association.

In a study of 23 patients with Graves' thyrotoxicosis, 65% of patients had pulmonary hypertension which normalized with definitive treatment, and a recent single-center cross-sectional study carried out in Ethiopia showed that 30% of patients with hyperthyroidism have echocardiographic evidence of pulmonary hypertension [4, 8]. Although the underlying pathophysiology for this complication is unclear, several mechanisms have been hypothesized: endothelial injury secondary to high cardiac output, immune-mediated endothelial damage, and enhanced metabolism of intrinsic pulmonary vasodilators [3, 9].

Increased expression of low-density lipoprotein (LDL) receptors and activity of lipoprotein lipase by thyroid hormones decrease the circulating levels of lipoproteins. Consequently, decreased levels of HDLC and LDLC are seen in patients with hyperthyroidism [10, 11]. The action of thyroid hormones in the liver is responsible for the reduction of LDLC levels, which is caused by enhanced transcription of LDL receptors in the liver. Therefore, the extent of LDLC level reduction is proportional to free thyroid hormone levels [11]. Hyperthyroidism is recognized as a significant cause of acquired hypocholesterolemia and unanticipated improvement of lipid levels in hyperlipidemic patients [12].

Thyrotoxicosis is an overlooked, reversible cause of pulmonary hypertension, and there is a high prevalence of pulmonary hypertension among hyperthyroid patients [13]. Thus, patients presenting with thyrotoxicosis and dyspnea should be screened for pulmonary hypertension [14]. All clinicians should be aware of this association, and this case highlights the importance of assessing thyroid function tests in patients with pulmonary hypertension.

## Abbreviations

LDLC: Low-density lipoprotein cholesterol
HDLC: High-density lipoprotein cholesterol
TSH: Thyroid-stimulating hormone
FT4: Free thyroxin
FT3: Free triiodothyronine.

## Consent

The authors obtained written informed consent from the patient to report and publish about her illness anonymously.

## Authors' Contributions

NLA Shyamali was involved in the history taking, examination, diagnosis, and management of the patient's condition and prepared the manuscript for publication. C Ponnamperuma performed and reported echocardiography and was involved in diagnosis and management of the patient's condition. All authors read and approved the final manuscript.

## Acknowledgments

The authors acknowledge the support from the staff of Asiri Medical Hospital, Sri Lanka, in the management of this patient's condition.

## References

[1] M. Shimazaki, T. Mitsuhashi, and K. Hasegawa, "Idiopathic pulmonary hypertension associated with hyperthyroidism—an autopsy case," *Nihon Rinsho. Japanese Journal of Clinical Medicine*, vol. 38, no. 3, pp. 1783–1786, 1980.

[2] M. Conradie, C. Koegelenberg, M. Conradie, B. Ascott-Evans, and F. Hough, "Pulmonary hypertension and thyrotoxicosis," *Journal of Endocrinology, Metabolism and Diabetes of South Africa*, vol. 17, no. 2, pp. 101–104, 2014.

[3] F. Rashidi, H. Sate, E. Faraji, and S. Tahsini Tekantapeh, "Thyrotoxicosis presenting as exertional dyspnea and pulmonary hypertension: case report and review of literature," *SAGE Open Medical Case Reports*, vol. 5, 2017.

[4] M. Marvisi, P. Zambrelli, M. Brianti, G. Civardi, R. Lampugnani, and R. Delsignore, "Pulmonary hypertension is frequent in hyperthyroidism and normalizes after therapy," *European Journal of Internal Medicine*, vol. 17, no. 4, pp. 267–271, 2006.

[5] M. J. Dougherty and E. Craige, "Apathetic hyperthyroidism presenting as tricuspid regurgitation," *Chest*, vol. 63, no. 5, pp. 767–772, 1973.

[6] S. L. Teasdale, W. J. Inder, M. Stowasser, and T. Stanton, "Hyperdynamic right heart function in Graves' hyperthyroidism measured by echocardiography normalises on restoration of euthyroidism," *Heart, Lung and Circulation*, vol. 26, no. 6, pp. 580–585, 2017.

[7] C. S. Singarayar, F. S. Hui, N. Cheong, and G. S. En, "Right ventricular dysfunction and pulmonary hypertension: a neglected presentation of thyrotoxicosis," *Endocrinology, Diabetes & Metabolism Case Reports*, vol. 2018, 2018.

[8] H. A. Mulatu, "Pattern and presentation of thyro-cardiac disease among patients with hyperthyroidism attending a tertiary hospital in Ethiopia: a cross sectional study," *Ethiopian Journal of Health Sciences*, vol. 29, no. 1, pp. 887–894, 2019.

[9] M. O. Hegazi, A. El Sayed, and H. El Ghoussein, "Pulmonary hypertension responding to hyperthyroidism treatment," *Respirology*, vol. 13, no. 6, pp. 923–925, 2008.

[10] Y. Chen, X. Wu, R. Wu et al., "Changes in profile of lipids and adipokines in patients with newly diagnosed hypothyroidism and hyperthyroidism," *Scientific Reports*, vol. 6, Article ID 26174, 2016.

[11] Y. Bonde, O. Breuer, D. Lütjohann, S. Sjöberg, B. Angelin, and M. Rudling, "Thyroid hormone reduces PCSK9 and stimulates bile acid synthesis in humans," *Journal of Lipid Research*, vol. 55, no. 11, pp. 2408–2415, 2014.

[12] C. V. Rizos, M. Elisaf, and E. Liberopoulos, "Effects of thyroid dysfunction on lipid profile," *The Open Cardiovascular Medicine Journal*, vol. 5, no. 1, pp. 76–84, 2011.

[13] E. Berta, I. Lengyel, S. Halmi et al., "Hypertension in thyroid disorders," *Frontiers in Endocrinology*, vol. 10, p. 482, 2019.

[14] S. Vallabhajosula, S. Radhi, R. Alalawi, R. Raj, K. Nugent, and C. Cevik, "Hyperthyroidism and pulmonary hypertension: an important association," *The American Journal of the Medical Sciences*, vol. 342, no. 6, pp. 507–512, 2011.

# 4

# Postpartum Pulmonary Hypertension Masquerading as Submassive Pulmonary Embolism

**Mahmood Mubasher ,[1] Amir Hanafi,[1] Tausif Syed,[1] Abir Zinal,[1] Ibrahim Y. Abubeker,[1] Mouhand F. H. Mohamed ,[2] Mohan Rao,[1] Ryan Hoefen,[1] and Mohammed Danjuma[2]**

[1]*Rochester Regional Health-Unity Hospital, Rochester, NY, USA*
[2]*Internal Medicine Department, Hamad General Hospital, Hamad Medical, Corporation, Doha, Qatar*

Correspondence should be addressed to Mouhand F. H. Mohamed; dr.m.oraiby@hotmail.com

Academic Editor: Inger F. Oey

Postpartum pulmonary hypertension (PPPHT) is an extremely rare disorder, with few reported cases. Late diagnosis and treatment are associated with significant morbidity and mortality. We present an 18-year-old female patient who presented four-week postpartum with a typical submissive pulmonary embolism picture subsequently diagnosed as postpartum pulmonary hypertension. The patient had an excellent response to treatment, with a dramatic improvement in her functional status. The authors aim to urge physicians to keep this rare disorder in mind as timely and accurate diagnosis is crucial for management—additionally, the importance of counseling patients about the imminent risks associated with planned future pregnancies.

## 1. Background

The sixth world symposium on pulmonary hypertension defines pulmonary hypertension (PHT) as the mean pulmonary artery pressure (mPAP) > 20 mmHg or pulmonary vascular resistance (PVR) > 3 Wood units [1]. Patients with PHT typically present with progressive fatigue and shortness of breath; this eventually leads to the development of right heart failure. PHT secondary to left heart disease (Type 2 PHT) continues to be the most common type of pulmonary hypertension [2, 3]. PPPHT is a rare variant of PHT. The period of the most considerable risk is within 30 days after delivery [4]. Clinical manifestations vary; presentation as acute massive pulmonary embolism was reported [4, 5]. Whilst its exact pathogenesis remains uncertain, the interaction of a host of factors may play a role in the evolution and progression of PPPHT. The most notable amongst these factors includes the role of cardiac output during pregnancy and delivery and autotransfusion from the uteroplacental circulation to the systemic circulation, along with the release of uterine pressure on the inferior vena cava after delivery suddenly increasing the preload [6, 7]. The second factor is a possible underlying placental hypoxia that induces the release of biological factors that impact on vascular remodeling and vasoconstriction through their effect on the endothelium and smooth muscles [8]. Thirdly (although not supported by robust evidence), amniotic fluid embolism during labor that inadvertently reached the pulmonary circulation could potentially induce an inflammatory reaction that leads to an increase in pulmonary vascular resistance [9]. Recent advances in clinical therapeutics of PTH have seen a significant reduction in maternal mortality attributable to it from 30-50% to 17-30% [10].

## 2. Case Presentation

An 18-year-old female patient with a past medical history significant for iron deficiency anemia presented four-week postpartum (first pregnancy) with a one-week history of chest pain and shortness of breath. The patient described a left-sided chest pain as not radiating, constant and stabbing in nature, moderate to severe, pleuritic, and not related to physical activity. The pain was associated with worsening shortness of breath and palpitations. The patient reported associated exertional dyspnea, dizziness, and fatigue that restricted her ability to take care of her baby. She denied fever, orthopnoea, paroxysmal nocturnal dyspnea, or lower limb swelling. The patient had recently returned from a twenty-eight-hour car journey. Apart from anemia, her pregnancy and delivery were both uneventful. The patient has no allergies, no family history of cardiovascular, or clotting disorders.

On examination, the patient was distressed, tachycardic, and tachypneic and had normal blood pressure. She required $FiO_2$ of 44% to maintain normal saturation. Heartbeat was regular: soft heart sounds without murmurs, gallops, or rubs. There was no parasternal heave and no clinical signs of fluid overload. Moreover, there were no clinical features of endocarditis. She had normal vesicular breath sounds bilateral, with no crackles or wheezes. Lower limb examination was normal without signs of deep vein thrombosis.

Her EKG showed sinus tachycardia with T wave inversion in leads V1-3 (Figure 1).

Biochemical investigations showed a D-dimer of 3331 ng/ml (<500 ng/ml), BNP of 1034 pg/ml (<125 pg/ml), mildly elevated troponin I, and microcytic anemia. Otherwise, renal function, electrolytes, liver function tests, and thyroid hormones were within normal limits. Transthoracic echocardiogram showed a severely dilated right ventricle with globally reduced right ventricular systolic function and a left ventricular ejection fraction of 45-50% (Figure 2). CT pulmonary angiogram showed a dilated pulmonary trunk with no evidence of pulmonary embolism (Figure 3). An extensive venous thromboembolic workup including ultrasound Doppler of both lower limbs, CT venogram of the pelvis and lower limbs, and V/Q scan was negative.

Cardiac MRI showed a severely dilated right ventricle with a strain pattern with significant global reduced right ventricular systolic function, no signs of dysplasia or myocarditis, normal coronary anatomy, and no septal defects. Coronary angiography showed no coronary artery disease or dissection. Right heart catheterization (RHC) revealed the following: right atrial pressure = 12 mmHg (normal range 1-8 mmHg), right systolic ventricular pressure = 45 mmHg (normal range 15-30 mmHg), mean pulmonary artery pressure = 31 mmHg (normal range 10-22), pulmonary capillary wedge pressure = 7 mmHg (normal range 6-15), cardiac output = 2.97 L/min (normal range00204-8 mmHg), and cardiac index of 1.74/min/$m^2$ (normal range 2.8-4.2), respectively.

Eventually, the patient was diagnosed with postpartum pulmonary hypertension. She was admitted and treated in the intensive care unit under the direct care of a pulmonary hypertension team. Her management was guided by a close follow-up of her hemodynamics. Given the high risk of sudden deterioration at any given point, inotropic support was considered and planned. Luckily, the patient's blood pressure remained normal. Good perfusion pressure was supported by normal lactate measures and absence of end-organ damage. Intravenous furosemide infusion was initiated with close monitoring of volume status, which was well tolerated without the need for inotropic support along with parenteral iron. The patient was discharged on torsemide and spironolactone.

## 3. Outcome and Follow-Up

On review three weeks postdischarge, her functional status was back to premorbid levels with improved exercise tolerance. Repeated transthoracic echocardiogram revealed no significant interval changes. Repeat right heart catheterization showed mild pulmonary hypertension, normal right and left ventricular filling pressures, and normalization of the cardiac output and index. The patient was counseled about the importance of contraception and the risks of pregnancy, given the associated mortality risk. However, a few months later, the patient became pregnant, and after a multidisciplinary meeting and recounseling, she underwent a therapeutic abortion. She remains to follow in the pulmonology clinic and is doing well.

## 4. Discussion

Postpartum pulmonary hypertension is an infrequent yet serious entity that can easily be overlooked. Keeping it in mind is very important as early diagnosis and appropriate treatment can have a significant impact on the patient's morbidity and mortality.

The presentation of our patient's submassive pulmonary embolism picture bore a resemblance to other published reports [4, 5]. As was the case with our patient, an extensive workup is usually advised to rule out venous thromboembolism. According to the PIOPED II trial [11], the sensitivity of CT pulmonary angiogram (CTPA) in this regard is about 83%. With high pulmonary embolism probability, the negative predictive value is 95% and increases to 97% if combined by negative CT venogram [11]. Even though amniotic fluid embolism is commonly seen during or immediately after labor, V/Q scan was done to rule it out as the diagnostic yield of CTPA with regard to amniotic fluid embolism is very low. Our patient had sex during the puerperium, which may have made her at risk of having air embolism, in which the penis is thought to act as a piston forcing air into the vagina [12–14]. However, the absence of air in echocardiogram made this unlikely. Coronary artery disease and dissection were ruled out by coronary angiography. Cardiac MRI ruled out myocarditis and arrhythmogenic right ventricular dysplasia as well as the unroofed coronary sinus. Right heart catheterization (RHC) confirmed the PHT as the primary cause of right heart strain, and the normal pulmonary capillary wedge pressure excluded a left ventricular cause of the PHT. The low cardiac output and low cardiac index are likely secondary to the decreased preload secondary to PHT.

It is difficult to know whether the pregnancy and labor-induced stress unmasked a preexisting PHT or if this is a new onset PHT. Owing to the absence of preexisting PHT in our patient, the lack of prior symptoms, the event-free pregnancy, and the start of symptoms three-

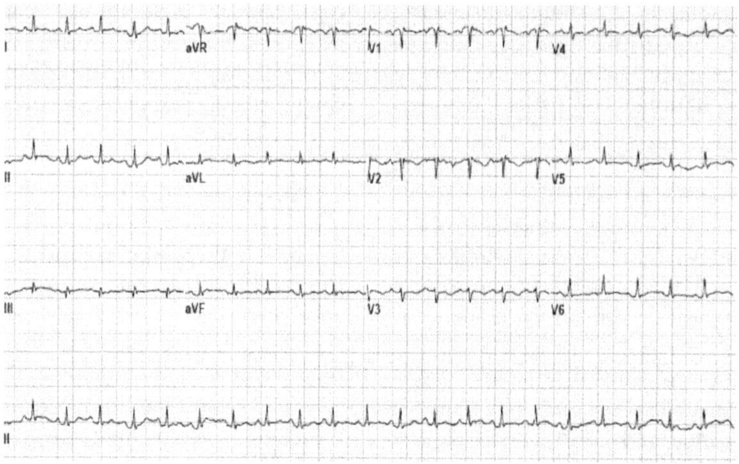


FIGURE 1: Electrocardiogram of the patient showing sinus tachycardia with T wave inversion in leads V1-3.

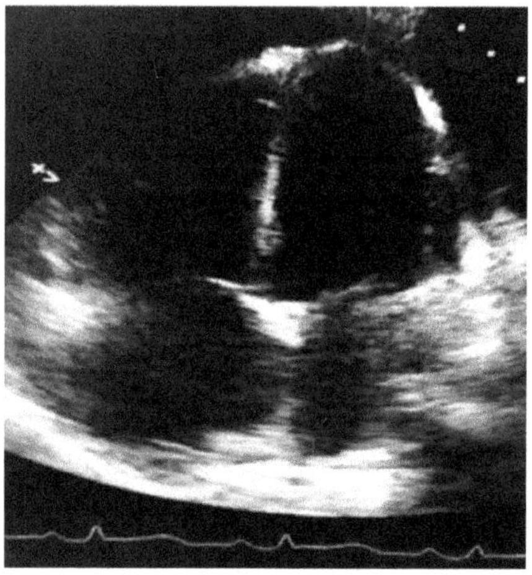

FIGURE 2: Transthoracic echocardiogram showing marked dilatation of right ventricle with globally reduced right ventricular systolic function.

week postpartum, we strongly believe that PPPHT is the correct diagnosis. Patients with PPPHT should be treated in intensive care units under the care of a pulmonary hypertension specialist team. Patients may require supplementary oxygen to maintain adequate oxygenation. Fluid overload should be treated with diuretics; however, the presence of right heart failure (RHF) makes treatment challenging. Patients often require an invasive assessment of hemodynamics to prevent loss of the preload the patient depends on to maintain cardiac output. Our patient had a dramatic improvement of symptoms and normalization of functional status with diuretics alone without the need for pulmonary hypertension-targeted treatments. Treatment of iron deficiency may help in controlling PHT, as previously reported in several studies, which showed that iron deficiency in patients with PHT was considered an important contributing factor [15].

In refractory cases, balloon atrial septostomy is considered a bridge for lung transplantation as it increases preload, cardiac output, and systemic oxygen transport [16]. However, this should be done in a stepwise manner to avoid refractory hypoxemia that may increase mortality [17, 18]. Lung transplant is indicated in the World Health Organization (WHO) functional class III or IV during escalating therapy, rapidly progressive disease, and the continuous need for parenteral targeted pulmonary hypertension therapy. The average five-year survival posttransplantation is around 45-50% [19]. Although the overall progression and prognosis of PPPHT are not well understood, dramatic response to diuretics, lack of need of parenteral targeted pulmonary hypertension therapy, and the normalization of functional status are all favorable prognostic factors.

Even in patients with a good prognosis, future pregnancies are contraindicated. Advice on effective contraceptive methods must be given. Progestogen-only methods and intrauterine devices can be used in women with PHT. Injectable progesterone-only methods and estrogen-containing contraceptives may increase the risk of venous thromboembolism [6, 20, 21]. Dual contraception is indicated in women taking Bosentan due to the interaction between the drug and progesterone-based methods of contraception [6, 16]. Although our understanding of the progression and prognosis of PPPHT is limited, the tough decision of therapeutic abortion was taken after a multidisciplinary meeting and a detailed discussion with the patient and was supported by the current pulmonary artery hypertension guidelines that recommend avoidance of pregnancy and termination of it if it happened [16].

## 5. Limitation

It is difficult to ascertain or conclude whether the pregnancy and labor-induced stress unmasked a preexisting PHT or if this is a new onset PHT. However, the favorable response to treatment is in keeping with new-onset PPPHT.

## 6. Conclusions

Postpartum pulmonary hypertension is an extremely rare disorder that has a significant impact on patients' morbidity and mortality. Early diagnosis and appropriate management

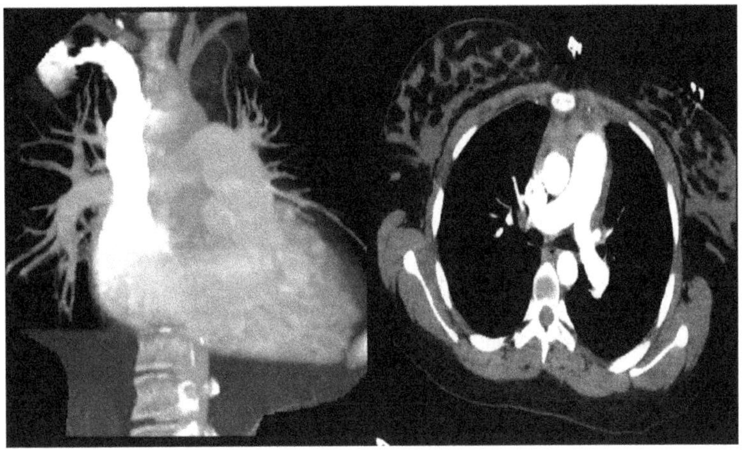

FIGURE 3: CT pulmonary angiogram showing dilated pulmonary trunk, with no evidence of pulmonary embolism.

under the direct supervision of pulmonary hypertension specialists are essential. Postpartum pulmonary hypertension is considered a relative contraindication for further pregnancies. Clinicians should counsel patients on adopting proper contraceptive plans.

## Authors' Contributions

MM is responsible for conceptualization, methodology, data curation, visualization, and project administration. MM and AH wrote and prepared the original draft. MM, AH, TS, AZ, IY, MFHM, MR, RH, and MD wrote the review and edited the file. MD performed the supervision. All authors have read and agreed to the published version of the manuscript.

## Acknowledgments

We acknowledge the Qatar National Library (QNL) for funding the publication of this article. We acknowledge the patient for allowing us to share the details of her case. We also acknowledge all the medical personnel involved in the care of this patient.

## References

[1] G. Simonneau, D. Montani, D. S. Celermajer et al., "Haemodynamic definitions and updated clinical classification of pulmonary hypertension," *European Respiratory Journal*, vol. 53, no. 1, article 1801913, 2019.

[2] G. Simonneau, I. M. Robbins, M. Beghetti et al., "Updated clinical classification of pulmonary hypertension," *Journal of the American College of Cardiology*, vol. 54, no. 1, pp. S43–S54, 2009.

[3] R. J. Oudiz, "Pulmonary hypertension associated with left-sided heart disease," *Clinics in Chest Medicine*, vol. 28, no. 1, pp. 233–241, 2007.

[4] J. P. Escalante, A. Diez, M. Figueroa Casas et al., "Postpartum pulmonary hypertension," *Medicina*, vol. 75, no. 1, pp. 44–47, 2015.

[5] E. Demerouti, A. Manginas, S. Rammos, G. Athanassopoulos, G. Karatasakis, and G. Pavlides, "Postpartum pulmonary arterial hypertension: two cases covering a wide spectrum of presentations," *Hellenic journal of cardiology*, vol. 53, no. 6, pp. 472-475, 2012.

[6] K. M. Olsson and X. Jais, "Birth control and pregnancy management in pulmonary hypertension," *Seminars in Respiratory and Critical Care Medicine*, vol. 34, no. 5, pp. 681–688, 2013.

[7] Endorsed by the European Society of Gynecology (ESG), the Association for European Paediatric Cardiology (AEPC), and the German Society for Gender Medicine (DGesGM), V. Regitz-Zagrosek, C. B. Lundqvist et al., "ESC guidelines on the management of cardiovascular diseases during pregnancy: the Task Force on the Management of Cardiovascular Diseases during pregnancy of the European Society of Cardiology (ESC)," *European Heart Journal*, vol. 32, no. 24, pp. 3147–3197, 2011.

[8] S. J. Sheppard and R. A. Khalil, "Risk factors and mediators of the vascular dysfunction associated with hypertension in pregnancy," *Cardiovascular & Hematological Disorders-Drug Targets*, vol. 10, no. 1, pp. 33–52, 2010.

[9] P. Olley and W. Whitaker, "Postpartum pulmonary hypertension," *Obstetrics and Gynecology*, vol. 29, no. 3, pp. 369–377, 1967.

[10] B. M. Weiss, L. Zemp, B. Seifert, and O. M. Hess, "Outcome of pulmonary vascular disease in pregnancy: a systematic overview from 1978 through 1996," *Journal of the American College of Cardiology*, vol. 31, no. 7, pp. 1650–1657, 1998.

[11] P. Reinartz, B. Nowak, J. Wildberger, W. Schaefer, and U. Buell, "PIOPED II in the diagnosis of pulmonary embolism: evolution or stagnation?," *Journal of Nuclear Medicine*, vol. 47, suppl 1, pp. 20P–20P, 2006.

[12] P. A. Batman, J. Thomlinson, V. C. Moore, and R. Sykes, "Death due to air embolism during sexual intercourse in the puerperium," *Postgraduate Medical Journal*, vol. 74, no. 876, pp. 612-613, 1998.

[13] B. D. Lifschultz and E. R. Donoghue, "Air embolism during intercourse in pregnancy," *Journal of Forensic Sciences*, vol. 28, no. 4, pp. 1021-1022, 1983.

[14] A. Truhlar, V. Cerny, P. Dostal et al., "Out-of-hospital cardiac arrest from air embolism during sexual intercourse: case report and review of the literature," *Resuscitation*, vol. 73, no. 3, pp. 475–484, 2007.

[15] E. Soon, C. M. Treacy, M. R. Toshner et al., "Unexplained iron deficiency in idiopathic and heritable pulmonary arterial hypertension," *Thorax*, vol. 66, no. 4, pp. 326–332, 2011.

[16] N. Galiè, M. M. Hoeper, M. Humbert et al., "Guidelines for the diagnosis and treatment of pulmonary hypertension: the task force for the diagnosis and treatment of pulmonary hypertension of the European Society of Cardiology (ESC) and the European Respiratory Society (ERS), endorsed by the International Society of Heart and Lung Transplantation (ISHLT)," *European Heart Journal*, vol. 30, no. 20, pp. 2493–2537, 2009.

[17] J. Sandoval, J. Gaspar, T. Pulido et al., "Graded balloon dilation atrial septostomy in severe primary pulmonary hypertension. A therapeutic alternative for patients nonresponsive to vasodilator treatment," *Journal of the American College of Cardiology*, vol. 32, no. 2, pp. 297–304, 1998.

[18] A. M. Keogh, E. Mayer, R. L. Benza et al., "Interventional and surgical modalities of treatment in pulmonary hypertension," *Journal of the American College of Cardiology*, vol. 54, no. 1, pp. S67–S77, 2009.

[19] E. P. Trulock, L. B. Edwards, D. O. Taylor et al., "Registry of the International Society for Heart and Lung Transplantation: Twenty-third Official Adult Lung and Heart-Lung Transplantation Report–2006," *The Journal of Heart and Lung Transplantation*, vol. 25, no. 8, pp. 880–892, 2006.

[20] A. R. Hemnes, D. G. Kiely, B. A. Cockrill et al., "Statement on pregnancy in pulmonary hypertension from the Pulmonary Vascular Research Institute," *Pulmonary Circulation*, vol. 5, no. 3, pp. 435–465, 2016.

[21] S. Mantha, R. Karp, V. Raghavan, N. Terrin, K. A. Bauer, and J. I. Zwicker, "Assessing the risk of venous thromboembolic events in women taking progestin-only contraception: a meta-analysis," *BMJ*, vol. 345, no. aug07 2, article e4944, 2012.

5

# Two Cases of Severe Hypertension in JAK2 Mutation-Positive Myeloproliferative Neoplasms

**Raunak Rao, Spoorthy Kulkarni, and Ian B. Wilkinson**

*Division of Experimental Medicine and Immunotherapeutics, University of Cambridge, Cambridge, UK*

Correspondence should be addressed to Raunak Rao; ramr2@cam.ac.uk
and Spoorthy Kulkarni; spoorthy.kulkarni@addenbrookes.nhs.uk

Academic Editor: Nilda Espinola-Zavaleta

*Background.* Myeloproliferative neoplasms are a heterogeneous group of disorders resulting from the abnormal proliferation of one or more terminal myeloid cells—established complications include thrombosis and haemorrhagic events; however, there is limited evidence to suggest an association with arterial hypertension. Herein, we report two independent cases of severe hypertension in JAK2 mutation-positive myeloproliferative neoplasms. *Case Presentations.* Case 1: a 39-year-old male was referred to our specialist hypertension unit with high blood pressure (BP) (200/120 mmHg), erythromelalgia, and headaches. We recorded elevated serum creatinine levels (146 $\mu$M) and panmyelosis. Bone marrow biopsy confirmed JAK2-mutation-positive polycythaemia vera. Renal imaging revealed renal artery stenosis. Aspirin, long-acting nifedipine, interferon-alpha 2A, and renal artery angioplasty were employed in management. BP reached below target levels to an average of 119/88 mmHg. Renal parameters normalised gradually alongside BP. Case 2: a 45-year-old male presented with high BP (208/131 mmHg), acrocyanosis, (vasculitic) skin rashes, and nonhealing ulcers. Fundoscopy showed optic disc blurring in the left eye and full blood count revealed thrombocytosis. Bone marrow biopsy confirmed JAK2-mutation-positive essential thrombocytosis. No renal artery stenosis was found. Cardiac output was measured at 5 L/min using an inert gas rebreathing method, providing an estimated peripheral vascular resistance of 1840 dynes/s/cm$^5$. BP was well-controlled (reaching 130/70 mmHg) with CCBs. *Conclusions.* These presentations highlight the utility of full blood count analysis in patients with severe hypertension. Hyperviscosity and constitutive JAK-STAT activation are amongst the proposed pathophysiology linking myeloproliferative neoplasms and hypertension. Further experimental and clinical research is necessary to identify and understand possible interactions between BP and myeloproliferative neoplasms.

## 1. Introduction

Myeloproliferative neoplasms (MPNs) are clonal disorders arising in the haematopoietic stem cell compartment. MPNs are mostly diagnosed in the age range of 50 to 60 years; however, presentations can occur in younger patients, especially with familial predisposition.

The most common MPN driver gene is Janus kinase 2 (JAK2), a cognate tyrosine kinase for both the erythropoietin and thrombopoietin receptors. JAK2-mutation-positive MPNs are associated with a higher rate of vascular complications. These include thrombotic events and occlusive vascular diseases. As of yet, there is limited evidence concerning a potential connection with arterial hypertension. However, several forms of vascular complications of MPNs have been described, including pulmonary hypertension [1], portal hypertension [2], and renovascular hypertension [3].

A retrospective analysis published in 2018 studying 1010 MPN patients in Malaysia demonstrated a significant association between JAK2 V617F mutation-positive MPNs and hypertension [4]. More recently, a study including 10 essential thrombocytosis patients with venous thrombosis found that all cases had concurrent arterial hypertension [5]. We report two cases of acute severe hypertension associated with JAK2 V617F mutation-positive MPNs. Earlier identification of MPNs in young, severely hypertensive patients may help in choosing the right treatment strategy leading to effective blood pressure (BP) control.

TABLE 1: Summary of case presentations.

| | Case 1 | Case 2 |
|---|---|---|
| Initial BP (mmHg) | 200/120 | 208/131 |
| Presenting symptoms | Erythromelalgia, occipital headaches, Vertigo, one episode of dyspnoea + eye floaters + syncope (1-2 minutes) | Acrocyanosis, Vasculitic skin rashes, nonhealing toe ulceration |
| Past medical history | Spondylolisthesis | Migraines with aura |
| Family history | Father: Vasovagal syncope, myocardial infarction | Unremarkable |
| Social history | Ex-smoker | 20 units of alcohol per week |
| Investigations and results | | |
| Fundus examination | Papilloedema with nasal margin blurring | Arteriovenous nipping with nasal margin blurring |
| Urine dipstick | Unremarkable | Unremarkable |
| FBC | WBC—$15.8 \times 10^9$/L; RBC—$6.20 \times 10^9$/L; Hct -0.534 L/L PLT $-953 \times 10^9$/L; Neutrophil count $-12.10 \times 10^9$/L | PLT -1096 x$10^9$/L |
| Liver function tests | Not indicated | Total bilirubin—38 $\mu$mol/L; ALT—42 U/L; Gamma GT—94 U/L |
| Electrocardiogram | Sinus rhythm 70 bpm, left axis deviation, biphasic T waves in leads V5 and V6 | Unremarkable |
| Echocardiogram | Moderate global left ventricular hypertrophy with 1.4 cm wall thickness | Mild aortic dilatation |
| Creatinine | 146 $\mu$M | 88 $\mu$M |
| Renin | 107 mU/L | 80 mU/L |
| Autoimmune screen | Negative | Negative |
| Vasculitic skin rash biopsy | N/A | Unremarkable |
| Contrast CT abdomen | N/A | Enlarged left adrenal gland, lower abdominal lymphadenopathy |
| Inert gas rebreathing studies (clinical research facility) | N/A | Peripheral vascular resistance -1840 dynes/s/$cm^5$ |
| Interventions | Renal artery angioplasty, aspirin 75 mg, intermittent venesection, interferon-alpha 2A | Aspirin 75 mg, long-acting nifedipine |
| Outcomes | Normalisation of BP and renal parameters, minor side effects from interferon therapy (decreased libido and reported thinning of hair), now managed with single dose of long-acting nifedipine | Normalisation of BP, no adverse outcomes reported, toe ulceration now healed |

## 2. Case Presentations

Summaries of Cases 1 and 2 are displayed in Table 1.

*2.1. Case 1 Polycythaemia Vera.* A detailed account of Case 1 is displayed in Table 1.

Presentation: A 39-year-old male was referred to our specialist hypertension unit with a high BP (200/120 mmHg), erythromelalgia, and headaches.

Investigations: We recorded elevated serum creatinine levels (146 $\mu$M), panmyelosis with raised haematocrit (0.534 L/L), white blood cell (WBC) ($15.8 \times 10^9$/L) and platelet (PLT) ($953 \times 10^9$/L) counts. Bone marrow biopsy confirmed JAK2-mutation-positive polycythaemia vera. Renal imaging revealed renal artery stenosis (Figure 1(a)).

Outcomes and follow-up: Aspirin, nifedipine, interferon-alpha 2A (cytoreductive therapy—under haematology), and renal artery angioplasty (Figure 1(b)) were employed in management. BP reached below target levels to an average of 119/88 mmHg (Figure 2(a)). Renal parameters normalised gradually alongside BP (Figure 2(b)).

*2.2. Case 2 Essential Thrombocytosis.* Presentation: A 45-year-old male presented with high BP (208/131 mmHg), acrocyanosis, vasculitic skin rashes (Figure 3(a)), and non-healing ulcers (Figure 3(b)).

Investigations: Fundoscopy showed optic disc blurring in the left eye and full blood count (FBC) revealed thrombocytosis (PLT $-953 \times 10^9$/L). Bone marrow biopsy confirmed JAK2-mutation-positive essential thrombocytosis.

Outcomes and follow-up—unlike our Case 1 patient, no renal artery stenosis was found. BP was well-controlled (reaching 130/70 mmHg) with nifedipine.

## 3. Discussion

Severely elevated BP (>180/120 mmHg) concomitant with new or progressive target organ dysfunction constitutes

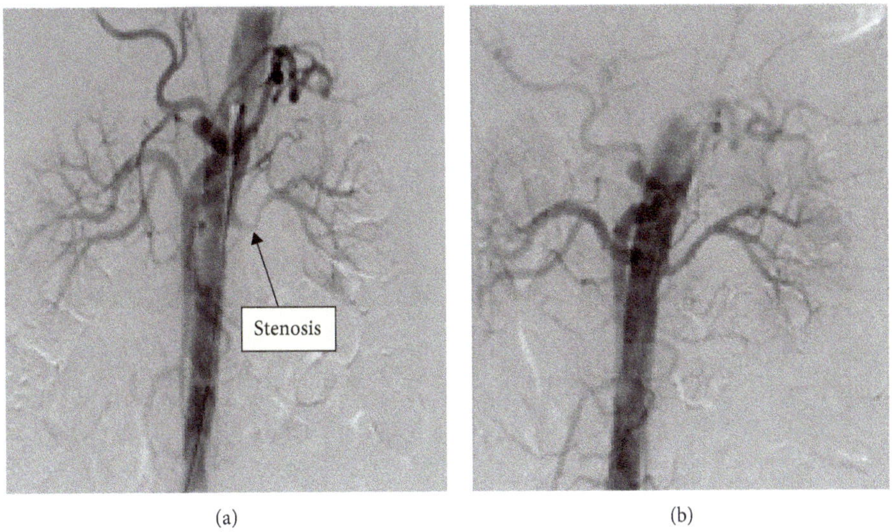


FIGURE 1: Case 1—(a) CT renal angiogram showing right renal artery before angioplasty. (b) CT renal angiogram showing right renal artery after angioplasty.

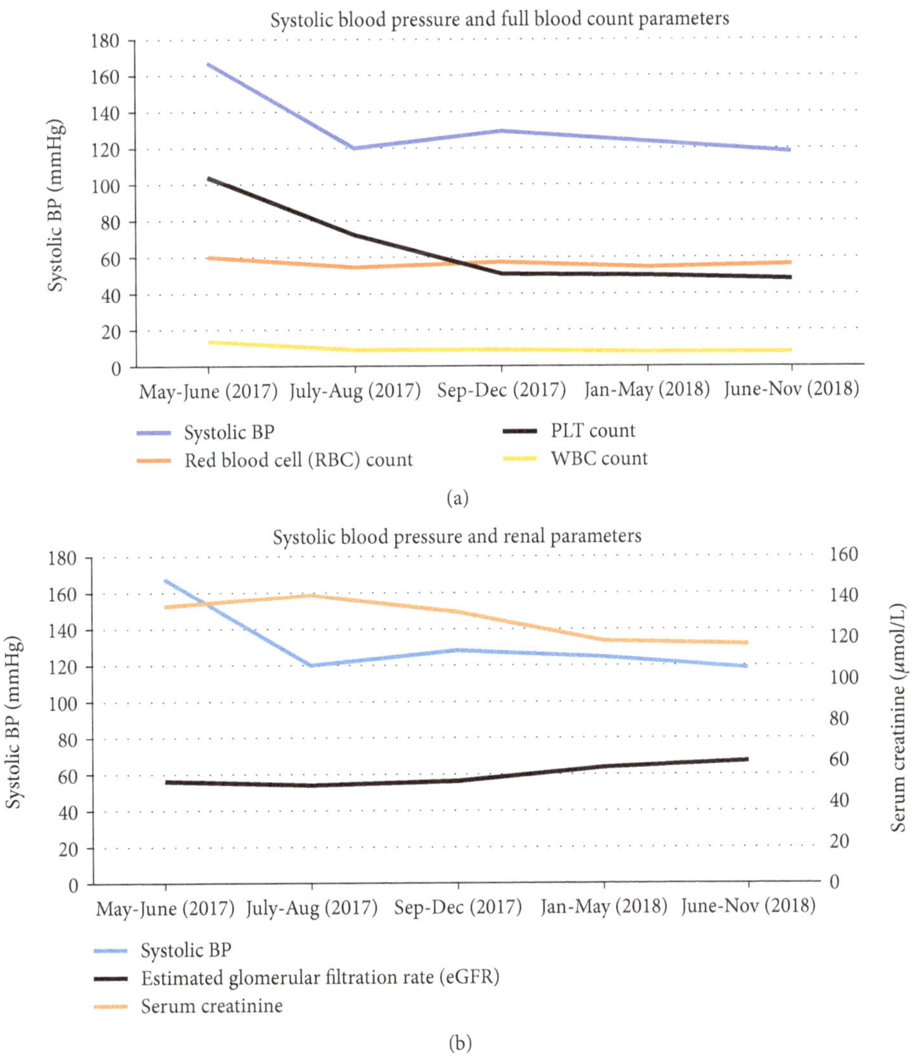


FIGURE 2: Case 1—(a) Changes in BP alongside FBC. (b) Changes in BP alongside renal parameters.

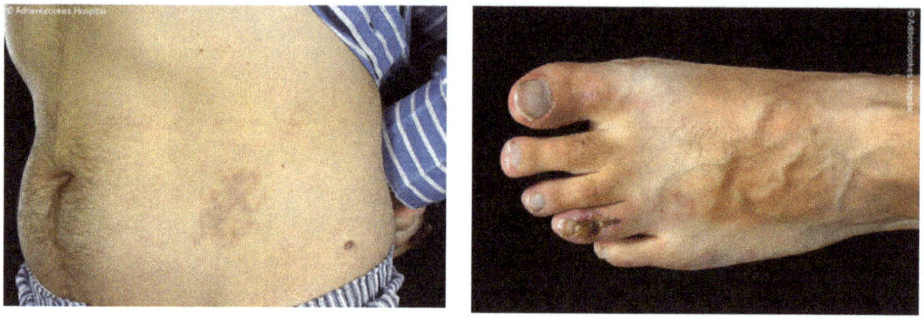

(a) (b)

FIGURE 3: Case 2—(a) Vasculitic skin rashes. (b) Nonhealing ulcers.

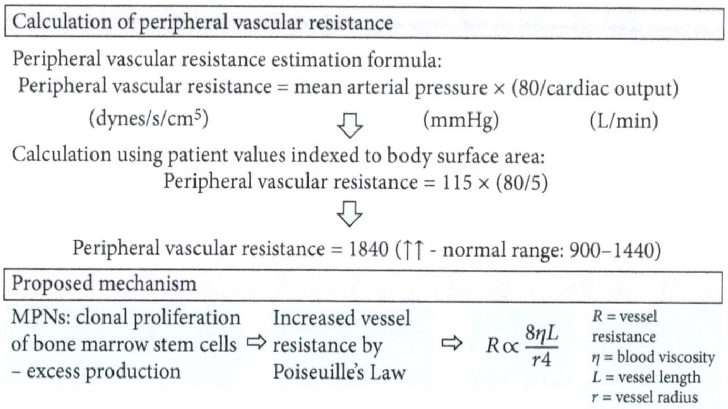


FIGURE 4: Case 2—Vessel resistance calculation and suggested mechanism for increase. Elevated peripheral vascular resistance with nonhealing ulcers could indicate vasoconstriction and microvascular rarefaction.

accelerated hypertension. Current practice overlooks FBC analysis when evaluating hypertension. Effective BP control was achieved in Case 1 and 2 with overlapping therapeutic interventions, suggesting a degree of similarity between the two pathophysiologies.

Both cases demonstrated good clinical responses to CCBs (over ACE inhibitor in Case 1), which cause direct vasodilatation through inhibition of calcium ion influx in vascular smooth muscle. This mechanism of action might be favourable in the context of hyperviscosity and elevated vascular resistance, as proposed in Figure 4. In Case 2, peripheral vascular resistance (PVR) was calculated from cardiac output and stroke volume measurements using an inert gas rebreathing method (Innocor) [6]. This provided an estimate of 1840 dynes/s/$cm^5$, considerably exceeding the normal range of 900-1440 dynes/s/$cm^5$, and that usually is seen in hypertension.

Raised PVR together with nonhealing ulceration could strongly suggest that vasoconstriction and microvascular rarefaction underly the hypotheses. A number of mechanisms may explain this in patients with essential thrombocytosis and polycythaemia vera. Increased haematocrit and platelet aggregation lead to whole blood hyperviscosity, which can add to both, the humoral and haemodynamic changes. Increased haematocrit increases the probability of adhesive wall collisions mediated by platelets. Platelets synthesise and discharge haemostatic mediators including thromboxane A2, PGF2 alpha, and serotonin, all of which are potent vasoconstrictors. These may lead to the activation of endothelial cells, resulting in increased expression of adhesion molecules and secretion of thrombogenic and angiogenic peptides from local inflammatory cells and procoagulant factors including von Willebrand factor (vWF). Endothelial injury/-dysfunction has been postulated to be one of the mechanisms by which raised haematocrit predisposes to thrombotic complications [7]. Flow-mediated dilation (FMD), a marker for endothelial function, was found to be reduced in a small study in MPN patients, demonstrating the role of endothelium dysfunction [8]. Endothelial damage further leads to arterial insufficiency and capillary rarefaction—particularly in the microcirculation where endothelial dysfunction is greatest. This leads to a vicious cycle of endothelial damage, accounting for the chronic ulceration displayed by our patient.

The haemodynamic effects of ACE inhibitors and CCBs are known to differ. Whilst ACE inhibitors antagonise the renin-angiotensin system and reduce sympathetic output, CCBs mediate dilatation of large conduit and resistance arteries. These differences might explain the preferential responsiveness exhibited in both cases. However, the true relevance for MPN patients remains unclear, particularly as there is conflicting evidence to demonstrate a direct correlation between blood viscosity and pressure in normotensive and hypertensive subjects [9, 10].

Case 1 indicates an additional renovascular component to the patient's presentation. Several factors are likely to have contributed to the stenotic lesion including raised haematocrit, dysregulated coagulation, and abnormal vascular endothelial functions. These mechanisms have been discussed by Tamura et al. in a previous description of two patients with hypertension secondary to renal artery stenosis with JAK2 V617F-positive MPNs, both of whom were successfully managed with angioplasty [11]. The utility of angioplasty is considered highly dependent on the pathogenesis of renal artery stenosis. In patients with atherosclerotic stenosis, angioplasty demonstrates no significant advantage over medical management in the regulation of BP [12]. In comparison, MPN-associated renovascular hypertension responds well to this intervention. The greater extent of unresolved ischaemia in atherosclerotic pathophysiology is thought to account for this difference, meaning that MPN patients with coexistent renovascular atherosclerosis might receive limited benefit from renal angioplasty [13]. However, the fact that both patients responded to vasodilatory medications could imply that the stenosis is a bystander or indeed a by-product here rather than the main driver for acute rise in blood pressure.

Constitutive JAK-STAT activation has been suggested to increase the activation of platelets, and recruitment of platelets and leukocytes in conjunction with accelerated vascular cell hyperplasia [7]. Furthermore, the activated JAK-STAT pathway is known to contribute to local synthesis of Angiotensin II (Ang II), and in turn, the progression of Ang II-dependent hypertension [14]. Ang II-activated JAK2 prompts phosphorylation of Arhgef1 in vascular smooth muscle cells [15]; consequently, Arhgef1 stimulates the RhoA-Rho kinase axis, resulting in BP augmentation. In support of these findings, pharmacological inhibition of JAK2 has been shown to reduce hypertension in Ang-II infused animal models [16, 17]. JAK-STAT signalling has also been implicated in renal injury, with hyperglycaemia inducing the pathway via Ang II in glomerular mesangial cells [18]. Consistent with this observation, JAK2 inhibition in rat models prevented proteinuria and hypertension in streptozotocin-induced diabetic nephropathy [19], as well as ameliorating renal ischaemia-reperfusion injury [20].

Further study of the relationship between haemorheology, haemodynamics, and the role of endothelial dysfunction in MPNs is needed.

## 4. Conclusion

This report highlights the importance of simple FBC analysis in severe hypertension and the potential therapeutic role of CCBs. Increased platelet counts, hyperviscosity, rarefaction of vasculature, and resultant release of vasoconstrictive mediators are amongst the proposed pathophysiologies linking MPNs and hypertension. Associated vascular complications like arterial and venous thrombosis may add to the burden of vascular damage. Further experimental and clinical evidence is required to identify mechanisms of interaction between JAK2 function and BP.

## Abbreviations

JAK2: Janus kinase 2
MPNs: Myeloproliferative neoplasms
BP: BP
WBC: White blood cell
PLT: Platelet
FBC: Full blood count
CT: Computerised tomography
RBC: Red blood cell
JAK-STAT: Janus kinase-signal transducer and activator of transcription
ACE: Angiotensin-converting enzyme
PVR: Peripheral vascular resistance
Ang II: Angiotensin II.

## Consent

Written informed consent was obtained from the patients for publication of their individual details and accompanying images in this manuscript. The consent form is held by the authors and is available for review by the Editor-in-Chief.

## Authors' Contributions

RR and SK drafted the manuscript. SK participated in patient care. IBW bore the overall responsibility of patient care, provided clinical expertise, and oversaw drafting. All authors read and approved the final manuscript.

## References

[1] T. Yi, W. Ma, J. Qiu, and W. Ding, "Pulmonary hypertension with massive megalosplenia: a case report," *Medicine*, vol. 98, no. 12, article e14594, 2019.

[2] A. Durivage, G. Le Templier, A. Cumyn, and N. Sauvé, "Pregnancy in a woman with latent myeloproliferative neoplasm induced chronic portal vein thrombosis, portal cavernoma, and gastric varices," *Case Reports in Obstetrics and Gynecology*, vol. 2019, Article ID 5702983, 4 pages, 2019.

[3] F. Z. Ha-Ou-Nou, D. Boumzebra, and L. Essaadouni, "Coexistence of renal artery stenosis, primary antiphospholipid syndrome and polycythaemia vera: an exceptional association," *Lupus*, vol. 23, no. 1, pp. 84–87, 2014.

[4] Y. Y. Yap, K. B. Law, J. Sathar et al., "The epidemiology and clinical characteristics of myeloproliferative neoplasms in Malaysia," *Experimental Hematology & Oncology*, vol. 7, no. 1, p. 31, 2018.

[5] I. Horvat, A. Boban, R. Zadro et al., "Influence of blood count, cardiovascular risks, inherited thrombophilia, and JAK2 V617F burden allele on type of thrombosis in patients with Philadelphia chromosome negative myeloproliferative neoplasms," *Clinical Lymphoma Myeloma and Leukemia*, vol. 19, no. 1, pp. 53–63, 2019.

[6] J. E. Middlemiss, A. Cocks, K. Paapstel et al., "Evaluation of inert gas rebreathing for determination of cardiac output: influence of age, gender and body size," *Hypertension Research*, vol. 42, no. 6, pp. 834–844, 2019.

[7] M. H. Kroll, L. C. Michaelis, and S. Verstovsek, "Mechanisms of thrombogenesis in polycythemia vera," *Blood Reviews*, vol. 29, no. 4, pp. 215–221, 2015.

[8] A. Yildiz, M. Güryildirim, M. S. Pepeler, M. Yazol, S. Ö. Oktar, and K. Acar, "Assessment of endothelial dysfunction with flow-mediated dilatation in myeloproliferative disorders," *Clinical and Applied Thrombosis/Hemostasis*, vol. 24, no. 7, pp. 1102–1108, 2018.

[9] G. Ciuffetti, L. Pasqualini, M. Pirro et al., "Blood rheology in men with essential hypertension and capillary rarefaction," *Journal of Human Hypertension*, vol. 16, no. 8, pp. 533–537, 2002.

[10] B. Y. S. Vázquez, "Blood pressure and blood viscosity are not correlated in normal healthy subjects," *Vascular Health and Risk Management*, vol. 8, pp. 1–6, 2012.

[11] K. Tamura, K. Haruhara, K. Azushima, T. Iwamoto, and H. Wakui, "Possible interesting link between Janus kinase 2 mutation and renovascular hypertension," *Journal of Clinical Hypertension*, vol. 20, no. 4, pp. 805-806, 2018.

[12] C. J. Cooper, T. P. Murphy, D. E. Cutlip et al., "Stenting and medical therapy for atherosclerotic renal-artery stenosis," *The New England Journal of Medicine*, vol. 370, no. 1, pp. 13–22, 2014.

[13] E. Mishima, T. Suzuki, Y. Takeuchi et al., "Renovascular hypertension associated with JAK2 V617F positive myeloproliferative neoplasms treated with angioplasty: 2 cases and literature review," *Journal of Clinical Hypertension*, vol. 20, no. 4, pp. 798–804, 2018.

[14] R. Satou and R. Gonzalez-Villalobos, "JAK-STAT and the renin-angiotensin system: the role of the JAK-STAT pathway in BP and intrarenal renin-angiotensin system regulation," *JAK-STAT*, vol. 1, no. 4, pp. 250–256, 2012.

[15] C. Guilluy, J. Brégeon, G. Toumaniantz et al., "The Rho exchange factor Arhgef1 mediates the effects of angiotensin II on vascular tone and blood pressure," *Nature Medicine*, vol. 16, no. 2, pp. 183–190, 2010.

[16] A. Kirabo, P. N. Kearns, Y. P. Jarajapu et al., "Vascular smooth muscle Jak2 mediates angiotensin II-induced hypertension via increased levels of reactive oxygen species," *Cardiovascular Research*, vol. 91, no. 1, pp. 171–179, 2011.

[17] A. K. L. Banes-Berceli, H. Al-Azawi, D. Proctor et al., "Angiotensin ii utilizes Janus kinase 2 in hypertension, but not in the physiological control of blood pressure, during low-salt intake," *American Journal of Physiology-Regulatory, Integrative and Comparative Physiology*, vol. 301, no. 4, pp. R1169–R1176, 2011.

[18] M. B. Marrero, A. K. Banes-Berceli, D. M. Stern, and D. C. Eaton, "Role of the JAK/STAT signaling pathway in diabetic nephropathy," *American Journal of Physiology - Renal Physiology*, vol. 290, no. 4, pp. F762–F768, 2006.

[19] A. K. Banes, S. Shaw, J. Jenkins et al., "Angiotensin II blockade prevents hyperglycemia-induced activation of JAK and STAT proteins in diabetic rat kidney glomeruli," *American Journal of Physiology-Renal Physiology*, vol. 286, no. 4, pp. F653–F659, 2004.

[20] N. Yang, M. Luo, R. Li et al., "Blockage of JAK/STAT signalling attenuates renal ischaemia-reperfusion injury in rats," *Nephrology, Dialysis, Transplantation*, vol. 23, no. 1, pp. 91–100, 2007.

6

# Subacute Thyroiditis Presenting as Idiopathic Intracranial Hypertension

**Kanyanatt Boonyatarp**,[1] **Kanoksri Samintharapanya**,[2] **Thanawat Vongchaiudomchoke**,[3] **and Nuttaya Wachiraphansakul**[4]

[1]*Department of Internal Medicine, Lampang Hospital, Lampang, Thailand*
[2]*Division of Neurology, Department of Internal Medicine, Lampang Hospital, Lampang, Thailand*
[3]*Division of Nephrology, Department of Internal Medicine, Lampang Hospital, Lampang, Thailand*
[4]*Division of Endocrinology and Metabolism, Department of Internal Medicine, Lampang Hospital, Lampang, Thailand*

Correspondence should be addressed to Nuttaya Wachiraphansakul; iewnuttaya@gmail.com

Academic Editor: Toshihiro Kita

*Background.* Several case reports have illustrated a rare neurological manifestation, idiopathic intracranial hypertension (IIH), in patients with thyrotoxicosis. However, none were diagnosed with thyroiditis. We report the case of a patient with subacute thyroiditis who presented with severe intractable headache due to IIH. *Case Presentation.* A 36-year-old woman visited Lampang Hospital in February 2021 complaining of neck pain and progressive severe intractable headache. Her vital signs and neurological examination were normal. Thyroid examination revealed a single 1 cm right thyroid nodule. A computed tomography (CT) scan of her brain illustrated diffuse brain edema. However, CT angiography and venography of the brain did not show abnormalities. The opening pressure of the cerebrospinal fluid was elevated (27 $cmH_2O$). The free triiodothyronine level was 6.19 pg/mL, free thyroxine was 2.32 ng/dL, and thyroid-stimulating hormone was 0.0083 $\mu$IU/mL. Anti-Tg was positive at a low titer, but anti-TPO was negative. TRAb was also negative. Methimazole and acetazolamide were prescribed and monitored. The symptoms resolved completely within 2 weeks of onset. Thyroid hormones had returned to normal by 8 weeks. *Conclusion.* This is the first case report of subacute thyroiditis presenting with IIH.

## 1. Introduction

Thyroiditis is the term used to describe thyroid gland inflammation that arises from any etiology. Therefore, there are variations in the clinical manifestations and course of thyroiditis. Its diagnosis is made by clinical symptoms of thyrotoxicosis with acute destruction of the thyroid gland, which leads to the release of the thyroid hormone into the systemic circulation. Thyroid gland tenderness is commonly found in cases of subacute thyroiditis and infectious thyroiditis but is rarely seen in Hashimoto's thyroiditis. However, no manifestations of idiopathic intracranial hypertension (IIH; also called pseudotumor cerebri) have been reported for the thyrotoxicosis stage. Here, we report the first case of subacute thyroiditis that presents as IIH.

## 2. Case Presentation

A 36-year-old woman visited Lampang Hospital in February 2021 complaining of a severe progressive intractable headache for 1 week. She also had dull aching shoulder and neck pain on the right side. These symptoms were not relieved with nonsteroidal anti-inflammatory drugs. She had no relevant medical history and was not taking any medications. On physical examination, her body temperature was 36.3°C. No clinical signs of hyperthyroidism were observed. Neurological examination was normal. There was no limitation of extraocular muscle movement, fundoscopic examination did not reveal papilledema, and the visual fields of both eyes were normal. Due to her painful neck, her thyroid function was evaluated on the first day of admission. The

Table 1: Symptoms, laboratory results, and treatment by day of illness, hospital day, and follow-up day.

| | Hospital day | | | | | Follow-up day | | | |
|---|---|---|---|---|---|---|---|---|---|
| | 1 | 2 | 3 | 4 | 11 | 24 | 38 | 68 | 218 |
| Day of illness | D8 | D9 | D10 | D11 | D18 | D31 | D45 | D85 | D225 |
| Neck pain | ■ | ■ | ■ | ■ | ■ | | | | |
| Headache | ■ | ■ | ■ | | | | | | |
| Vomiting | ■ | ■ | ■ | | | | | | |
| Body temperature (°C) | 36.3 | 36.7 | 37.2 | 36.9 | 36.9 | 36.2 | 37.0 | 36.5 | 36.5 |
| Hemoglobin (g/dL) | 10.2 | 9.9 | 11.3 | | 12.7 | 12.0 | 12.9 | 12.7 | |
| White blood cell count (/cu.mm) | 5400 | 7400 | 6900 | | 5500 | 5500 | 4700 | 4800 | |
| Neutrophil (%) | 76 | 74 | 67 | | 61 | 71 | 60 | 55 | |
| Lymphocyte (%) | 17 | 18 | 22 | | 27 | 22 | 32 | 34 | |
| Platelet count ($\times 10^3$/cu.mm) | 287,000 | 269,000 | 346,000 | | 399,000 | 317,000 | 324,000 | 273,000 | |
| Free T3 (pg/mL) (1.71–3.71) | 6.19 | | | | 7.07 | 2.86 | 2.15 | 2.07 | 2.23 |
| Free T4 (ng/dL) (0.70–1.48) | 2.32 | | | | 2.20 | 1.18 | 0.66 | 0.87 | 0.98 |
| TSH ($\mu$IU/mL) (0.350–4.940) | 0.0083 | | | | 0.0040 | 0.0047 | 2.18 | 4.39 | 3.16 |
| Anti-Tg (IU/mL) | 10.13 | | | | | | | | 5.28 |
| Anti-TPO (IU/mL) | <3.00 | | | | | | | | 0.25 |
| TRAb (IU/L) | <0.8 | | | | | | | | |
| ESR (mm/hr) | | 51 | | | | | | | 6 |
| hs-CRP (mg/L) | | 41.4 | | | | | | | |
| BUN (mg/dL) | 15 | 15 | 13 | | 120 | | | | |
| Creatinine (mg/dL) | 0.57 | 0.49 | 0.70 | | 0.54 | 0.54 | | | |
| Sodium (mmol/L) | 143 | 142 | 138 | | 139 | 140 | | | |
| Potassium (mmol/L) | 4.1 | 3.8 | 3.8 | | 3.8 | 3.7 | | | |
| Chloride (mmol/L) | 110 | 111 | 111 | | 110 | 107 | | | |
| Bicarbonate (mmol/L) | 28 | 24 | 18 | | 16 | 25 | | | |
| CSF opening pressure ($cmH_2O$) | 27 | | 18 | | | | | | |
| Glucose CSF | 52 | | | | | | | | |
| Protein CSF | 23.9 | | | | | | | | |
| Color | Colorless | | | | | | | | |
| RBC | No RBC | | | | | | | | |
| Cell count | No cell | | | | | | | | |
| Therapy | | | | | | | | | |
| Methimazole | 15 mg/day | | 10 mg/day | | | 5 mg/day | | | |
| Acetazolamide | 500 mg/day | 750 mg/day | | | 500 mg/day × 14 days | | | | |

Anti-Tg: antithyroglobulin antibody; anti-TPO: antithyroid peroxidase antibody; BUN: blood urea nitrogen; CSF: cerebrospinal fluid; ESR: erythrocyte sedimentation rate; hs-CRP: high-sensitivity C-reactive protein; T3: triiodothyronine; T4: thyroxine; TRAb: antithyroid receptor antibody.

tests revealed primary hyperthyroidism: a free triiodothyronine level of 6.19 pg/mL (1.71–3.71 pg/mL), a free thyroxine level of 2.32 ng/dL (0.70–1.48 ng/dL), and a thyroid-stimulating hormone level of 0.0083 $\mu$IU/mL (0.35–4.94 $\mu$IU/mL) (Table 1). The results of a brain computed tomography (CT) scan illustrated a diffuse absence of cortical sulci, which was consistent with diffuse brain edema. Nevertheless, CT angiography and venography of her brain did not demonstrate abnormalities (Figure 1). The opening pressure of the cerebrospinal fluid (CSF) was elevated (27 $cmH_2O$), and the CSF had normal levels of glucose and protein without cells. The erythrocyte sedimentation rate was high (51 mm/h). A workup was then conducted to determine the cause of thyrotoxicosis. A neck ultrasound showed a single 1 cm right thyroid nodule (Figure 2). However, she did not undergo thyroid scintigraphy due to recent administration of contrast media. While waiting for thyroid antibody results, methimazole (15 mg/day) and acetazolamide (750 mg/day) were prescribed. Potential etiologies of IIH were excluded by blood and CSF analyses (Table 1). Immunological investigation revealed a slightly elevated level of antithyroglobulin antibody (anti-Tg; 10.13 IU/ml). Antithyroid peroxidase antibody (anti-TPO) and antithyroid receptor antibody (TRAb) were both negative. With neck pain accompanied by thyrotoxicosis and a high erythrocyte sedimentation rate, subacute thyroiditis was the most likely diagnosis. Her headache gradually improved without the addition of steroid treatment, and it disappeared after 1 week. Acetazolamide was continued for 2 weeks, and she returned to the euthyroid state. Methimazole was tapered and discontinued after 6 weeks. Six months after the onset of thyrotoxicosis, her thyroid function was still normal, and her thyroid sonographic results did not reveal nodularity. A steady decline in the anti-Tg level was observed over the 6-month period, supporting the diagnosis of subacute thyroiditis (Table 1).

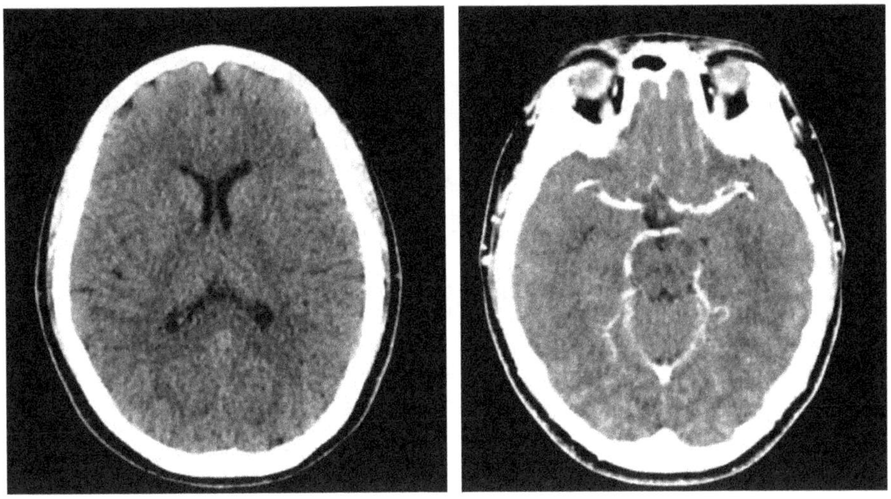

Figure 1: Brain computed tomography and venography revealed diffuse absence of cortical sulci without venous obstruction, consistent with diffuse cerebral edema.

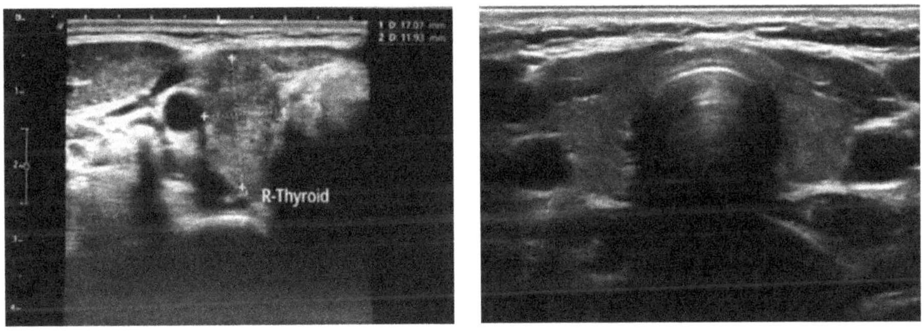


(a) (b)

Figure 2: (a) A neck ultrasound showed a solitary 1 cm right thyroid nodule. (b) Follow-up neck ultrasound revealed no nodularity.

## 3. Discussion and Conclusions

Subacute thyroiditis, also known as de Quervain's thyroiditis, is believed to be caused by postviral inflammation that causes inflammation of the thyroid gland. The clinical course of subacute thyroiditis usually shows 3 consecutive phases that unfold over approximately 6 months. During the first weeks after the onset of symptoms, transient thyrotoxicosis is found as preformed thyroid hormones are released from the damaged gland. Within a few weeks, many patients enter a hypothyroid phase, which is later followed by euthyroid restoration [1]. Tenderness and goiter are common manifestations in most cases [2, 3]. A thyroid antibody workup should be performed to exclude Hashimoto's thyroiditis, which is one of the most common causes of thyroiditis [2]. Differential diagnosis between Graves' disease is also mandatory. In addition, TRAb levels must be measured as treatments for thyroiditis and Graves' disease differ [4].

The presentation in our case involved a painful thyroid enlargement without specific signs of Graves' disease. There was no exposure to contrast media before the first thyroid function workup. The TRAb results were negative. Although a low anti-Tg titer was found, subacute thyroiditis was the most likely diagnosis due to the clinical symptoms and the decrease in the thyroid titer over time.

Aside from tremor and mild agitation, neurological manifestations of thyroiditis are rarely seen. Steroid-responsive encephalopathy, known as Hashimoto encephalopathy, has been reported in individuals with cognitive or neuropsychiatric involvement accompanied by positive anti-TPO [5]. In our case, we demonstrated another neurological manifestation that was found simultaneously with thyroiditis: IIH. This combination of thyroiditis and IIH has not been previously reported.

IIH is not common, with an incidence rate of 0.9 cases per 100,000 population [6]. In nearly 90% of cases, no clearly identifiable etiology could be found. Thus, to make a diagnosis of IIH, other secondary causes of increased intracranial pressure must be investigated and ruled out. Brain magnetic resonance venography should be performed to exclude cerebral venous sinus thrombosis. The most well-known theory of IIH development is venous outflow obstruction or stenosis without thrombosis. Other theories, such as an increased CSF production rate or loss of cerebral autoregulation, have also been proposed [7–9].

There are only a few case reports of thyroid disorders and IIH. Two cases of Graves' disease were reported [10, 11].

Levothyroxine treatment of chronic hypothyroidism in children followed by the development of IIH was also reported [12]. Another 2 cases of levothyroxine treatment accompanied by the occurrence of IIH were reported in 2 patients with thyroid carcinoma after thyroidectomy [13].

Two mechanisms of thyroid hormone action and IIH have been postulated. First, thyroxine replacement might alter CSF flow due to normalization of excess water in body fluid composition, leading to correction of hyponatremia in the chronic hypothyroid state. Normalization of excess fluid in the CSF might alter the dynamics of the CSF and predispose patients to IIH [11]. Second, thyrotoxicosis leads to decreased cerebral vascular resistance, increased cerebral venous blood flow, and elevated venous blood pressure. As a consequence, failure of adequate drainage of the CSF from the subarachnoid space occurs, and IIH develops [11, 14].

In the present case, a postulated second mechanism is that transient overt thyrotoxicosis may have decreased cerebral vascular resistance and increased cerebral venous volume. Genetic susceptibility and structural abnormalities in venous drainage might also have played an important role, but they are still under investigation.

There are limitations to the investigations in this case. First, thyroid scintigraphy and fine-needle aspiration of thyroid tissue were not performed to definitively diagnose subacute thyroiditis. However, the diagnosis of subacute thyroiditis was the most likely cause of thyrotoxicosis in this patient due to the presence of a painful thyroid goiter in the first manifestation. Furthermore, there were no clinical clues of Graves' disease, and the TRAb level was normal. In the literature, a low positive titer (less than 100 IU/mL) of anti-Tg was also reported for subacute thyroiditis [15]. In the future, interval follow-ups of the clinical manifestations and the thyroid antibody levels should be carried out to determine the cause of thyroiditis. Second, to diagnose IIH, brain magnetic resonance venography was not performed in this case to assess cerebral venous drainage as it could detect venous stasis or early venous thrombosis. Brain CT venography was performed instead due to its widespread availability and acceptable sensitivity for detecting venous thrombosis (approximately 90%) [16, 17].

In conclusion, we demonstrated the first case of the thyrotoxicosis phase of thyroiditis with the unusual neurological manifestation of IIH. The mechanism and causal relationship between the 2 conditions are still unclear; however, these might be established by further investigations in the future.

## Ethical Approval

This study protocol was reviewed and approved by the Lampang Hospital Ethics Committee (approval no. EC ID 71/64).

## Consent

The patient was deidentified and provided written informed consent to publish her case (including publication of images).

## Authors' Contributions

KB, TV, and NW designed the study and wrote the manuscript. KB, KS, TV, and NW contributed to data acquisition. KB, KS, and NW interpreted the data. NW was responsible for supervision or mentorship. Each author contributed important intellectual content to the content of this manuscript, and all authors approved the final version of the manuscript.

## Acknowledgments

The authors would like to thank Sakda Sathirareuangchai and David Park for English language editing.

## References

[1] R. M. Ruggeri, A. Campennì, D. Deandreis et al., "SARS-COV-2-related immune-inflammatory thyroid disorders: facts and perspectives," *Expert Review of Clinical Immunology*, vol. 17, no. 7, pp. 737–759, 2021.

[2] J. Slatosky, B. Shipton, and H. Wahba, "Thyroiditis: differential diagnosis and management," *American Family Physician*, vol. 61, no. 4, pp. 1047–1054, 2000.

[3] G. A. Brent and A. P. Weetman, "Hypothyroidism and thyroiditis," *Williams Textbook of Endocrinology*, Elsevier, Amsterdam, Netherlands, pp. 416–448, 2016.

[4] R. M. Ruggeri, A. Campennì, G. Giuffrida et al., "Endocrine and metabolic adverse effects of immune checkpoint inhibitors: an overview (what endocrinologists should know)," *Journal of Endocrinological Investigation*, vol. 42, no. 7, pp. 745–756, 2019.

[5] R. S. Ransing, K. K. Mishra, and D. Sarkar, "Neuropsychiatric manifestation of Hashimoto's encephalopathy in an adolescent and treatment," *Indian Journal of Psychological Medicine*, vol. 38, no. 4, pp. 357–360, 2016.

[6] A. J. Degnan and L. M. Levy, "Pseudotumor cerebri: brief review of clinical syndrome and imaging findings," *American Journal of Neuroradiology*, vol. 32, no. 11, pp. 1986–1993, 2011.

[7] H. Suzuki, J. Takanashi, K. Kobayashi, K. Nagasawa, K. Tashima, and Y. Kohno, "MR imaging of idiopathic intracranial hypertension," *American Journal of Neuroradiology*, vol. 22, no. 1, pp. 196–199, 2001.

[8] R. I. Farb, I. Vanek, J. N. Scott et al., "Idiopathic intracranial hypertension: the prevalence and morphology of sinovenous stenosis," *Neurology*, vol. 60, no. 9, pp. 1418–1424, 2003.

[9] J. N. P. Higgins, J. H. Gillard, B. K. Owler, K. Harkness, and J. D. Pickard, "MR venography in idiopathic intracranial hypertension: unappreciated and misunderstood," *Journal of Neurology, Neurosurgery & Psychiatry*, vol. 75, no. 4, pp. 621–625, 2004.

[10] E. Coutinho, A. M. Silva, C. Freitas, and E. Santos, "Graves' disease presenting as pseudotumor cerebri: a case report," *Journal of Medical Case Reports*, vol. 5, no. 1, p. 68, 2011.

[11] M. Gutch, A. Bhattacharjee, S. Kumar, and D. Pushkar, "Graves' disease and idiopathic intracranial hypertension,"

*Medical Journal of Dr. D. Y. Patil University*, vol. 10, no. 3, pp. 290–292, 2017.

[12] C. Van Dop, F. A. Conte, T. K. Koch, S. J. Clark, S. L. Wilson-Davis, and M. M. Grumbach, "Pseudotumor cerebri associated with initiation of levothyroxine therapy for juvenile hypothyroidism," *New England Journal of Medicine*, vol. 308, no. 18, pp. 1076–1080, 1983.

[13] N. Panza, M. De Rosa, G. Lombardi, and M. Salvatore, "Pseudotumor cerebri and thyroid-replacement therapy in patients affected by differentiated thyroid carcinoma," *Journal of Endocrinological Investigation*, vol. 8, no. 4, pp. 357-358, 1985.

[14] W. Sensenbach, L. Madison, S. Eisenberg, and L. Ochs, "The cerebral circulation and metabolism in hyperthyroidism and myxedema," *Journal of Clinical Investigation*, vol. 33, no. 11, pp. 1434–1440, 1954.

[15] E. Nishihara, N. Amino, T. Kudo et al., "Moderate frequency of anti-thyroglobulin antibodies in the early phase of subacute thyroiditis," *European Thyroid Journal*, vol. 8, no. 5, pp. 268–272, 2019.

[16] P. Chiewvit, S. Piyapittayanan, and N. Poungvarin, "Cerebral venous thrombosis: diagnosis dilemma," *Neurology International*, vol. 3, no. 3, p. e13, 2011.

[17] G. Saposnik, F. Barinagarrementeria, R. D. Brown Jr. et al., "Diagnosis and management of cerebral venous thrombosis: a statement for healthcare professionals from the American Heart Association/American Stroke Association," *Stroke*, vol. 42, no. 4, pp. 1158–1192, 2011.

# 7

# Congenital Cytomegalovirus Infection Manifesting as Neonatal Persistent Pulmonary Hypertension

**Elizabeth Walter-Nicolet,[1] Magali Leblanc,[2] Marianne Leruez-Ville,[3] Philippe Hubert,[4] and Delphine Mitanchez[1]**

[1] *Service de Néonatologie, Hôpital Armand Trousseau, AP-HP, Faculté de Médecine, Université Pierre et Marie Curie, 75012 Paris, France*
[2] *Service de Réanimation Néonatale, Hôpital Universitaire D'Angers, 49033 Angers, France*
[3] *Laboratoire de Virologie, Hôpital Necker-Enfants Malades, AP-HP, Faculté de Médecine, Université Paris-Descartes, 75015 Paris, France*
[4] *Service de Réanimation Polyvalente Pédiatrique et Néonatale, Hôpital Necker-Enfants Malades, AP-HP, Faculté de Médecine, Université Paris-Descartes, 75015 Paris, France*

Correspondence should be addressed to Delphine Mitanchez, delphine.mitanchez@trs.aphp.fr

Academic Editor: Dimitris Georgopoulos

Various neonatal symptoms can lead to a diagnosis of congenital CMV infection. We report two cases of persistent pulmonary hypertension in relation with congenital CMV infection following maternal primary infection and reinfection, respectively. Both infants had severe refractory hypoxemia, requiring high-frequency ventilation, inhaled nitric oxide and inotropic support. One of them required extracorporeal membrane oxygenation for five days. Ganciclovir therapy was attempted in the two cases on day 12 postnatal. One of the infant died on day 15 postnatal. The other survived and is developing uneventfully at 15 months of age. *Conclusion*: Neonatal persistent pulmonary hypertension can be the consequence of congenital CMV infection. Intensive respiratory support and IV ganciclovir are indicated in case of life-threatening condition.

## 1. Introduction

Cytomegalovirus (CMV) is one of the most common causes of congenital infection in the developed countries, affecting approximately 1% of all live births. Most of infected infants will remain asymptomatic, but about 10% of infected newborns will have symptomatic disease and 10–15% will develop problems during the first 6 years of life [1]. Symptoms include growth restriction, microcephaly, seizures, cerebral ventriculomegaly, chorioretinis, hepatitis syndrome, thrombocytopenia, anemia, and pneumonitis [2]. Preconceptional maternal immunity does not provide complete protection to the fetus, and congenital CMV infection may occur in infants of mother who are seropositive for CMV prior to pregnancy. The outcome of recurrent maternal infection may be severe [3, 4]. The benefit of antiviral therapy in congenital CMV infection is still controversial [5, 6]. We present two cases of congenital CMV disease presenting with severe persistent pulmonary hypertension (PPH).

*Case 1.* A 30-year-old woman in her second normal pregnancy delivered vaginally a 2940 g (25th percentile) female infant with a head circumference of 34 cm (50th percentile) at 39 weeks gestation. Maternal asthenia and fever complicated the antenatal course at 31-week gestation. No prenatal abnormal ultrasonographic finding was recorded. Apgar score was 10 at 1 and 5 minutes. Mechanical ventilation was initiated in the first hour of life for acute respiratory distress. Chest X-Ray showed alveolo-interstitial pneumonitis. Antibiotic therapy including amoxicillin, cefotaxime, and amikacin was initiated. Despite mechanical ventilation, refractory hypoxemia developed within 12 hours of life. Echocardiogram showed a structurally normal heart and diagnosed pulmonary hypertension (peak velocity of tricuspid regurgitation at 4 m/sec, pure right-to-left shunt at both atrial and ductal level, and reduced mean pulmonary blood velocity at 0.19 m/sec). Despite high-frequency ventilation (HFV), inhaled nitric oxide (NO) (20 ppm), inotropic support (dobutamine 10 $\mu$g/kg/min), and surfactant therapy (Curosurf 200 mg/kg), the infant's condition deteriorated. Hepatomegaly and splenomegaly were noted on day 5. Biological abnormalities included elevated C-reactive protein (80 mg/L), thrombocytopenia (61 $\times$ $10^9$/L), neutropenia (0.37 $\times$ $10^9$/L), elevated conjugated bilirubinemia (total serum bilirubin 285 $\mu$mol/L; direct bilirubin 185 $\mu$mol/L), and aspartate aminotransferase (207 UI/L). Cultures for bacteria and fungi were negative. CMV was isolated in the urines and in the blood plasma by PCR performed on day 12. Intravenous ganciclovir treatment (12 mg/kg/d) and polyclonal immunoglobulin G (Octagam 1 g/kg every 24 hours for 2 days) were initiated. Severe hypoxemia persisted with progressive hypercapnia. Chest X-ray found severe pulmonary interstitial emphysema. The patient died on day 15. Parents declined postmortem examination and percutaneous lung biopsy. Maternal seroconversion during the seventh month of pregnancy was confirmed by retrospective analysis of maternal serum sample taken monthly for toxoplasmosis testing (IgG $< 0.4$ UI/l and IgM $< 0.9$ UI/l on the 7th month of gestation and IgG $= 0.7$ UI/l and IgM $= 2.9$ UI/l one month latter) with ETI-CMV-G and ETI-CMV-M assays (DiaSorin, France).

*Case 2.* A 33-year-old woman in her second normal pregnancy delivered vaginally a 2520 g (20th percentile) male infant, with a head circumference of 32 cm (10th percentile) at 37 weeks gestation. Apgar score was of 7 and 8 at 1 and 5 minutes, respectively, and the infant required mechanical ventilation for persistent cyanosis. Chest radiographs showed moderate alveolar syndrome. Echocardiography confirmed an anatomically normal heart and pulmonary hypertension (pure right-to-left shunt at both atrial and ductal level, hypertrophy of right ventricle, and intermittent tricuspid regurgitation). Blood cell count showed marked thrombocytopenia (20 $\times$ $10^9$/L) with normal leucocytes count. Amoxicillin and gentamicin therapy was initiated.

Despite HFV, adjunction of NO (20 ppm), and inotropic support (dobutamine 20 $\gamma$/kg/min, epinephrine 0.5 $\gamma$/kg/min), PPH worsened and was associated with refractory hypoxemia. The infant required extracorporeal membrane oxygenation support for 5 days. He tolerated the withdrawal of NO on day 4 and weaning of ECMO on day 8. FiO2 was decreased to 50%. Echocardiogram revealed infrasystemic pulmonary hypertension and moderate hypertrophy of the right ventricle. After transient respiratory improvement, echocardiogram confirmed severe exacerbation of PPH. HFV, 100% FiO2, adjunction of NO (20 ppm), and pulmonary vasoactive agent (prostacyclin 40 ng/kg/min) were required.

Blood culture and gastric swab were negative for bacteria and fungi. Because of neonatal thrombocytopenia, urine was screened for cytomegalovirus (CMV) on day 1 and confirmed congenital CMV infection (17 500 copies/ml). CMV DNA was detected by PCR in blood sample and bronchoalveolar lavage (BAL) on day 12 (resp., 500 copies/mL and 1520 copies/mL). Simultaneously, the patient presented jaundice and hepatosplenomegaly. Conjugated hyperbilirubinemia (total serum bilirubin 101 $\mu$mol/L; direct bilirubin 73 $\mu$mol/L) was noted. Platelet count was normal (238 $\times$ $10^9$/L). Intravenous ganciclovir (10 mg/kg/d) was initiated on day 13 and prolonged for 6 weeks with no side effect. CMV DNA amplification became negative in bronchoalveolar lavage, blood, and urine within two weeks, and the respiratory status slowly improved. NO was progressively decreased until withdrawal at day 25. The infant was successfully weaned of the ventilator on day 32, and oxygen therapy was needed until day 56. Cholestasis progressively resolved. Neurological status remained normal. Ophthalmologic examination ruled out CMV retinitis. Head CT scan showed bilateral subependymal cysts without calcifications. The infant was discharged at 2 months. Echocardiogram was normal from the 3rd month of life and remained normal at 9 months. Clinical and neurological examination at 15 months was normal. Auditory brainstem evoked responses were normal at 10-month followup.

Positive CMV-specific IgG (46 U/mL) of high avidity (96%) (VIDAS CMV IgG, BioMérieux, France) and negative IgM (VIDAS CMV IgGM) detected on maternal serum collected at 20 weeks of gestation were in favour of preexisting immunity. CMV-specific IgG antibody levels were comparable between the serum sample collected at 29-week gestation and at birth.

## 2. Discussion

We report two cases of congenital cytomegalovirus infection presenting at birth with PPH and refractory hypoxemia. Neonatal PPH is usually associated with perinatal asphyxia, meconium aspiration syndrome, hyaline membrane disease, or bacterial infection. These causes were excluded in these two cases, and PPH was most probably a direct complication of CMV congenital pneumonitis. Pneumonitis is rarely the only manifestation of congenital CMV disease in neonate [7] and its incidence is low [8]. To our knowledge, only one case of congenital CMV infection presenting as severe PPH was previously reported [9].

CMV spreads into the lungs following fetal viremia. Usual pathological findings in congenitally infected fetal lungs are immature and dystelectatic lungs associated with interstitial oedema, the absence of cellular reaction, or purulent inflammation [10, 11]. Vasculitis is another suspected pathogenic mechanism leading to neonatal demise [12, 13]. In allogenic transplant recipients, CMV pneumonitis was described as an immunopathogenic mechanism due to a T-cell response to viral antigens expressed on lung cells [14]. However, a case of extensive CMV infection presented with severe pulmonary hypertension has been reported in an adult with acquired immune deficiency syndrome [15]. Post-mortem examination showed infection in the lung endothelial cells. Enlarged CMV-infected endothelial cells protruded into and compromised the lumens of the small vessels, leading to a significant increase in pulmonary arterial resistances. According to these pathologic features, pulmonary hypertension may be transient if specific antiviral therapy is initiated. Respiratory support including mechanical ventilation, NO, and ECMO should be initiated and maintained as long as pulmonary hypertension persists. These measures may help to control respiratory status as long as antiviral therapy may be effective.

Antiviral treatment options are limited. Ganciclovir was first used in children over 20 years ago, but the optimal dose, duration, and route of administration remain poorly evidence based [6]. The benefits of early treatment with ganciclovir in congenital CMV infection, especially on sensorineural hearing loss, remain controversial [16, 17]. However, congenitally infected infants with severe organ disease such as pneumonitis, oesophagitis, persistent severe thrombocytopenia, and active sight-threatening chorioretinitis appeared to benefit from ganciclovir therapy [5, 18]. In the first case reported here, respiratory status was severely affected when ganciclovir was initiated. This precluded expecting a significant improvement. In the second case, when ganciclovir therapy was associated with respiratory support, respiratory status improved and the patient recovered. We did not observe any side effect although ganciclovir-related severe but reversible neutropenia has been reported in two-thirds of the treated infants [16]. This suggests that the administration of antiviral therapy is appropriate in severe condition attributed to CMV infection. However, larger studies should be designed to drive further evidence on clinical benefit of this treatment.

Polyclonal globulins in association with ganciclovir were used in the first case. Specific anti-CMV immunoglobulins are not available in France. CMV immunoglobulin therapy has not been directly evaluated for the treatment of neonates with symptomatic congenital CMV disease, but it may be effective in case of transfusion-acquired CMV infection [18]. The benefit of using CMV immunoglobulins has been evaluated in the prevention of CMV disease after lung transplantation but failed to improve outcome [19]. In CMV seropositive autologous hematopoietic stem cell recipients, the outcome of CMV pneumonia remains poor despite treatment with ganciclovir and CMV hyperimmune globulin administration [20].

Preconceptional immunity to CMV provides incomplete protection, and congenital CMV infection can occur in infants following both primary and recurrent infection in the mother [21]. Although the latter is less prevalent, the prognosis of fetal infection is similar to that following primary infection [3, 4, 21]. Recurrent infection is caused either by reinfection with a new CMV strain or reactivation of a latent infection [18]. Reactivation of CMV infection during pregnancy is reported in 10–30% of seropositive women, and the risk of transmitting the virus is about 1–3% [22]. In the second case, we reported CMV-positive urine on the first day of life excluded a postnatal CMV infection. In case of maternal recurrent infection, we can hypothesize that maternal antibodies in association with antiviral therapy may help to recovery.

## 3. Conclusion

This report highlights the potential implication of congenital CMV in severe PPH, even in case of recurrent maternal CMV infection. PPH should be systematically investigated by echocardiography in cases of congenital CMV pneumonitis. Severe neonatal PPH with no obvious aetiology should imply searching for congenital CMV infection. In cases with life-threatening PPH, the administration of antiviral therapy appears appropriate, associated with respiratory support including extracorporeal ventilation, as long as severe neurological impairment has been excluded. The severity of the clinical condition and progressive end-organ disease outweigh the potential toxicity of this treatment.

## References

[1] M. G. Michaels, "Treatment of congenital cytomegalovirus: where are we now?" *Expert Review of Anti-Infective Therapy*, vol. 5, no. 3, pp. 441–448, 2007.

[2] S. B. Boppana, R. F. Pass, W. J. Britt et al., "Symptomatic congenital cytomegalovirus infection: neonatal morbidity and mortality," *Pediatric Infectious Disease Journal*, vol. 11, no. 2, pp. 93–99, 1992.

[3] M. A. Gaytant, G. I. Rours, E. A. Steegers et al., "Congenital cytomegalovirus infection after recurrent infection: case reports and review of the literature," *European Journal of Pediatrics*, vol. 162, no. 4, pp. 248–253, 2003.

[4] U. G. Ergun, S. Bakaris, H. Ucmak et al., "Fatal congenital cytomegalovirus infection following recurrent maternal infection after a 7-year interval," *Saudi Medical Journal*, vol. 28, no. 2, pp. 264–267, 2007.

[5] G. J. Demmler, "Congenital cytomegalovirus infection treatment," *Pediatric Infectious Disease Journal*, vol. 22, no. 11, pp. 1005–1006, 2003.

[6] M. Sharland, S. Luck, P. Griffiths et al., "Antiviral therapy of CMV disease in children," *Advances in Experimental Medicine and Biology*, vol. 697, pp. 243–260, 2011.

[7] S. Stagno, "Cytomegalovirus," in *Infectious Diseases of the Fetus and Newborn Infant*, J. S. Remington and J. O. Klein, Eds., pp. 312–353, W. B. Saunders, Philadelphia, Pa, USA, 4th edition, 1995.

[8] Z. Shen, S. Q. Shang, C. C. Zou et al., "The detection and clinical features of human cytomegalovirus infection in infants," *Fetal and Pediatric Pathology*, vol. 29, no. 6, pp. 393–400, 2010.

[9] P. C. Ng, T. F. Fok, C. H. Lee et al., "Congenital cytomegalovirus infection presenting as severe persistent pulmonary hypertension of the newborn," *Journal of Perinatology*, vol. 18, no. 3, pp. 234–237, 1998.

[10] A. L. Bissinger, C. Sinzger, E. Kaiserling et al., "Human cytomegalovirus as a direct pathogen: correlation of multiorgan involvement and cell distribution with clinical and pathological findings in a case of congenital inclusion disease," *Journal of Medical Virology*, vol. 67, no. 2, pp. 200–206, 2002.

[11] J. Piazze, G. Nigro, M. Mazzocco et al., "The effect of primary cytomegalovirus infection on fetal lung maturity indices," *Early Human Development*, vol. 54, no. 2, pp. 137–144, 1999.

[12] S. Stagno and R. J. Whitley, "Herpesvirus infections of pregnancy. Part I: cytomegalovirus and Epstein-Barr virus infections," *New England Journal of Medicine*, vol. 313, no. 20, pp. 1270–1274, 1985.

[13] S. L. Zeichner and S. A. Plotkin, "Mechanisms and pathways of congenital infections," *Clinics in Perinatology*, vol. 15, no. 2, pp. 163–188, 1988.

[14] J. E. Grundy, J. D. Shanley, and P. D. Griffiths, "Is cytomegalovirus interstitial pneumonitis in transplant recipients an immunopathological condition?" *Lancet*, vol. 2, no. 8566, pp. 996–999, 1987.

[15] F. B. Smith, J. H. Arias, T. H. Elmquist et al., "Microvascular cytomegalovirus endothelialitis of the lung: a possible cause of secondary pulmonary hypertension in a patient with AIDS," *Chest*, vol. 114, no. 1, pp. 337–340, 1998.

[16] D. W. Kimberlin, C. Y. Lin, P. J. Sánchez et al., "Effect of ganciclovir therapy on hearing in symptomatic congenital cytomegalovirus disease involving the central nervous system: a randomized, controlled trial," *Journal of Pediatrics*, vol. 143, no. 1, pp. 16–25, 2003.

[17] M. G. Michaels, D. P. Greenberg, D. L. Sabo et al., "Treatment of children with congenital cytomegalovirus infection with ganciclovir," *Pediatric Infectious Disease Journal*, vol. 22, no. 6, pp. 504–508, 2003.

[18] S. P. Adler, G. Nigro, and L. Pereira, "Recent advances in the prevention and treatment of congenital cytomegalovirus infections," *Seminars in Perinatology*, vol. 31, no. 1, pp. 10–18, 2007.

[19] R. M. Kruger, S. Paranjothi, G. A. Storch et al., "Impact of prophylaxis with cytogam alone on the incidence of CMV viremia in CMV-seropositive lung transplant recipients," *Journal of Heart and Lung Transplantation*, vol. 22, no. 7, pp. 754–763, 2003.

[20] M. Boeckh, "Current antiviral strategies for controlling cytomegalovirus in hematopoietic stem cell transplant recipients: prevention and therapy," *Transplant Infectious Disease*, vol. 1, no. 3, pp. 165–178, 1999.

[21] S. B. Boppana, L. B. Rivera, K. B. Fowler et al., "Intrauterine transmission of cytomegalovirus to infants of women with preconceptional immunity," *New England Journal of Medicine*, vol. 344, no. 18, pp. 1366–1371, 2001.

[22] G. Malm and M. L. Engman, "Congenital cytomegalovirus infections," *Seminars in Fetal and Neonatal Medicine*, vol. 12, no. 3, pp. 154–159, 2007.

# 8

# Multifactorial Etiology Pulmonary Hypertension in a Patient with Sarcoidosis

**Barreto Ana Terra Fonseca,[1] Barreto Lucas Vinícius da Fonseca,[1] Cavalcante Felipe Naze Rodrigues,[2] Oliveira Joselina Luzia Menezes,[1,3,4] Almeida-Santos Marcos Antônio,[2,3] Garcez Juliane Dantas Seabra,[1,3] Barreto-Filho José Augusto Soares,[1,3,4] and Sousa Antônio Carlos Sobral[1,3,4,5]**

[1]*Departamento de Medicina, Universidade Federal de Sergipe (UFS), São Cristóvão, SE, Brazil*
[2]*Departamento de Medicina, Universidade Tiradentes, Aracaju, SE, Brazil*
[3]*Centro de Ensino e Pesquisa da Fundação Lucas, Aracaju, SE, Brazil*
[4]*Núcleo de Pós-Graduação em Medicina da UFS, São Cristóvão, SE, Brazil*
[5]*The American College of Cardiology, New York, NY, USA*

Correspondence should be addressed to Barreto Ana Terra Fonseca; anaterrafbarreto@yahoo.com.br

Academic Editor: Nurten Sayar

Differential diagnosis between pre- and postcapillary pulmonary hypertension (PH) in patients with diastolic heart failure (DHF) is a challenge in clinical practice. The presence of PH is implicated in worse prognosis in patients with this disease. This case report approaches the process of investigation of pulmonary hypertension in adult patient with DHF, double mitral lesion, and sarcoidosis with poor clinical outcome.

## 1. Introduction

Pulmonary hypertension (PH) is characterized by pulmonary artery medium pressure (PAPm) ≥25 mmHg at rest, measured by right heart catheterization. It could be due to a primary increase in the pulmonary arterial system (PAH) or, when secondary, to the increase in the venous system pressure as well within the pulmonary capillary (pulmonary venous hypertension). Also, it can happen in association with a series of clinical conditions [1]. In clinical practice, however, its interpretation, etiologic diagnosis, and therapeutic approach are still a challenge for clinicians.

The pathogenesis of PH is complex and, in most cases, multifactorial. Pulmonary arterial hypertension (PH group 1) is a proliferative vasculopathy of pulmonary arteriolar musculature. On the other hand, the pathophysiology of PH secondary to left heart failure (HF), PH postcapillary or group 2, is less understood. However, it is established that there may be an overlap of these PH etiologies since vascular remodeling and increased pulmonary vascular resistance are common features in both groups. For this group, more studies to evaluate the real benefit of therapy for PH are necessary [2].

Among the most emblematic diagnostic challenges, we could cite patients in whom left HF does not explain the degree of PH or when there is a second potential etiology.

In sarcoidosis (PH group 5), pathological mechanisms of PH are also multiple and complex: pulmonary fibrosis and hypoxemia, granulomatous involvement of arterioles or pulmonary veins, and compression of the proximal pulmonary arteries by hilar lymph nodes [3].

We describe a case report of a dialytic patient, with association of pulmonary sarcoidosis, HF with preserved ejection fraction (HFpEF), PH, and mitral valve disease refractory to optimal medical treatment.

## 2. Case Report

A male patient, 53 years old, was admitted to the internal medicine ward of the University Hospital of the Federal University of Sergipe on 31/3/15 with dyspnea at rest, orthopnea, nocturnal paroxystic dyspnea, and edema of the lower limbs during one month. He reported dyspnea related to moderate to intense efforts, starting 18 years earlier (when pulmonary sarcoidosis was suspected and confirmed through transbronchial lung biopsy). In the last 4 years, he mentioned mild effort dyspnea/leg edema. The echocardiography exam presented moderate mitral stenosis with severe calcification of the valve and subvalve apparatus, in spite of the lack of a rheumatic disease history. Among the comorbidities, he presented signs and symptoms of severe chronic renal failure for the earlier six years (actually, he was under dialysis for about 4.5 years) and epilepsy (about 15 years). He was a former smoker (15 packs/year) and referred to previous exposure to dust in work place.

He took regularly metoprolol 50 mg/day, Amlodipine 2.5 mg/day, Sildenafil 20 mg q8 hr, hemodialysis q2 days, prednisone 10 mg/day, Sevelamer 800 mg q8 hr, Phenobarbital 100 mg/day, and the folic acid/calcitriol. He reported episodes of symptomatic hypotension, a fact that do not allow drug optimization of heart failure (HF) and motivated hospitalization for clinical compensation.

On physical examination, his skin was pale, albeit hydrated. In the cardiac auscultation, there was a regular rhythm, presence of premature beats, grade III mitral, and tricuspid systolic murmur, accentuated second sound. The heart rate was 92 beats per minute and the blood pressure was 92 × 58 mmHg. We also noticed jugular venous distension, even while standing. In the lung auscultation, murmurs were present in both sides, but markedly decreased at right lower lobe. The respiratory rate was 28 breaths per minute. The abdomen was flat, and we could touch the inferior boarder of the liver at four centimeters from the costal margin (painful on palpation). There was evidence of edema within the abdominal wall. The skin was hot and dry, there was ankle pitting, and we could classify the degree of edema as 3+ (maximum = 4) in the tibiae. The peripheral pulse was present and symmetric.

The chest radiography (Figure 1) showed an increased cardiac area, middle arch rectification, left atrial increase, bilateral calcified hilar lymphadenopathy, and Kerley B lines. The electrocardiogram presented sinus rhythm with heart rate of 92 bpm, right axis deviation, divisional posterior inferior blocking, and increased P (biatrial overload) and T waves (secondary changes in ventricular repolarization). The evolutionary findings of EchoDopplercardiograms (ED) transthoracic revealed progression of mitral stenosis (mitral valve opening evolved from 1.35 $cm^2$ to 1 $cm^2$), extensive calcification of the mitral valve (score of Wilkin's 15 points), moderate aortic and tricuspid insufficiency, and normo-functioning pulmonary valve. The systolic pulmonary artery pressure (PASP) worsened (48 mmHg to 79 mmHg) and micronodular hyperechoic images were noted diffusely in left ventricle myocardium. Comparative description of diameters and ejection fraction are shown in Table 1.

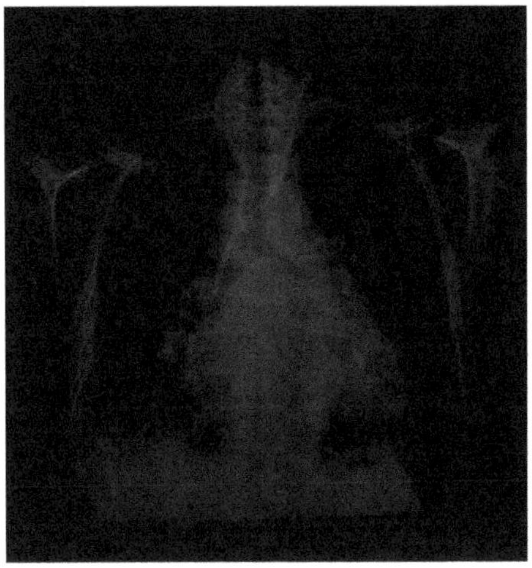

FIGURE 1: Increased cardiac area, middle arch rectification, left atrial increase, bilateral hilar lymphadenopathy, and calcified and Kerley B lines.

TABLE 1: Transthoracic echocardiograms.

| | 09/04/15 (admission) | 07/11/13 |
|---|---|---|
| Aorta/left atrium (cm) | 3.1/6.1 (volume = 78 mL/$m^2$) | 3.2/5.5 |
| Right chambers | Enlarged | Normal |
| Left ventricle (diastole/systole) (cm) | 3.8/2.2 | 4.1/2.3 |
| Ejection fraction (Simpson) | 74% | 76% |

Hemodialysis was instituted daily in order to improve clinical status. The doses of metoprolol (150 mg/day) and prednisone (40 mg/day) were increased. However, the approaches adopted have not accomplished any success.

The right heart catheterization was performed for the investigation of pulmonary arterial hypertension with nitroprusside 200 $\mu$g/mL at a dose of 2.8 mcg/kg/min for 1 h. The following pressures were obtained: (a) before vasodilator: pulmonary artery pressure, 76/30 mmHg (mean 51) and Aorta, 96/76 mmHg (mean 85); (b) after vasodilator: pulmonary artery, 65/31 mmHg (mean 49) and Aorta, 104/53 mmHg (mean 70 mmHg). The end-diastolic pressure of the left ventricle was 20 mmHg and coronary angiography revealed only mild diffuse parietal irregularities.

A few days later, the patient developed drowsiness, tachypnea, use of accessory respiratory muscles, 94% of arterial oxygen saturation on supplemental oxygen 3 L/min, blood pressure 70×50 mmHg, heart rate 112 beats per minute, worsening of mitral systolic murmur (grade IV) and mitral diastolic murmur, cold and clammy skin, and weak pulse. He was transferred to the intensive care unit to receive hemodynamic support with vasoactive drugs, but he evolved with refractory shock and death.

## 3. Discussion

The PH is a common complication of left HF; usually its manifestation often overlaps with those of underlying condition and implicates more severe clinical presentation. In clinical practice, the diagnosis is usually done indirectly, through transthoracic ED. However, their interpretation, main diagnosis, and therapeutic approach still are a challenge for clinician [4].

The comparative analysis of ED showed unfavorable evolution of mitral stenosis, valve area reduction, left atrial enlargement, worsening of PSAP, and right chambers enlargement. These data corroborate the etiology of postcapillary PH in this patient (group 2 PH, associated with left heart disease) [5].

The postcapillary PH is more common in HFpEF which consists of abnormality in active relaxation and active stiffness (diastolic dysfunction) with preserved left ventricular ejection fraction. When HFpEF occurs, it results in more severe symptoms and worsening of exercise tolerance, hallmark of the patient in question [4, 6].

As there was not found satisfactory reduction in PAPm under vasodilator testing (pulmonary reactivity criteria: fall PAPm to <49 mmHg, reduction of at least 10 mmHg, or maintenance/increase in cardiac output) and the estimated pulmonary capillary wedge pressure was 20 mmHg, it infers fix PH with postcapillary component probably secondary to valve heart disease. The differential diagnosis between PH modalities before and after capillary in patients with HFpEF is a challenge in daily clinical practice and it entails difficulty on treating this subgroup of patients. However, the literature states that group 2 PH patients can have precapillary component, featuring a mixed PH [2]. Thus, it was decided to maintain the treatment with phosphodiesterase 5 inhibitors even after the above examinations do not corroborate primary etiology. However, more studies are needed to evaluate the benefit of therapy for PH in this group.

The diagnosis of PH, by itself, cannot exclude the possibility of it being due to mitral valve disease in this patient. However, the prescription of sildenafil started long before the clinical presentation of the valve disease and, at that early phase, the treatment improved the patient condition. Notwithstanding, we must acknowledge that sildenafil could potentially contribute to the clinical deterioration of the patient. Indeed, due to an increase of symptoms a few weeks before the fatal event, the use of sildenafil was put to a halt.

Myocardial infiltration, sarcoidosis characteristic, viewed at ED probably did not contribute to the clinical presentation, as usually it manifests itself with restrictive cardiomyopathy, ventricular aneurysm, pericardial disease, infiltrative valve dysfunction, ventricular tachycardia, and supraventricular arrhythmias [3].

In this case the surgical approach of mitral valve was not possible. The patient did not have favorable valve anatomical conditions to mitral stenosis percutaneous repair and also had high surgical risk (severe pulmonary hypertension and disorders of right ventricle and kidneys) to mitral valve replacement. There was no possibility to carry out more radical therapies like cardiac transplantation because of severe fixed pulmonary hypertension and atrial septostomy because of high mortality inherent to it [7].

It is very difficult to determine the time when HF patient care should be palliative. Anguita and Ojeda [8] defined a few points to guidance in making this decision: class functional III-IV despite optimal treatment, absence of triggering factors or advanced treatable comorbidities that limit survival, hypotension, renal failure, and frequent decompensation despite maximum tolerated treatment. All these prognostic factors were presented in this case and it was featured as terminal HF.

## Ethical Approval

The authors state that for this investigation there has been no experience in humans and/or animals.

## Consent

The authors state that they followed the protocols of their work center on the publication of patient data and all patients in the study have been sufficiently informed and gave their informed consent in writing to participate in this study. The authors declare having received written consent from the relatives of patient. The corresponding author is in possession of this document.

## References

[1] M. M. Hoeper, H. J. Bogaard, R. Condliffe et al., "Definitions and diagnosis of pulmonary hypertension," *Journal of the American College of Cardiology*, vol. 62, no. 25, pp. D42–D50, 2013.

[2] J. L. Vachiery, Y. Adir, J. A. Barbera et al., "Pulmonary hypertension due to left heart diseases," *Journal of the American College of Cardiology*, vol. 62, pp. 100–108, 2013.

[3] R. Sulica, A. S. Teirstein, S. Kakarla, N. Nemani, A. Behnegar, and M. L. Padilla, "Distinctive clinical, radiographic, and functional characteristics of patients with sarcoidosis-related pulmonary hypertension," *Chest*, vol. 128, no. 3, pp. 1483–1489, 2005.

[4] J. C. Fang, T. DeMarco, M. M. Givertz et al., "World Health Organization Pulmonary Hypertension Group 2: pulmonary hypertension due to left heart disease in the adult - a summary statement from the Pulmonary Hypertension Council of the International Society for Heart and Lung Transplantation," *Journal of Heart and Lung Transplantation*, vol. 31, no. 9, pp. 913–933, 2012.

[5] D. B. Taichman, J. Ornelas, L. Chung et al., "Pharmacologic therapy for pulmonary arterial hypertension in adults: CHEST guideline and expert panel report," *Chest*, vol. 146, no. 2, pp. 449–475, 2014.

[6] J. A. C. Teixeira, P. S. Teixeira, and A. C. L. da Nóbrega, "Exercício na insuficiência cardíaca de fração de ejeção normal," *Revista Brasileira de Cardiologia*, vol. 26, no. 4, pp. 303–312, 2013.

[7] V. V. McLaughlin, S. J. Shah, R. Souza, and M. Humbert, "Management of pulmonary arterial hypertension," *Journal of the American College of Cardiology*, vol. 65, no. 18, pp. 1976–1997, 2015.

[8] S. M. Anguita and P. S. Ojeda, "Tratamiento médico de la insuficiencia cardiaca por disfunción diastólica," *Revista Española de Cardiología*, vol. 6, pp. 53F–58F, 2006.

# 9

# Malignant Hypertension Causing a Pulmonary-Renal Syndrome

**Bryan Yong**[1] **and David A. Power**[2]

[1] *Clinical School, University of Melbourne, Parkville, Victoria, Australia*
[2] *Department of Nephrology, Austin Health, Studley Road, Heidelberg 3084, Victoria, Australia*

Correspondence should be addressed to David A. Power; david.power@austin.org.au

Academic Editor: Theodore I. Steinman

*Background.* Pulmonary-renal syndrome is characterised by acute kidney injury, haematuria, and haemoptysis and is a well-recognised presentation of diseases such as ANCA vasculitis that require urgent immunosuppression. *Case Presentation.* A patient presented with a brief history of haemoptysis, acute renal failure, microscopic haematuria, and severe hypertension. The diagnosis was initially not clear so he was treated with antihypertensives, renal replacement therapy, and immunosuppression. Renal biopsy subsequently showed evidence of malignant hypertension. Autoantibodies were uniformly negative. *Conclusions.* This case demonstrates that malignant hypertension can present as pulmonary-renal syndrome.

## 1. Background

Pulmonary haemorrhage with acute kidney injury and References is classically caused by immunologically mediated diseases such as ANCA-associated vasculitis, anti-GBM disease, which is also known as Goodpasture's syndrome, or systemic lupus erythematosus [1]. In the acute clinical setting, it is often necessary to treat patients with immunosuppressive agents and plasma exchange prior to accurate diagnosis. We present an unusual case of haemoptysis and acute kidney injury, treated with initial immunosuppression, where hypertension was found to be the causative problem.

## 2. Case Summary

A thirty-three-year-old Indian gentleman presented with a two-week history of haemoptysis and a three-day history of fever, epigastric discomfort, nausea, and headache. This occurred on a background of hypertension, diagnosed 8 years previously. He was a smoker with a 5 pack-year smoking history. He took no regular or over the counter medications.

At presentation, he was markedly hypertensive (225/145 mmHg) and tachycardic (110 bpm). He was afebrile with normal oxygen saturations and had dual heart sounds with a loud P2. Clinical examination indicated euvolemic fluid status. There were bilateral mid and lower zone inspiratory crackles and he had small volume haemoptysis. There were no focal neurological signs. Optic fundoscopy revealed flame haemorrhages and cotton wool spots, consistent with grade 3 hypertensive retinopathy (Figure 1). An electrocardiogram revealed high amplitude QRS complexes in V1 and V6 consistent with left ventricular hypertrophy. The echocardiogram showed normal left ventricular size but moderate to severe left ventricular wall thickness.

On admission, he had a normocytic anaemia (Hb 75 g/L, RR = 130-180 g/L) and thrombocytopenia (platelets 98 $\times 10^9$/L, RR = 150-400 $\times 10^9$/L). The serum creatinine was elevated at 810 $\mu$mol/L (RR = 62-106 $\mu$mol/L), with an estimated glomerular filtration rate (eGFR) of 7 mL/min (RR = $\geq$90 mL/min) (Table 1). The haemolysis screen revealed a bilirubin of 46 $\mu$mol/L (RR = <18 $\mu$mol/L), reticulocyte count of 333 $\times 10^9$/L (RR = 20-100 $\times 10^9$/L), lactate dehydrogenase (LDH) of 1177 IU/L (RR = 135-225 IU/L), and a haptoglobin of <0.1 mg/L (RR = 0.3-2.0 mg/L). The peripheral blood smear showed moderate schistocytosis and moderate polychromasia, in keeping with haemolysis (Table 1). A dipstick was positive for proteinuria (2+) and haematuria (2+). Urine microscopy showed 40 $\times 10^6$ erythrocytes (RR < 40 $\times 10^6$). Ultrasound revealed normal sized kidneys without hydronephrosis. Corticomedullary differentiation was normal. The chest

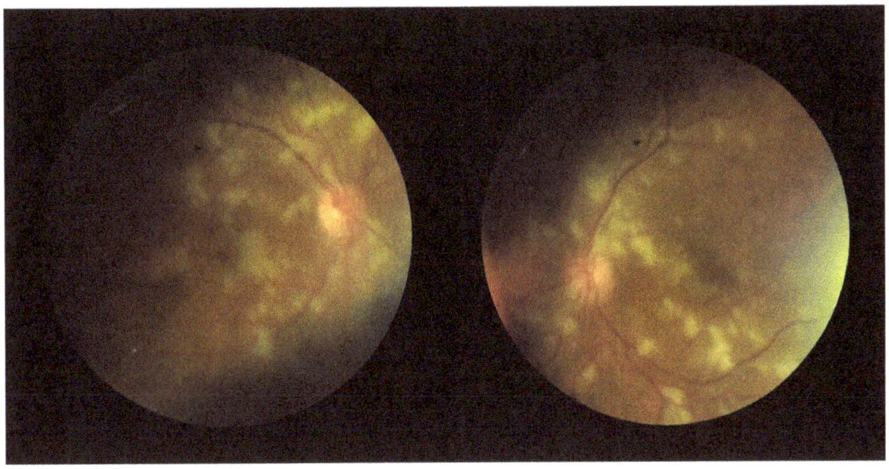

FIGURE 1: Right and left funduscopic images showing flame haemorrhages and cotton wool spots, consistent with grade 3 hypertensive retinopathy.

TABLE 1: Laboratory results.

| FBC | Hb | MCV | WCC | Platelets | |
|---|---|---|---|---|---|
| | 75 | 87 | 11.3 | 98 | |
| *Ref. range* | *130-180 g/L* | *80-96 FL* | *4-11 x $10^9$/L* | *150-400 x $10^9$/L* | |
| **UEC** | **Na** | **K** | **Cr** | **eGFR** | |
| | 135 | 2.5 | 810 | 7 | |
| *Ref. range* | *136-145 mmol/L* | *3.5-5.1 mmol/L* | *62-106 μmol/L* | *≥90 mL/min* | |
| **Haemolysis screen** | **Bilirubin** | **Reticulocytes** | **LDH** | **Haptoglobin** | |
| | 46 | 333 | 1177 | <0.1 | |
| *Ref. range* | *<18 μmol/L* | *20-100 x $10^9$/L* | *135-225 IU/L* | *0.3-2.0 mg/L* | |
| **Blood smear** | Moderate schistocytosis and polychromasia | | | | |
| **Serology** | **ANA** | **ANCA** | **Anti-GBM** | **ENA panel** | **ADAMTS13** |
| | Negative | Negative | <5 | Negative | 52 |
| *Ref. range* | | | *<20 U/mL* | | *40-130%* |

X-ray showed cardiomegaly, patchy bilateral airspace opacities that were worse on the right side.

The clinical suspicion was that of an ANCA vasculitis or anti-GBM disease, with a differential diagnosis that included complement mediated haemolytic uraemic syndrome (HUS), thrombotic thrombocytopaenic purpura (TTP), and malignant hypertension.

The hypertension was treated with metoprolol, methyldopa, and hydralazine to achieve a BP of 150/100. Pulse methylprednisolone therapy, followed by cyclophosphamide, and plasma exchange were commenced. The headache, haemoptysis, and evidence of haemolysis rapidly resolved following this treatment. Renal biopsy was initially delayed due to hypertension and was subsequently performed on day 3 (Figure 2). The biopsy contained 18 glomeruli. Most glomeruli showed a consolidated, bloodless appearance with obscuration of capillary loops by endothelial cell swelling and subendothelial zone expansion. Staining for IgA, IgM, IgG, fibrinogen, C3c, and C1q was negative. The biopsy suggested malignant hypertensive nephropathy as the underlying cause of the acute kidney injury. Therapy with steroids, cyclophosphamide, and plasma exchange was ceased once the renal biopsy results became available. Furthermore, the autoimmune screening panel which included antinuclear antibodies (ANA), antinuclear cytoplasmic antibodies (ANCA), anti-GBM antibodies, extractable nuclear antibodies (ENA), and complement levels was normal. The ADAMTS13 levels in addition were later found to be normal and did not suggest complement mediated HUS.

Control of hypertension was associated with resolution of the biochemical evidence of haemolysis. CT angiogram showed no evidence of renal artery stenosis. The patient remained dialysis dependent for 7 months and then regained sufficient renal function to cease dialysis. Fourteen months after presentation, the BP is 127/87 with serum creatinine 337 μmol/L and eGFR 19 ml/min. Current medications are perindopril, indapamide, carvedilol, frusemide, calcitriol, and rosuvastatin. A recent echocardiogram shows left ventricular hypertrophy and low normal systolic function. He remains under regular review by cardiology and nephrology.

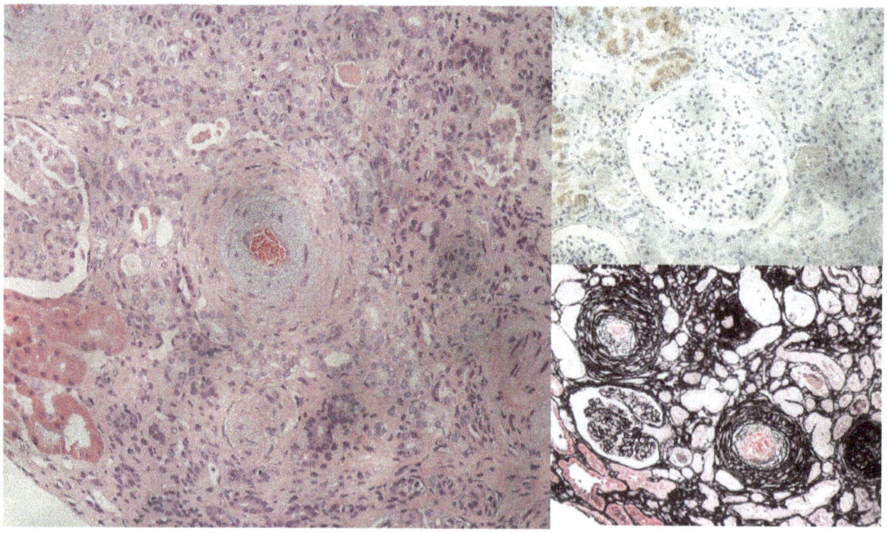

Figure 2: Renal biopsy. Left: arteriolar thickening and myxoid changes. Top right: negative immunofluorescence staining. Bottom right: onion skinning of arterioles on silver staining.

## 3. Discussion

Pulmonary haemorrhage with acute kidney injury is classically caused by immunologically mediated diseases such as ANCA associated vasculitis, Goodpasture's syndrome, or systemic lupus erythematosus [1]. The combination of hypertension, hypertensive changes on fundoscopy, laboratory evidence of microangiopathic haemolytic anaemia, and a renal biopsy consistent with thrombotic microangiopathy suggested that the unifying diagnosis in this case was malignant hypertension. Renal biopsy findings and negative ANCA, anti-GBM, and ANA serologies were supportive of a nonimmunological cause. Clinical and biochemical improvements with strict hypertension control also supported the diagnosis of malignant hypertension.

Malignant hypertension typically presents with nonspecific symptoms such as agitation, an altered conscious state, chest discomfort, and headache. It is a rare cause of pulmonary-renal syndrome [2–5]. As we were unable to perform a kidney biopsy due to hypertension, it was difficult to exclude an immunological cause for the pulmonary-renal syndrome. The patient presented on the weekend and it proved impossible to obtain emergency serology, which might have helped to exclude several of the diagnoses entertained. This would likely have spared the patient unnecessary immunosuppression. It is also worth noting that severe hypertension is unusual in patients with anti-GBM disease and ANCA vasculitis, which is described in a few case series [6, 7].

This patient had clear evidence of intravascular haemolysis. There were schistocytes observed in the peripheral blood smear, which would support a diagnosis of atypical HUS. Pulmonary haemorrhage is considered quite unusual in aHUS. The diagnosis was considered possible, however, until the prompt resolution of haemolysis with control of blood pressure suggested that aHUS was unlikely. The appearances of malignant hypertension on renal biopsy are similar to that of aHUS when thrombotic microangiopathy (TMA) is present. In TMA, the appearances on renal biopsy include intravascular and glomerular thrombi as well as mesangial changes. In malignant hypertension, however, more severe vascular changes in small arterioles would be expected.

The mechanism of haemoptysis in malignant hypertension is unclear. Malignant hypertension may cause pulmonary haemorrhage via direct vascular endothelial injury from mechanical stress. Elevated left ventricular pressure and pulmonary oedema causing pulmonary haemorrhage may be an alternate mechanism. It was reported that 63% of patients with malignant hypertension had renal impairment on presentation [8]. Renal survival was notably found to be 84% and 72% at five and ten years, respectively.

While immunological causes of pulmonary-renal syndrome are more common, malignant hypertension should be considered in the differential diagnosis in the correct clinical setting. Hypertension management alone may result in improvement in haemolysis markers and pulmonary symptoms; however long term renal outcome remains poor.

## References

[1] C. McCabe, Q. Jones, A. Nikolopoulou, C. Wathen, and R. Luqmani, "Pulmonary-renal syndromes: An update for respiratory physicians," *Respiratory Medicine*, vol. 105, no. 10, pp. 1413–1421, 2011.

[2] H. S. Park, Y. A. Hong, B. H. Chung et al., "Malignant hypertension with an unusual presentation mimicking the immune mediated pulmonary renal syndrome," *Yonsei Medical Journal*, vol. 53, no. 6, pp. 1224–1227, 2012.

[3] S. Aithal, N. Marley, and G. Venkat-Raman, "An unusual nonimmunological cause of renal pulmonary syndrome," *Clinical Nephrology*, vol. 72, no. 4, pp. 322–325, 2009.

[4] P. Dalal, G. Phadke, A. Gill et al., "A patient with hemoptysis and renal failure," *International Journal of Hypertension*, vol. 2011, Article ID 268370, 3 pages, 2011.

[5] K. Hida, J. Wada, M. Odawara et al., "Malignant hypertension with a rare complication of pulmonary alveolar hemorrhage," *American Journal of Nephrology*, vol. 20, no. 1, pp. 64–67, 2000.

[6] M. J. Gutiérrez-Sánchez, V. Petkov-Stoyanov, and J. A. Martín-Navarro, "Reversible posterior leukoencephalopathy syndrome in Goodpasture's syndrome," *Nefrología*, vol. 32, no. 4, pp. 540-541, 2012.

[7] J. Odaka, T. Kanai, T. Ito et al., "Renal-limited necrotizing granulomatous vasculitis in a pediatric patient," *Pediatrics International*, vol. 57, no. 4, pp. 777–780, 2015.

[8] R. González, E. Morales, J. Segura, L. M. Ruilope, and M. Praga, "Long-term renal survival in malignant hypertension," *Nephrology Dialysis Transplantation* , vol. 25, no. 10, pp. 3266–3272, 2010.

# 10

# Deoxycorticosterone Producing Tumor as a Cause of Resistant Hypertension

**Saurabh Gupta,[1] Jose Melendez,[1] and Apurv Khanna[2]**

[1] *University of Connecticut Health Center, Farmington, CT 06030, USA*
[2] *SUNY Upstate Medical University, Syracuse, NY 13210, USA*

Correspondence should be addressed to Apurv Khanna, khannaa@upstate.edu

Academic Editor: Gerald S. Supinski

We describe a young woman with longstanding resistant hypertension. Evaluation for renal artery stenosis and primary aldosteronism was unrevealing. In this setting of a suppressed plasma aldosterone concentration (PAC) and a suppressed plasma renin activity (PRA), a differential diagnosis of a deoxycorticosterone (DOC) producing tumor was entertained. Biochemical and imaging studies confirmed this diagnosis. Rare and novel DOC producing tumors are an important cause of resistant hypertension.

## 1. Introduction

Hypertension is a ubiquitous health problem. The overall worldwide prevalence of hypertension in the adult population is around 26% [1]. A significant proportion of these individuals have hypertension that is difficult to control with conventional treatment. Such patients are more likely to have an underlying identifiable cause of hypertension [2]. Identification of these causes is therefore acquiring greater therapeutic importance for the clinician.

## 2. Case Presentation

A 35-year-old African American female presented to the University Clinic for evaluation of resistant hypertension. She had onset of hypertension at the age of 17 years and since then had suboptimally controlled blood pressure despite the use of 4 antihypertensive medications including a diuretic. When first seen in the clinic, she was 3 weeks post partum from delivery of a preterm infant due to preeclampsia. Her only complaint in the office was that of fatigue which was present even before pregnancy. Family history was positive for hypertension in her mother and maternal grandfather, developing in middle age. Medications included Lisinopril 20 mg daily, Hydrochlorthiazide 25 mg daily, Amlodipine 10 mg daily, and Doxazosin 1 mg at bedtime.

On examination, her blood pressure was 150/90 mmHg with a heart rate was 88. Physical examination was unremarkable other than trace pedal edema. There were no cushingoid features or virilisation noted on exam. Pertinent laboratory values included a serum sodium of 135 (137–144 meq/L), serum potassium 3.1 (3.6–5.1 meq/L), serum bicarbonate of 26 (22–26 meq/L), blood urea nitrogen 9 (8–24 mg/dL), and serum creatinine of 0.8 (0.6–1.2 mg/dL). At this first visit the patient received oral potassium supplementation, Lisinopril dose was increased to 40 mg daily and Amiloride 5 mg twice daily was added to the regimen. Despite these measures patient continued to have poorly controlled blood pressure.

Prior to referral to us, for evaluation of uncontrolled hypertension accompanied by hypokalemia in a young female, Magnetic Resonance Angiography (MRA) of the renal arteries to look for fibromuscular dysplasia was ordered by her treating physician. The MRA did not show any evidence of renal artery stenosis. The MRA also did not show any adrenal mass, though this investigation was done primarily to screen for a vascular lesion and would not define a mass as well as a conventional MRI. As we will highlight in the following sections, based on the results of her biochemical studies, this diagnosis was in fact, less likely and this would not have been our initial screening test. On evaluation by us, to screen for primary aldosteronism,

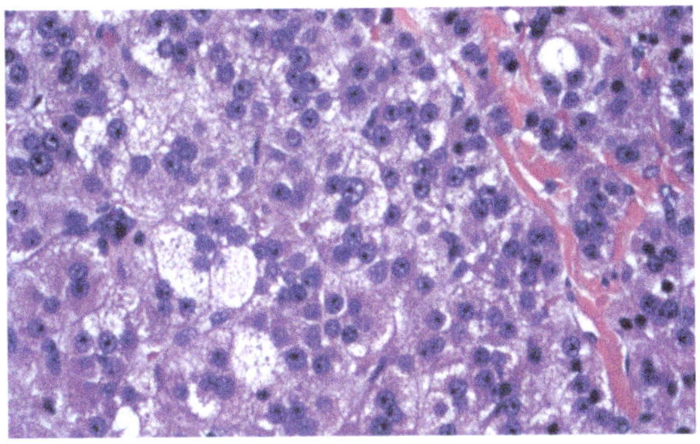

FIGURE 1: Adrenal cortical adenoma demonstrating focal high grade nuclear atypia.

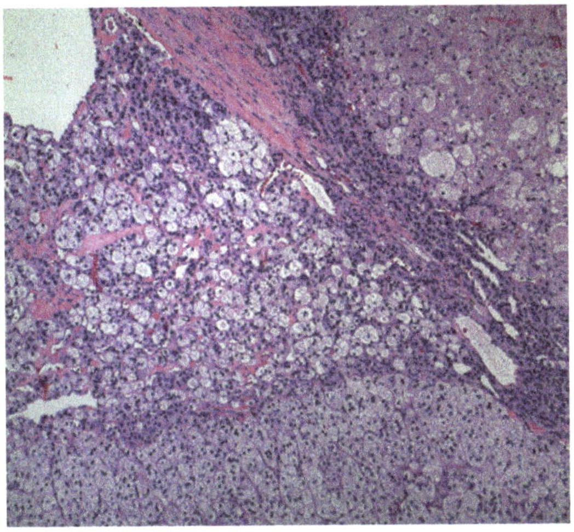

FIGURE 2: Adrenal cortical adenoma with areas of focal necrosis.

plasma aldosterone concentration (PAC), and plasma renin activity (PRA) levels were ordered. The PAC was suppressed at <4.0 ng/dL and the PRA level was also suppressed at <0.6 ng/mL/hr (0.6–4.0). In view of the suppressed PAC and PRA levels, the patient underwent a 24-hour urine collection for free cortisol and a plasma deoxycorticosterone (DOC) level was checked. The 24-hour urine collection was significant for an elevated free cortisol level of 219 (<45.0 mcg/day). The plasma deoxycorticosterone (DOC) levels were also markedly elevated at 65 (1.6–5.6 ng/dL). This leads us to suspect the presence of a cortisol and deoxycorticosterone cosecreting adrenal tumor. Subsequently a CT scan of the abdomen with intravenous contrast was done. It showed a 5.3 cm × 4.5 cm × 7 cm mass inferior to the right adrenal gland. The patient underwent a laparoscopic partial right adrenalectomy.

Histology revealed a right adrenal cortical adenoma on frozen section. While there was focal high grade nuclear atypia and focal necrosis, the findings were below the threshold for malignancy (see Figures 1 and 2). Three months postresection, patient had normalization of DOC and urine free cortisol levels. She also exhibited marked improvement in blood pressure control and was tapered off all her hypertensive medications. Her blood pressure was recorded at 100/50 mmHg at followup.

## 3. Discussion

Our approach towards patients with resistant hypertension involves obtaining a plasma renin activity (PRA) and a plasma aldosterone concentration (PAC) as an initial step. This helps separate patients into one of three categories:

(1) Those with a high PAC : PRA ratio; (2) those with a high PAC and high PRA, and (3) those with a low PAC and PRA levels. This is based on a high PAC : PRA ratio defined as >20 [3], and a high PAC value of ≥16 ng/dL [4].

(1) *High PAC : PRA Ratio.* The principal diagnosis here is of primary aldosteronism. The high PAC : PRA ratio is a good screening test but it is not diagnostic of this disorder. Further confirmation is provided by the aldosterone suppression test. Patients are salt-loaded either by mouth for 3 days or intravenously. The 24-hour urinary sodium excretion should be >200 mEq to document adequate sodium repletion. Urinary aldosterone excretion >12 mg/24 hours is consistent with hyperaldosteronism [3]. Once confirmed, patients need further testing with selective adrenal venous sampling for aldosterone to distinguish unilateral aldosterone producing adenomas (APA) from bilateral idiopathic hyperaldosteronism (IHA) [5]. The treatment of IHA is pharmacologic with use of mineralocorticoid receptor blockers while APA is treated surgically with unilateral total adrenalectomy.

(2) *High PAC : High PRA.* Patients presenting with a high PAC accompanied by a high PRA are further worked up for the presence of a unilateral renal artery stenosis or more rarely for a renin-secreting tumor. Renal arteriography remains the gold standard for diagnosis renal artery stenosis. Patients with fibromuscular disease respond better to angioplasty than those with atherosclerotic disease [6]. Renin secreting tumors are rare entities arising from the juxtaglomerular cells and are detected by radiologic imaging of the abdomen [7].

(3) *Low PAC : Low PRA.* The presence of a low PAC accompanied by a low PRA, as was present in our patient leads to differential diagnosis of bilateral renal artery stenosis, Cushing's syndrome, congenital adrenal hyperplasia (CAH), apparent mineralocorticoid excess (AME), deoxycorticosterone (DOC) producing tumors, and Liddle's syndrome. Cushing's syndrome can be caused either by excess endogenous cortisol or iatrogenically by excess steroid administration. A urinary-free cortisol level four times greater than normal is diagnostic of this disorder [8]. Apparent mineralocorticoid excess (AME) is a rare disorder causing a severe form of early onset hypertension. It is transmitted as an autosomal recessive trait. Patients suffer from a deficiency of 11$\beta$-hydroxysteroid dehydrogenase type 2 enzyme. This enzyme normally converts the more active cortisol to the inactive cortisone. In conditions of enzyme

deficiency, cortisol continues to flood the mineralocorticoid receptor causing sodium retention, potassium wasting, and hypertension. This syndrome is commonly found in settings of familial consanguinity and there is extensive target organ damage, nephrocalcinosis, and renal failure [9]. Our patient did not have these clinical features including consanguinity and renal failure. If urine cortisol levels are not elevated, then as the next step, we check serum deoxycorticosterone (DOC) levels. If elevated, as was present in this case, the differential is that of CAH versus a DOC producing tumor. CAH is most commonly caused due to 21 hydroxylase deficiency and this is not associated with hypertension. CAH due to deficiency of 11$\beta$-hydroxylase is seen most in the Middle East and is characterized by virilization of the infant and 17-hydroxylase enzyme deficiency is often manifest at birth and is also mainly seen in pediatric populations. However, partial enzyme deficiencies have been observed in hirsute women [10]. Thus in adult patients, congenital enzymatic defects are less likely compared to the likelihood of a DOC-producing tumor. This is investigated further with imaging of the abdomen. In the literature, DOC-producing tumors have been described only in a handful of cases [11]. In our patient, CT scan of the abdomen did indeed reveal an adrenal mass. Finally, if all testing is negative, the diagnosis of Liddle's syndrome is entertained. These patients have a mutation of the $\beta$ or $\gamma$ subunit of the renal epithelial sodium channel, causing is increased sodium reabsorption in the distal nephron [12]. This leads to manifestations similar to mineralocorticoid excess, such as hypertension, hypokalemia, and metabolic alkalosis. However, plasma renin activity and plasma aldosterone concentrations are secondarily suppressed in these patients. Treatment consists of blocking distal nephron sodium channels with drugs like amiloride and triamterene. In conclusion, in patients with resistant hypertension accompanied by low PRA and low PAC, Cushing's syndrome is an important diagnosis to be considered. If, however, Cushing's syndrome is ruled out, then in adult patients, rare deoxycorticosterone producing tumors are a distinct possibility.

## References


[1] P. M. Kearney, M. Whelton, K. Reynolds, P. Muntner, P. K. Whelton, and J. He, "Global burden of hypertension: analysis of worldwide data," *Lancet*, vol. 365, no. 9455, pp. 217–223, 2005.

[2] J. F. Setaro and H. R. Black, "Current concepts: refractory hypertension," *The New England Journal of Medicine*, vol. 327, no. 8, pp. 543–547, 1992.

[3] W. F. Young Jr. and M. J. Hogan, "Renin-independent hypermineralocorticoidism," *Trends in Endocrinology and Metabolism*, vol. 5, no. 3, pp. 97–106, 1994.

[4] W. F. Young Jr., "Primary aldosteronism: management issues," *Annals of the New York Academy of Sciences*, vol. 970, pp. 61–76, 2002.

[5] J. L. Doppman, J. R. Gill Jr., D. L. Miller et al., "Distinction between hyperaldosteronism due to bilateral hyperplasia and unilateral aldosteronoma: reliability of CT," *Radiology*, vol. 184, no. 3, pp. 677–682, 1992.

[6] D. P. Slovut and J. W. Olin, "Fibromuscular dysplasia," *The New England journal of medicine*, vol. 350, no. 18, pp. 1862–1871, 2004.

[7] K. O. Min, H. J. Kwon, S. J. Ahn et al., "Juxtaglomerular cell tumor of the kidney: a case report," *Journal of Korean Medical Science*, vol. 16, no. 2, pp. 233–236, 2001.

[8] H. Raff and J. W. Findling, "A physiologic approach to diagnosis of the cushing syndrome," *Annals of Internal Medicine*, vol. 138, no. 12, pp. 980–991, 2003.

[9] W. Chemaitilly, R. C. Wilson, and M. I. New, "Hypertension and adrenal disorders," *Current Hypertension Reports*, vol. 5, no. 6, pp. 498–504, 2003.

[10] A. W. Lucky, R. L. Rosenfield, and J. McGuire, "Adrenal androgen hyperresponsiveness to adrenocorticotropin in women with acne and/or hirsutism: adrenal enzyme defects and exaggerated adrenarche," *Journal of Clinical Endocrinology and Metabolism*, vol. 62, no. 5, pp. 840–848, 1986.

[11] H. Shibata, "Deoxycorticosterone-producing adrenal tumor," *Nippon Rinsho*, vol. 1, pp. 641–644, 2006.

[12] M. Furuhashi, K. Kitamura, M. Adachi et al., "Liddle's syndrome caused by a novel mutation in the proline-rich PY motif of the epithelial sodium channel $\beta$-subunit," *Journal of Clinical Endocrinology and Metabolism*, vol. 90, no. 1, pp. 340–344, 2005.

# 11

# Prevalence and Associated Factors of Portopulmonary Hypertension in Patients with Portal Hypertension

**Yueming Shao**,[1] **Xin Yin**,[2] **Tingting Qin**,[1] **Ruihua Zhang**,[1] **Yu Zhang**,[1] **and Xiaoyu Wen**[1]

[1]*Department of Hepatology, First Hospital of Jilin University, Xinmin Street, No. 71, Changchun, Jilin Province 130021, China*
[2]*Center for Infectious Diseases, West China Hospital of Sichuan University, Chengdu, Sichuan Province 610041, China*

Correspondence should be addressed to Xiaoyu Wen; xywen@jlu.edu.cn

Academic Editor: Zhaohui Bai

*Background and Aims.* There are few studies on the prevalence and clinical characteristics of portopulmonary hypertension (POPH) in patients with portal hypertension. In addition, invasive right heart catheterization further limits the clinical diagnosis of POPH patients. *Methods.* From January 2018 to December 2019, 1004 patients with portal hypertension were treated in the Department of Hepatology, the First Hospital of Jilin University. Based on the inclusion and exclusion criteria, 188 patients with portal hypertension were finally included. We collected complete clinical data, laboratory examinations, and imaging examinations. Patients were divided into a POPH group and a non-POPH group based on echocardiographic results. We calculated the prevalence of POPH in patients with portal hypertension. The differences in clinical characteristics of the two groups of patients were compared. *Results.* The prevalence of POPH in patients with portal hypertension was 2.8%. Among the 188 patients with portal hypertension with fingertip oxygen saturation < 95% at rest, 28 patients had POPH (12 males and 16 females), with an average age of 63 ± 8, and 160 patients did not have POPH (110 males, 50 women), with an average age of 59 ± 11. The proportion of women in the POPH group ($P < 0.01$) and patients without liver cancer ($P = 0.044$) was high. Compared to patients without POPH, patients with POPH had lower hemoglobin (related to the severity of anemia, $P < 0.01$), higher creatinine ($P < 0.05$), and lower partial pressure of oxygen and carbon dioxide ($P < 0.05$). Patients with POPH had a higher incidence of atrial enlargement, ventricular enlargement, mitral valve regurgitation, tricuspid regurgitation, pulmonary artery widening, pericardial effusion, and aortic regurgitation than those without POPH. The risk of POPH did not increase with the aggravation of the Child-Pugh classification. *Conclusion.* The prevalence of POPH in patients with portal hypertension is 2.8%. The proportion of women and nonliver cancer in POPH patients was higher than that in non-POPH patients. In addition, the POPH group had higher creatinine and lower hemoglobin, and echocardiography showed that POPH patients had more cardiac structural changes. In patients with portal hypertension, the risk in patients with POPH has nothing to do with the Child-Pugh classification and MELD score.

## 1. Introduction

Portopulmonary hypertension is defined as pulmonary hypertension formed on the basis of portal hypertension, which is common in liver cirrhosis, bile duct obstruction, and cholestatic diseases. The diagnosis of POPH relies on right heart catheterization. According to the latest guidelines, mean pulmonary artery pressure (mPAP) is higher than 20 mmHg (1 mmHg = 0.133 KPa), pulmonary vascular resistance (PVR) is higher than 240 dyn s cm$^{-5}$ (=3 Wood units), and pulmonary capillary wedge pressure (PCWP) is less than 15 mmHg [1].

Due to the low incidence of the disease, the current understanding of the disease remains unclear. On account of the limited clinical data, descriptions of the clinical features of the disease are rare and inconsistent. The prevalence

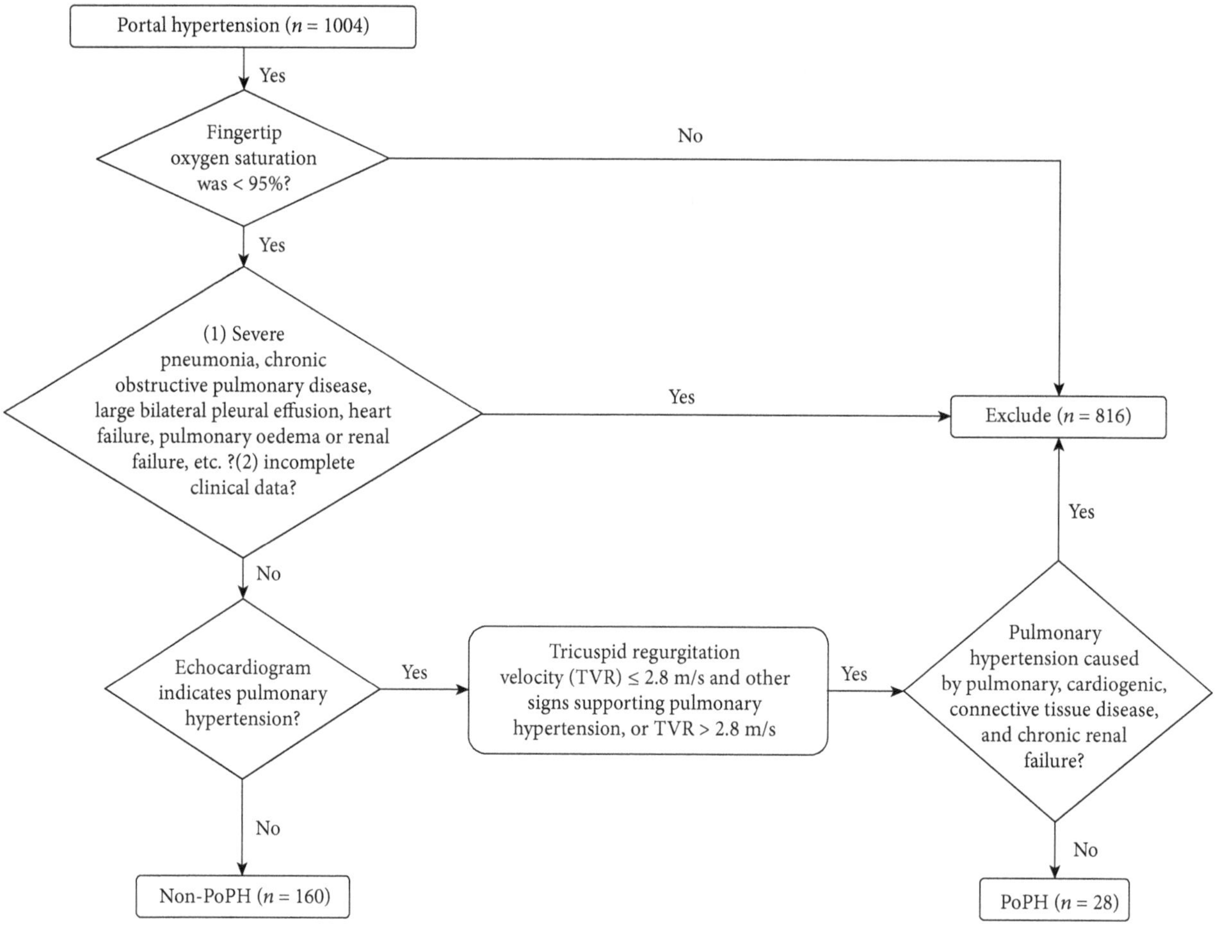


Figure 1: Study screening flowchart.

of POPH in patients with portal hypertension ranges from approximately 1% to 2% [2], and the prevalence of POPH in liver transplant patients increases from 5% to 8% [3]. The pathogenesis of POPH is not yet clear. At present, the mechanism generally acknowledged by scholars is the imbalance of vasoactive substances [4–6]. Diastolic vasoactive substances decreased, while systolic vasoactive substances increased, resulting in the balance being broken. The clinical manifestations of POPH are nonspecific. The main manifestation is different degrees of dyspnoea. One-third of patients may experience transient syncope. Owing to the invasion of right heart catheterization, echocardiography is often used clinically as a screening tool, and its sensitivity and specificity are shown to be high [7]. The treatment of POPH is mainly targeted therapy of pulmonary hypertension and liver transplantation. The 5-year survival rate of untreated POPH patients is 14.2% [8]. At present, the prognosis of POPH has been improved after liver transplantation and targeted therapy of pulmonary hypertension. The incidence of POPH is relatively low, and there are currently few reports on the clinical features and risk factor analysis of the disease in China. One previous study performed in China was focused on POPH in liver transplant recipients [8]. We conducted two consecutive years for patients with portal hypertension, whose study population is broader. Screening was performed to further clarify the incidence and clinical characteristics of POPH. We hope to provide clinical guidance for the early diagnosis of POPH through this research and to improve clinicians' understanding of POPH.

## 2. Materials and Methods

*2.1. Study Population.* From January 2018 to December 2019, 188 patients with portal hypertension (selected from 1004 patients with portal hypertension) who were admitted to the Department of Hepatology, the First Hospital of Jilin University, whose fingertip oxygen saturation was less than 95%, were enrolled in this research (Figure 1). The exclusion criteria were as follows: (1) patients with nonportal hypertension; (2) patients with severe pneumonia, chronic obstructive pulmonary disease, large bilateral pleural effusion, heart failure, pulmonary oedema, renal failure, etc., whose fingertip blood oxygen saturation was less than 95% in the resting state; (3) patients with pulmonary hypertension caused by pulmonary, cardiogenic, and connective tissue disease and chronic renal failure; and (4) patients with incomplete clinical data. The research protocol of this study was approved by the Ethics Committee of the First Hospital of Jilin University and was conducted in accordance with the Declaration of Helsinki (No. 2020-592). Informed consent was waived by the Institutional Review Board due to the retrospective nature of the study with no more than minimal risk.

*2.2. Data Collection.* We collected general information (sex, age, etiology, etc.) of the above patients, laboratory tests (complete blood count, coagulation function, liver function, renal function, etc.), and auxiliary examinations (echocardiography, abdominal computed tomography (CT) examination, chest CT, etc.). Echocardiography was performed according to the recommendations of the American Society of Echocardiography in 2015, and the patients were divided into the POPH group and the non-POPH group according to the 2015 ESC/ERS pulmonary hypertension diagnosis and treatment guidelines. We compared the differences in clinical characteristics, laboratory tests, and echocardiography between the two groups.

*2.3. Diagnosis of POPH.* The diagnosis of POPH is based on the 2015 ESC/ERS pulmonary hypertension guidelines. Patients with echocardiography indicating medium-to-high risk (tricuspid regurgitation velocity ≤ 2.8 m/s and other signs supporting pulmonary hypertension or tricuspid regurgitation velocity > 2.8 m/s) and excluding other causes of pulmonary hypertension were included in the POPH group, and the remaining patients were included in the non-POPH group.

*2.4. Statistical Analysis.* All data were statistically analyzed using SPSS 22.0 software (IBM ® Corporation, USA). Measurement data conforming to a normal distribution were described by the mean ± standard deviation. Comparisons between the two groups were performed by *t*-tests. Data not conforming to a normal distribution were taken as the median. The number and interquartile range P50 (P25-P75) were also used for description. The Mann-Whitney *U* test was used between these two groups. The enumeration data and grade data were described by the composition ratio, and the chi-square test was used for the comparison of the enumeration data between the two groups. The chi-square test was used to compare the grade data between the two groups. The correlation of grade data was analyzed by the trend chi-square test, and $P < 0.05$ indicated statistical significance.

Table 1: Analysis of demographic situation of the POPH group and non-POPH group.

| Variables | POPH ($n = 28$) | Non-POPH ($n = 160$) | $\chi^2/t$ | $P$ |
|---|---|---|---|---|
| Age (years) | 63 ± 8 | 59 ± 11 | -1.541 | 0.125 |
| Gender $N$ (%) | | | | |
| Male | 12 (42.9) | 110 (68.7) | 7.017 | <0.01 |
| Female | 16 (57.1) | 50 (31.3) | | |
| Etiology $N$ (%) | | | | |
| HBV | 10 (35.7) | 71 (44.4) | 0.729 | 0.393 |
| HCV | 2 (7.1) | 21 (13.1) | — | 0.537 |
| Alcohol | 9 (32.1) | 37 (23.1) | 1.049 | 0.306 |
| Drug | 1 (3.6) | 6 (3.8) | — | 1.00 |
| Autoimmune | 3 (10.7) | 14 (8.8) | — | 0.723 |
| Liver cancer $N$ (%) | | | | |
| Yes | 4 (14.3) | 51 (31.9) | 3.562 | 0.059 |
| No | 24 (85.7) | 109 (68.1) | | |
| Hypertension $N$ (%) | | | | |
| Yes | 5 (17.9) | 22 (13.7) | — | 0.563 |
| No | 23 (82.1) | 138 (86.3) | | |
| Diabetes $N$ (%) | | | | |
| Yes | 3 (10.7) | 30 (18.8) | — | 0.422 |
| No | 25 (89.3) | 130 (81.3) | | |
| Splenectomy $N$ (%) | | | | |
| Yes | 6 (21.4) | 21 (13.1) | — | 0. 249 |
| No | 22 (78.6) | 139 (86.9) | | |
| Portal vein thrombosis $N$ (%) | | | | |
| Yes | 4 (14.3) | 21 (13.1) | — | 0.771 |
| No | 24 (85.7) | 139 (86.9) | | |

The diagnosis of portal hypertension in this study is based on the 2016 Practice Guidance by the AASLD on Portal Hypertensive Bleeding in Cirrhosis [9]. All patients had manifestations of liver cirrhosis and portal hypertension confirmed by abdominal imaging (ultrasound, CT, or MRI), and most patients had complications of portal hypertension at the time of admission, such as portal hypertensive bleeding and ascites.

## 3. Results and Discussion

*3.1. Clinical Features.* In this study, a total of 1004 patients with portal hypertension were screened, and 188 patients with portal hypertension with fingertip oxygen saturation less than 95% were included. Twenty-eight of these were diagnosed with POPH. The patients were not targeted for pulmonary hypertension treatment before and after diagnosis. The proportion of female patients and patients without liver cancer in the POPH group was higher than that in the non-POPH group, and there was no significant difference in other aspects (Table 1). Data are provided as number of cases (%) (HBV: hepatitis B virus, HCV: hepatitis C virus).

*3.2. Laboratory Examination.* A statistical analysis of the laboratory test results of the two groups showed that the proportion of patients with anemia in the POPH group was higher than that of patients without POPH. The two groups also had differences in the distribution of anemia, and the mean corpuscular hemoglobin (MCH) and mean corpuscular hemoglobin concentration (MCHC) in the POPH group were lower. However, the mean corpuscular volume (MCV) of the non-POPH group was not significantly different from that of the POPH group. In addition, the POPH group had lower partial pressure of oxygen ($PaO_2$), partial pressure of carbon dioxide ($PaCO_2$), and potassium ions and higher creatinine (CREA) values than patients without POPH (Table 2). Data are provided as the median (IQR) and number of cases (%) (ALT: alanine aminotransferase, AST: aspartate aminotransferase, ALB: albumin, TBiL: total bilirubin, PT: prothrombin time, CREA: creatinine, $PaO_2$: partial pressure of oxygen, $PaCO_2$: partial pressure of carbon dioxide, PLT: platelet, HGB: hemoglobin, MCV: mean corpuscular volume, MCH: mean corpuscular hemoglobin, MCHC: mean corpuscular hemoglobin concentration, MELD: model for end-stage liver disease; normal ranges: AST 15-40 U/L; ALT 9-50 U/L; ALP: 45-135 U/L; ALB: 40-55 g/L; TBiL: 0-26.0 $\mu$mol/L; PT 9-13 s; CREA: 41-73 $\mu$mol/L; $PaO_2$: 83-

Table 2: Analysis of laboratory examination of the POPH group and non-POPH group.

| Variables | POPH ($n = 28$) | Non-POPH ($n = 160$) | $z/t$ | $P$ |
|---|---|---|---|---|
| ALT (U/L) | 21.8 (14.3-21.8) | 33.9 (19.6-59.9) | -1.451 | 0.147 |
| AST (U/L) | 43.9 (30.9-64.7) | 53.7 (34.2-91.9) | -1.043 | 0.297 |
| ALB (g/L) | 27.6 ± 5.7 | 28.4 ± 5.9 | 0.701 | 0.484 |
| TBiL ($\mu$mol/L) | 34.8 (18.5-95.4) | 40.7 (24.1-101.6) | -1.065 | 0.287 |
| PT (s) | 15.5 (13.6-19.3) | 15.0 (13.2-18.9) | -0.776 | 0.438 |
| CREA (mmol/l) | 80.0 (59.0-99.0) | 65.1 (52.3-80.0) | -2.091 | 0.037 |
| $PaO_2$ (mmHg) | 67.3 (58.0-77.9) | 72.7 (65.4-81.8) | -2.166 | 0.030 |
| $PaCO_2$ (mmHg) | 31.0 (27.7-32.9) | 33.0 (31.0-36.0) | -2.524 | 0.012 |
| Potassium ion (mmol/l) | 3.6 (3.2-3.8) | 3.9 (3.5-4.2) | -2.810 | <0.01 |
| Sodium ion (mmol/l) | 136.1 (133.6-138.9) | 135.9 (132.4-139.0) | -0.631 | 0.528 |
| PLT ($\times 10^9$/L) | 84.0 (51.0-121.0) | 86.0 (60.0-127.0) | -0.346 | 0.729 |
| HGB (g/L) | 95.2 ± 25.5 | 112.3 ± 31.0 | 2.744 | <0.01 |
| MCV (fl) | 93.0 (86.3-98.1) | 96.1 (90.6-101.8) | -1.771 | 0.077 |
| MCH (pg) | 31.4 (27.8-33.5) | 32.6 (30.7-35.5) | -2.235 | 0.025 |
| MCHC (g/L) | 330.0 (315.3-343.5) | 341.0 (329.3-350.0) | -2.457 | 0.014 |
| The degree of anemia $N$ (%) | | | | |
| Normal | 5 (17.8) | 79 (49.4) | -2.740 | <0.01 |
| Mild anemia | 11 (39.3) | 39 (24.4) | | |
| Moderate anemia | 11 (39.3) | 34 (21.3) | | |
| Severe anemia | 1 (3.6) | 8 (5.0) | | |
| Child-Pugh classification $N$ (%) | | | | |
| A | 4 (14.3) | 25 (15.6) | -0.012 | 0.990 |
| B | 14 (50) | 76 (47.5) | | |
| C | 10 (35.7) | 59 (36.9) | | |
| MELD score | 12.5 (10.0-18.5) | 11.0 (8.0-17.0) | -0.932 | 0.351 |

108 mmHg; $PaCO_2$: 35-48 mmHg; potassium ion: 3.5-4.5 mmol/L; sodium ion: 136-145 mmol/L; PLT: 125-350 × $10^9$/L; HBG: 115-150 g/L; MCV: 82-100 fL; MCH: 27-34 pg; MCHC: 316-354 g/L).

Calculation formulas are as follows: MELD = 3.8 × ln (bilirubin mg/dl) + 11.2 × ln (INR) + 9.6 × ln (creatinine mg/dl) + 6.4 × (etiology : 0 if cholestatic or alcoholic, 1 otherwise) [10].

*3.3. Echocardiography.* The echocardiography results between the POPH group and the non-POPH group are shown in Table 3. Compared to the non-POPH group, patients in the POPH group showed enlarged atrial and ventricular echocardiography, as well as mitral, tricuspid, and aortic regurgitation, pulmonary artery widening, and pericardial effusion ($P < 0.05$). There were no significant differences between the two groups in terms of pulmonary regurgitation, severity of diastolic function, and systolic function (left ventricular short-axis contraction rate and ejection fraction) ($P > 0.05$).

*3.4. Correlation between the Risk of Portopulmonary Hypertension and the Child-Pugh Classification and MELD Score.* Among 188 patients whose fingertip blood oxygen saturation was less than 95% at rest, 28 cases of POPH were screened. Among them, 16 were intermediate-risk patients, and 12 were high-risk patients. In other words, 4 were Child-Pugh A patients, 14 were Child-Pugh B patients, and 10 were Child-Pugh C patients. The above data were analyzed by the chi-square test trend (Table 4), and it was found that the risk of POPH did not increase with the aggravation of the Child-Pugh classification ($P = 0.382$). The MELD score of patients in the intermedium-risk group was 14.3 ± 8.0, while the MELD score in the high-risk group was 12.4 ± 7.1. The difference in MELD scores between the two groups could not be considered statistically significant ($t = 0.655$, $P = 0.518$) (Table 5).

## 4. Discussion

With the continuous development of current medical technology, the diagnosis of POPH has entered the field of a wide range of clinicians. However, the pathogenesis of POPH is not yet fully understood, and further study and exploration are needed. POPH is more commonly seen in patients with decompensated liver cirrhosis. How to effectively screen for POPH among the huge population of liver cirrhosis patients in China plays a particularly important role in their prognosis. Therefore, we hope to screen key patients through this study to further deepen people's understanding of the disease.

TABLE 3: Analysis of laboratory examination of the POPH group and non-POPH group.

| Echocardiography | POPH ($n = 28$) | Non-POPH ($n = 160$) | $\chi^2/z$ | $P$ |
|---|---|---|---|---|
| Enlargement of the left atrium $N$ (%) | | | | |
| Normal | 10 (35.7) | 132 (82.5) | 28.224 | <0.01 |
| Enlargement | 18 (64.3) | 28 (17.5) | | |
| Enlargement of the left ventricle $N$ (%) | | | | |
| Normal | 22 (78.6) | 153 (95.6) | — | <0.01* |
| Enlargement | 6 (21.4) | 7 (4.4) | | |
| Enlargement of the right atrium $N$ (%) | | | | |
| Normal | 13 (46.4) | 165 (96.9) | — | <0.01* |
| Enlargement | 15 (53.6) | 5 (3.1) | | |
| Enlargement of the right ventricle $N$ (%) | | | | |
| Normal | 25 (89.3) | 158 (98.8) | — | 0.024* |
| Enlargement | 3 (10.7) | 2 (1.2) | | |
| Pericardial effusion $N$ (%) | | | | |
| Yes | 12 (42.9) | 12 (7.5) | — | <0.01* |
| No | 16 (57.1) | 148 (92.5) | | |
| Mitral regurgitation $N$ (%) | | | | |
| Yes | 16 (57.1) | 25 (15.6) | 24.088 | <0.01 |
| No | 12 (42.9) | 135 (84.4) | | |
| Aortic regurgitation $N$ (%) | | | | |
| Yes | 8 (28.6) | 17 (10.6) | — | 0.016* |
| No | 20 (71.4) | 143 (89.4) | | |
| Pulmonary regurgitation $N$ (%) | | | | |
| Yes | 1 (3.6) | 1 (0.6) | — | 0.276* |
| No | 27 (96.4) | 159 (99.4) | | |
| Tricuspid regurgitation $N$ (%) | | | | |
| Yes | 26 (92.9) | 37 (23.1) | 52.006 | <0.01 |
| No | 2 (96.4) | 123 (76.9) | | |
| Pulmonary artery widening $N$ (%) | | | | |
| Yes | 10 (35.7) | 0 (0) | — | <0.01* |
| No | 18 (64.3) | 160 (100.0) | | |
| Diastolic function $N$ (%) | | | | |
| Normal | 2 (7.1) | 28 (17.5) | -1.781 | 0.075 |
| Suspicious reduction | 6 (21.4) | 45 (28.2) | | |
| Reduction | 20 (57.5) | 87 (54.3) | | |
| Left ventricular short-axis contraction rate (%) | 32 (31-33) | 32 (30-33) | -1.008 | 0.313 |
| Ejection fraction (%) | 60 (59-64) | 60 (60-63) | -0.653 | 0.514 |

*Fisher's exact test.

TABLE 4: Correlation between the risk of portal hypertension and Child-Pugh classification.

| Risk level | Child-Pugh A ($n = 4$) | Child-Pugh B ($n = 14$) | Child-Pugh C ($n = 10$) | $P$ |
|---|---|---|---|---|
| Medium | 2 | 7 | 7 | 0.382 |
| High | 2 | 7 | 3 | |

TABLE 5: Correlation between the risk of portal hypertension and MELD score.

| Risk level | Medium ($n = 16$) | High ($n = 12$) | $P$ |
|---|---|---|---|
| MELD score | 14.3 ± 8.0 | 12.4 ± 7.1 | 0.518 |

The study included 1004 patients, of which 188 subjects were the main study subjects. The prevalence of POPH among people with portal hypertension who did not undergo liver transplantation was 2.8%. There is no clear report of the incidence in patients with liver cirrhosis, and in patients with advanced liver cirrhosis, the incidence can be as high as 8.5% [11]. Although our research proves that there is no relationship between the risk of POPH and the

Child-Pugh classification and MELD score of patients, studies have shown that the correlation between POPH and the severity of liver disease is weak [12]. The mechanism of POPH risk in patients with advanced liver disease may be related to genetic polymorphisms of oestrogen-related genes and other pathways involving cell growth/apoptosis and oxidative stress [13]. The POPH group was more common in female patients, which may be related to the involvement of oestrogen in the disease [14]. Previous studies have proven that woman can be a risk factor for POPH [15].

Anemia is more common in patients in the POPH group. This may be because patients with chronic anemia require higher resting cardiac output to compensate for the decreased oxygen-carrying capacity, so pulmonary hypertension may also occur in hemolytic diseases [16]. A study is consistent with our results, showing that anemia is an independent risk factor for POPH [17]. Patients with liver cirrhosis and POPH show more valve regurgitation, enlargement of the atria and ventricles, and widening of the pulmonary artery on echocardiography. Therefore, when using echocardiography for POPH screening, attention should be paid to the abovementioned positive results of patients, and the screening and follow-up of the disease should be strengthened.

In patients with portohypertension whose fingertip oxygen saturation is less than 95% in the resting state, the partial pressure of oxygen and carbon dioxide in the POPH group is significantly lower than that in the non-POPH group, which is related to the increased alveolar-arterial oxygen gradient. In addition, the creatinine value and number of nonliver cancer patients in the POPH group were higher than those in the non-POPH group. The correlation between creatinine and liver cancer history and POPH has not been reported, but the increase in creatinine caused by increased visceral circulation load in POPH patients is not excluded, and a large sample is needed for further confirmation.

Our study found that there were no differences in liver function, Child-Pugh classification, MELD score, or etiology between the POPH group and the non-POPH group. This is consistent with the results of a previous study that the Child-Pugh classification is not related to POPH [18]. Studies have shown that increased MELD scores in POPH patients before transplantation are associated with poor survival after transplantation [19], and we need to confirm this conclusion with long-term follow-up observation. Foreign studies have reported that hepatitis C is a protective factor for POPH, but we did not find this in our research. Considering the differences in etiology between China and Western countries, the main cause of the population in China is viral hepatitis B. The main cause of the disease in the country is hepatitis C and alcoholic hepatitis, so the results between the two are not the same [20]. Patients with POPH often have hypoxia. To reduce the economic burden of hospitalized patients, we used fingertip blood oxygen saturation < 95% as the screening index in the resting state. Because a relevant research reported screened population whose arterial blood oxygen pressure was less than 60 mmHg, the sensitivity and specificity of fingertip blood oxygen saturation < 95% in the resting state can be as high as 100% and 93% [21]. The limitations of this study include the following points: (1) the sample size of samples is insufficient, so the number of positive patients is small, and the conclusions drawn need to be confirmed by further expanding the sample size, and (2) the diagnostic standard used in this study is echocardiography. Due to various reasons, right heart catheterization could not be performed for further confirmation.

In summary, to further clarify the clinical characteristics and predisposing factors of POPH patients, we still need to increase the sample size to analyze whether there are real differences in clinical characteristics between the two populations, and the reasons for the differences need to be further explored. In addition, in future research, we will further expand the sample size, explore the correlation between POPH and portal hypertension parameters, and deepen our understanding of POPH.

## 5. Conclusions

Our study provides estimates of the prevalence of POPH in patients with portal hypertension. The proportion of women with nonliver cancer in POPH patients is higher than that in non-POPH patients. The POPH group had higher creatinine and lower hemoglobin. Echocardiography showed greater changes in the heart structure of POPH patients.

## Authors' Contributions

Yueming Shao and Xin Yin contributed equally to this work.

## Acknowledgments

We thank all of the study participants. We also appreciate the contributions of the nurses and doctors at the Department of Hepatology, the First Hospital of Jilin University, to this study. This work was supported by the Foundation of Science and Technology Commission of Jilin Province (grant No. 20190201065JC).

## References

[1] G. Simonneau, D. Montani, D. S. Celermajer et al., "Haemodynamic definitions and updated clinical classification of pulmonary hypertension," *European Respiratory Journal*, vol. 53, no. 1, p. 1801913, 2019.

[2] L. Mancuso, F. Scordato, M. Pieri, E. Valerio, and A. Mancuso, "Management of portopulmonary hypertension: new perspectives," *World Journal of Gastroenterology*, vol. 19, no. 45, pp. 8252–8257, 2013.

[3] R. Rodríguez-Roisin, M. J. Krowka, P. Hervé, M. B. Fallon, and ERS Task Force Pulmonary-Hepatic Vascular Disorders (PHD) Scientific Committee, "Pulmonary-hepatic vascular disorders (PHD)," *The European Respiratory Journal*, vol. 24, no. 5, pp. 861–880, 2004.

[4] S. Raevens, A. Geerts, C. van Steenkiste, X. Verhelst, H. van Vlierberghe, and I. Colle, "Hepatopulmonary syndrome and portopulmonary hypertension: recent knowledge in pathogenesis and overview of clinical assessment," *Liver International*, vol. 35, no. 6, pp. 1646–1660, 2015.

[5] J. A. Talwalkar, K. L. Swanson, M. J. Krowka, J. C. Andrews, and P. S. Kamath, "Prevalence of spontaneous portosystemic shunts in patients with portopulmonary hypertension and effect on treatment," *Gastroenterology*, vol. 141, no. 5, pp. 1673–1679, 2011.

[6] T. Thevenot, D. Weil, and V. di Martino, "What is the true relationship between spontaneous portosystemic shunts and portopulmonary hypertension in cirrhotic patients?," *Gastroenterology*, vol. 155, no. 5, pp. 1647-1648, 2018.

[7] I. O. Colle, R. Moreau, E. Godinho et al., "Diagnosis of portopulmonary hypertension in candidates for liver transplantation: a prospective study," *Hepatology*, vol. 37, no. 2, pp. 401–409, 2003.

[8] J. Li, Q. Zhuang, X. M. Zhang et al., "Prevalence and prognosis of portopulmonary hypertension in 223 liver transplant recipients," *Canadian Respiratory Journal*, vol. 2018, Article ID 9629570, 6 pages, 2018.

[9] G. Garcia-Tsao, J. G. Abraldes, A. Berzigotti, and J. Bosch, "Portal hypertensive bleeding in cirrhosis: risk stratification, diagnosis, and management: 2016 practice guidance by the American Association for the study of liver diseases," *Hepatology*, vol. 65, no. 1, pp. 310–335, 2017.

[10] P. S. Kamath, R. H. Wiesner, M. Malinchoc et al., "A model to predict survival in patients with end-stage liver disease," *Hepatology*, vol. 33, no. 2, pp. 464–470, 2001.

[11] M. A. Ramsay, B. R. Simpson, A. T. Nguyen, K. J. Ramsay, C. East, and G. B. Klintmalm, "Severe pulmonary hypertension in liver transplant candidates," *Liver Transplantation and Surgery*, vol. 3, no. 5, pp. 494–500, 1997.

[12] M. J. Krowka, K. L. Swanson, R. P. Frantz, M. D. McGoon, and R. H. Wiesner, "Portopulmonary hypertension: results from a 10-year screening algorithm," *Hepatology*, vol. 44, no. 6, pp. 1502–1510, 2006.

[13] K. E. Roberts, M. B. Fallon, M. J. Krowka et al., "Genetic risk factors for portopulmonary hypertension in patients with advanced liver disease," *American Journal of Respiratory and Critical Care Medicine*, vol. 179, no. 9, pp. 835–842, 2009.

[14] N. Al-Naamani, M. J. Krowka, K. A. Forde et al., "Estrogen signaling and portopulmonary hypertension: the Pulmonary Vascular Complications of Liver Disease Study (PVCLD2)," *Hepatology*, vol. 73, no. 2, pp. 726–737, 2020.

[15] S. M. Kawut, M. J. Krowka, J. F. Trotter et al., "Clinical risk factors for portopulmonary hypertension," *Hepatology*, vol. 48, no. 1, pp. 196–203, 2008.

[16] E. E. Lin, M. T. Gladwin, and R. F. Machado, "Pulmonary hypertension in patients with hemoglobinopathies: could a mechanism for dysfunction provide an avenue for novel therapeutics?," *Haematologica*, vol. 90, no. 4, pp. 441–444, 2005.

[17] H. S. CHEN, S. R. XING, W. G. XU et al., "Portopulmonary hypertension in cirrhotic patients: prevalence, clinical features and risk factors," *Experimental and Therapeutic Medicine*, vol. 5, no. 3, pp. 819–824, 2013.

[18] M. Atsukawa, A. Tsubota, M. Hatano et al., "Prevalence and characteristics of portopulmonary hypertension in cirrhotic patients who underwent both hepatic vein and pulmonary artery catheterization," *Hepatology Research*, vol. 50, no. 11, pp. 1244–1254, 2020.

[19] R. J. Salgia, N. P. Goodrich, H. Simpson, R. M. Merion, and P. Sharma, "Outcomes of liver transplantation for portopulmonary hypertension in model for end-stage liver disease era," *Digestive Diseases and Sciences*, vol. 59, no. 8, pp. 1976–1982, 2014.

[20] A. al-Harbi, K. Abdullah, A. al-Abdulkareem, A. Alghamdi, and H. al-Jahdali, "Prevalence of portopulmonary hypertension among liver transplant candidates in a region highly endemic for viral hepatitis," *Annals of Transplantation*, vol. 19, pp. 1–5, 2014.

[21] M. R. Arguedas, H. Singh, D. K. Faulk, and M. B. Fallon, "Utility of pulse oximetry screening for hepatopulmonary syndrome," *Clinical Gastroenterology and Hepatology*, vol. 5, no. 6, pp. 749–754.e1, 2007.

# 12

# Central Systolic Hypertension in Patients with Well-Controlled Hypertension

**Jozef Bulas,[1] Mária Potočárová,[1] Ján Murín,[1] Katarína Kozlíková,[2] Ján Luha,[3] and Martin Čaprnda[1]**

[1] *1st Department of Internal Medicine, Comenius University, Faculty of Medicine, Mickiewiczova 13, 813 69 Bratislava, Slovakia*
[2] *Institute of Medical Physics, Biophysics, Informatics and Telemedicine, Comenius University, Faculty of Medicine, Sasinkova 2, 813 72 Bratislava, Slovakia*
[3] *Institute of Medical Biology, Genetics and Clinical Genetics, Comenius University, Faculty of Medicine, Sasinkova 4, 813 72 Bratislava, Slovakia*

Correspondence should be addressed to Jozef Bulas; jozef2bulas@gmail.com

Academic Editor: Shigehiko Ogoh

*Background.* Central systolic blood pressure (CSBP) has prognostic significance and simplified devices for its estimation have been introduced recently. The aim of this study was to assess the achievement of the target CSBP in treated hypertensive patients. *Subjects and Methods.* One hundred patients with well-controlled hypertension were analysed. For CSBP estimation, we used the Arteriograph (TensioMed Ltd.), which uses one cuff for all measurements, the "single-point measurement" approach. *Results.* We found that 62% of patients had CSBP ≥ 130 mmHg, the suggested cut-off value for hypertension. When sex-specific classification was employed (CSBP ≥ 137 mmHg for female and CSBP ≥ 133 mmHg for male), only 13% of patients (mainly women) remained in the hypertensive range. We also found that 55% of patients had a CSBP higher than brachial pressure. Multiple analyses showed that CSBP was significantly associated with sex, height, and return time. *Conclusions.* A high proportion of treated hypertensive patients had CSBP levels that exceeded their brachial BP. CSBP positively correlated with lower height and shorter return time of the reflected pressure wave and was significantly higher in females compared to males. These findings suggest that, for CSBP classification, it is important to take height and sex-specific differences into account.

## 1. Introduction

Arterial hypertension is the most important modifiable cardiovascular risk factor. Blood pressure (BP) measurement has been extensively used for more than a century, and brachial cuff BP has been used for the diagnosis and treatment of hypertension. Consequently, guidelines and classifications are based on this approach [1, 2].

Systolic BP is a result of the interaction between ejected stroke volume and the dampening function of large arteries and propagative and reflected pressure waves. Both pulse pressure and systolic pressure increase due to pulse pressure amplification as pressure waves propagate from the heart to the periphery, and from where the pressure waves reflect back to the heart [3, 4].

Early return of reflected pressure waves (in the case of stiffer arteries) may increase central systolic pressure in the aortic root during late systole and may increase the workload of the left ventricle [5]. Standard BP measurement using the brachial artery does not allow for the estimation of central BP and the ascertainment of the real work of the left ventricle [6, 7].

Central systolic blood pressure (CSBP) is considered an important haemodynamic parameter, and several large studies indicate that it is an important prognostic risk factor [8]. Cardiovascular events decrease with lower CSBP levels, and this finding explains the differences between patient subgroups with similar brachial BP but different CSBP; lower CSBP levels resulted in more favourable clinical outcomes [9–11].

The standard for noninvasive central BP estimation is generally accepted to be applanation tonometry, in which pulse waves on the radial or carotid arteries are detected by a sensitive probe. The pulse wave curve obtained requires calibration, and this is achieved by entering the BP values from brachial BP measurements and is corrected by the transfer factor. The peripheral pressure waveform is then intertwined with the wave in the ascending aorta [3, 12]. Such an examination is methodologically challenging (needs specialized equipment and training) and time-consuming and requires a high degree of expertise [12, 13].

Newer and simpler methods rely on cuff-based waveform analyses, in which pressure waves and BP measurements are taken by a single BP cuff on the arm. This technique, called single-point measurement, is operator-independent and such devices have shown some promise for routine clinical use [14]. The obtained pressure wave curve has a typical pattern that facilitates the analysis of BP changes and the evaluation of heart cycle timing.

For the research and clinical implication of vascular stiffness measurement, it is important to standardise the methodology of examination of arterial stiffness. Methodological aspects of stiffness measurements, wave reflections, central pulse pressure, and aortic pressure estimation are discussed in the Recommendation of the American Heart Association (AHA) 2015 [14]. Papers concerning "reference values" of pulse wave velocity (PWV, a marker of arterial stiffness) and of CSBP have been published recently [15–17]. Although the routine clinical use of CSBP measurement is under debate, growing evidence of the prognostic significance of such an approach supports its implementation in practice [18–20]. The continued improvement of the accuracy and reliability and the standardisation of methodology suggest that CSBP measurement will become more common in daily practice [7, 18].

In this study, we aimed to identify the potential benefits of CSBP measurement in the management of patients with hypertension in clinical practice. Thus, we analysed a group of patients who visited our outpatient department that specializes in providing care for patients with high BP. We also assessed how successful we were in achieving the recommended CSBP level according to data in the current literature and to compare CSBP readings to brachial BP in treated hypertensive patients.

## 2. Materials and Methods

For this analysis, we retrospectively selected data from 100 patients with well-controlled hypertension (brachial blood pressure below 140/90 mmHg) from a group of 199 consecutive patients referred to our outpatient department for further investigation or for a follow-up examination from May 2008 to December 2015. The patients were originally involved in a research project studying central haemodynamics and preclinical cardiovascular disease, which was approved by Ethical committee of University Hospital Commenius University Bratislava. The patients signed an informed consent form after we explained to them the nature and aim of this type of noninvasive BP measurement, which was added to our usual set of examinations devoted to the search for preclinical cardiovascular diseases in patients diagnosed with hypertension. The patients selected for this analysis had undergone a basic clinical examination and a recent echocardiographic examination. They had a blood pressure (measured by arteriography) below 140/90 mmHg and their current medication list was known. The exclusion criteria were as follows: atrial fibrillation, systolic or diastolic BP above the target values, left ventricular systolic dysfunction, heart failure, unstable angina or clinically significant valve disease, advanced renal failure [glomerular filtration rate (GFR) < 60 ml/(min·m$^2$)], and/or significantly increased liver function test values (liver function test values greater than 3 times the upper normal limit).

Each patient underwent standard clinical evaluation, measurement of anthropometric parameters, laboratory tests including lipid profile, and echocardiography with the measurement of basic parameters such as left ventricular wall thickness and dimensions, systolic function, calculated left ventricular mass (LVM) according to Devereux et al. [21], LVM indexed to the body surface area ($LVM_i$), relative wall thickness, and diastolic function. The threshold for left ventricular hypertrophy (LVH) was considered as the left ventricular mass index, $LVM_i \geq 95\,g/m^2$ for women and $LVM_i \geq 115\,g/m^2$ for men [1]. Specifically, patients with well-controlled BP, below 140/90 mmHg, at the time of examination (recommended goal arm BP) were included in the analysis.

The invasively and noninvasively validated instrument, Arteriograph Tensiomed Ltd. (H-1103 Budapest, Hungary), was used to estimate the central BP [20, 22–25]. It works based on the oscillometric principle, using only one cuff for both BP measurement and waveform detection for pressure wave analysis (one measurement site, single-point analysis) [14]. The cuff for BP and central haemodynamic evaluation was tightly fastened on the dominant arm above the elbow as recommended in the user's manual [26]. The pressure wave is self-calibrated using the brachial pressure, which is obtained during the same measurement cycle [26]. One measurement cycle lasts 2 to 3 minutes. Patients were examined after 5 to 10 minutes of rest in the supine position. After placing the cuff in the proper position on the arm, the actual measurement is automated and operator-independent, and results of measurements depend solely on the measuring device. Because of the inherent variability of blood pressure, [13] some differences were expected between repeated measurements. A two-way ANOVA on these repeated measurements revealed significant differences between the first and third measurements, but not between the second and third of the three repeated measurements in one session. For evaluation of the reliability of measurements, we measured the concordance of the direction of the differences between the CSBP and sBP-brachial (higher or lower CSBP). From 41 tested measurements, only five patients showed a divergence in the direction of differences. In our cohort, 88% of all patients showed concordance in the direction of the differences between CSBP and sBP-brachial (all three values of CSBP measured in one patient were either higher or lower than values of sBP-brachial). The opposite direction of differences was present mainly in patients with small (near to zero) CSBP to sBP-brachial differences.

Table 1: Basic clinical characteristics of the subjects.

| | All | Males | Females | $p$ value |
|---|---|---|---|---|
| Number of patients ($n$) | 100 | 38 | 62 | |
| Age (years) | 64.0 ± 10.7 | 60.6 ± 11.0 | 66.1 ± 10.0 | $p = 0.018$ |
| Height (cm) | 169.3 ± 9.2 | 178.4 ± 5.0 | 163.6 ± 6.1 | $p < 0.001$ |
| Weight (kg) | 80.2 ± 15.4 | 93.3 ± 13.0 | 72.2 ± 10.7 | $p < 0.001$ |
| BMI (kg/m$^2$) | 27.9 ± 3.9 | 29.3 ± 3.8 | 27.0 ± 3.7 | $p = 0.010$ |
| BSA (m$^2$) | 1.9 ± 0.2 | 2.1 ± 0.1 | 1.8 ± 0.1 | $p < 0.001$ |
| sBP-brachial (mmHg) | 123.6 ± 10.1 | 122.5 ± 10.7 | 124.2 ± 9.8 | $p = 0.414$ |
| dBP-brachial (mmHg) | 74.9 ± 6.9 | 75.3 ± 6.9 | 74.7 ± 7.0 | $p = 0.803$ |
| PP-brachial (mmHg) | 48.8 ± 7.3 | 47.2 ± 6.7 | 49.8 ± 7.5 | $p = 0.137$ |
| Heart rate (b/min) | 62.6 ± 8.5 | 62.6 ± 9.0 | 62.6 ± 8.3 | $p = 0.899$ |

Data are given as mean ± standard deviation.
sBP: systolic blood pressure, dBP: diastolic blood pressure, and PP: pulse pressure.
BMI: body mass index. BSA: body surface area.

The Arteriograph Tensiomed provides several parameters of peripheral and central haemodynamics; the most important are brachial systolic and diastolic pressure, pulse pressure, heart rate, CSBP, brachial and aortic augmentation indexes, duration of left ventricular ejection, diastolic reflection area, and systolic and diastolic area indexes (see Abbreviations).

We classified CSBP according to the values published by Cheng et al. in 2013 [16]. The threshold for optimal central BP was less than 110/80 mmHg, for prehypertension it was 110–129/80–89 mmHg, and for hypertension it was greater than or equal to 130/90 mmHg. For the cut-off value for normal PWV, we used a speed of 10 m/s as recommended in the 2013 ESC/ESH guidelines [1].

For data processing, we used the mean values from two to three subsequent measurements or the measurement with the lowest standard deviation of PWVao value provided by the Arteriograph. Obtained data were submitted for statistical evaluation (IBM SPSS Statistics 23), testing first for normality of distribution using the Shapiro-Wilk test. For comparisons of nonnormally distributed data, we used the Mann–Whitney $U$-test, $\chi^2$ test in contingency tables, and Fisher's exact test. For comparisons of selected parameters, we used the $t$-test. For testing of relationships between selected parameters we used Pearson and Spearman's correlation. Multivariate stepwise regression analysis was used for verifying significant correlation of CSBP with important parameters. A $p$ value < 0.05 was selected as the threshold for significant differences.

## 3. Results

*3.1. Patient's Characteristics.* We evaluated 100 patients (38 males and 62 females) with an average age of 64.0 ± 10.7 years. Women were significantly older than men were, were shorter, had a lower body mass index (BMI), and had nonsignificantly higher systolic brachial BP than men (Table 1). Basic laboratory values can be found in Table 2. LVH according to the sex-specific scale for LVM$_i$ was significantly more prevalent in females (Table 3).

Risk factors for cardiovascular diseases, such as dyslipidemia (in 89% of patients), impaired glucose tolerance (21%), type 2 diabetes mellitus (T2DM, 24%), and obesity (31%), were relatively common (Table 4). Frequently occurring comorbidities were stable coronary artery disease (43%), mild renal dysfunction [GFR, 60–90 mL/(min·m$^2$)] in 31%, history of transient ischaemic attack or stroke (10%), and PAD (4%) (Table 4). All patients were treated mostly by a combination of antihypertensive drugs; angiotensin converting enzyme inhibitors (ACEI), calcium channel blockers (CCB), hydrochlorothiazide-type diuretics (D), and beta-adrenergic blocking drugs (BB) were the most frequently used antihypertensives (Table 5).

Table 2: Basic laboratory values.

| | Mean ± SD |
|---|---|
| S_glucose (mmol/l) | 5.7 ± 1.2 |
| S_creatinine ($\mu$mol/l) | 77.1 ± 17.2 |
| S_urea (mmol/l) | 5.9 ± 1.7 |
| S_uric acid ($\mu$mol/l) | 312.3 ± 78.9 |
| GFR (ml/(min·m$^2$)) | 81.3 ± 23.3 |
| S_total cholesterol (mmol/l) | 4.9 ± 1.0 |
| S_LDL cholesterol (mmol/l) | 3.3 ± 2.1 |
| S_HDL cholesterol (mmol/l) | 1.4 ± 0.4 |
| S-TAG cholesterol (mmol/l) | 1.5 ± 1.1 |

S: serum, LDL: low-density lipoprotein, HDL: high-density lipoprotein, TAG: triglyceride, GFR: glomerular filtration rate.

*3.2. Central Systolic BP and Aortic Stiffness.* All patients in the study group were well-treated and achieved the recommended goal for brachial BP (<140/90 mmHg), as measured by the Arteriograph in each measurement cycle. Mean systolic brachial BP in the whole group was 123.6 ± 10.1 mmHg; the values for women were higher than those for men, but the differences were not significant. CSBP was significantly higher in females compared to males (Table 6).

The mean value of the estimated CSBP in the aorta was 123.2 ± 12.1 mmHg, but almost two-thirds of patients (62%) had CSBP ≥ 130 mmHg consistent with central hypertension according to the proposed classification for central BP

Table 3: Basic echocardiographic parameters.

| Parameter | Males | Females | $p$ value |
|---|---|---|---|
| Left ventricular dimension (cm) | 5.1 ± 0.4 | 4.7 ± 0.4 | n/a |
| LVM (g) | 230.5 ± 45.6 | 172.8 ± 45.6 | n/a |
| $LVM_i$ ($g/m^2$) | 108.7 ± 18.1 | 96.8 ± 22.8 | n/a |
| Relative wall thickness. RWT | 0.41 ± 0.05 | 0.39 ± 0.05 | $p = 0.205$ |
| Left ventricular EF (%) | 58.6 ± 4.4 | 60.3 ± 4.1 | $p = 0.024$ |
| Left ventricular hypertrophy, LVH | 11 patients (29%) | 33 patients (53%) | $p = 0.023$ |

Data are given as mean ± standard deviation.
LVM: left ventricular mass, $LVM_i$: left ventricular mass per $m^2$ of body surface area ($g/m^2$), RWT: relative wall thickness-ratio of wall thickness to internal dimension of left ventricle (RWT = IVS + LVPW/LVID), LVH: left ventricular hypertrophy-$LVM_i \geq 95\,g/m^2$ in women or $LVM_i \geq 115\,g/m^2$ in men, and n/a: not applicable due to sex differences of reference values.

Table 4: Cardiovascular risk factors and comorbidities.

| | Incidence |
|---|---|
| *Cardiovascular risk factors* | |
| Dyslipidemia | 89% |
| Obesity (BMI > 30 kg/m$^2$) | 31% |
| Renal dysfunction [GF 60–90 ml/(min·m$^2$)] | 31% |
| Impaired glucose tolerance (IGT) | 21% |
| Diabetes mellitus type 2 (T2DM) | 24% |
| Combination of IGT + T2DM | 45% |
| Smoking | 5% |
| *Comorbidities* | |
| Coronary artery disease | 43% |
| Transient ischaemic attack/stroke | 10% |
| Retinopathy | 11% |
| Chronic heart failure | 8% |
| Peripheral obliterative artery disease (PAD) | 4% |

BMI: body mass index.

Table 5: Antihypertensive and hypolipidemic treatment.

| Number of drugs per patient ($n$, mean ± SD) | 2.6 ± 1.2 |
|---|---|
| Percentage distribution of antihypertensive drugs used | |
| ACE inhibitors, ACEI (%) | 55 |
| Calcium channel blockers (dihydropyridines), CCB (%) | 55 |
| Diuretics, D (%) | 54 |
| Beta-blockers, BB (%) | 52 |
| Angiotensin II receptor blockers (ARBs) (%) | 21 |
| Centrally acting antihypertensives (%) | 12 |
| Calcium channel blocker nondihydropyridine, verapamil (%) | 9 |
| Alpha-adrenoreceptor blocking drugs, AB (%) | 6 |
| Urapidil (%) | 6 |
| Statin therapy (%) | 53 |
| Fibrate therapy (%) | 11 |

published in JACC 2013 [16]. The mean CSBP in the central hypertensive subgroup was 130.6 ± 7.5 mmHg while that in the central nonhypertensive subgroup was CSBP 111.0 ± 7.1 mmHg (Table 7, part A).

When we used another, sex-specific (but more complex) classification suggested by a "Working Group for Central Systolic Blood Pressure" published in EHJ 2014 [17], only 13% of patients remained in the hypertensive level. Dividing patients into subgroups according to these cut-off values for hypertension (men: CSBP ≥ 133 mmHg; women: CSBP ≥ 137) showed that patients with higher CSBP had lower height and weight and were nonsignificantly older; these characteristics were more prevalent in women (Table 7, part B). PWVao was nonsignificantly faster (10.2 m/s versus 9.4 m/s) and the aortic and brachial augmentation indexes were significantly higher among hypertensive patients. The brachial systolic BP-to-central systolic BP ratio was significantly lower in the hypertensive patients (Table 7, part B). Using simple analysis we found a significant correlation of CSBP with lower height ($r = -0.299$, $p = 0.003$), shorter RT ($r = -0.324$, $p = 0.001$), and higher PVVao ($r = 0.223$, $p = 0.026$). Multiple analyses (model with age, height, weight, RT, PWVao, and sex) showed that CSBP was significantly dependent on sex and return time. After removing sex from the model, the height became a significant parameter. After dividing patients according to sex, the PWVao was significant in both sexes, the RT was significant in women, and age was significant in males (Table 8).

When we compared the central and brachial systolic BPs, we discovered that more than half of our patients (55%) had a higher central systolic BP than brachial BP; mean central systolic BP values in these subgroups were 129 ± 10.3 mmHg for the subgroup with higher central systolic than brachial BP versus 116 ± 10.1 mmHg for the subgroup with lower central systolic than brachial BP (Table 7, part C). The PWVao in the subgroup with higher central than brachial systolic BP was faster (9.8 ± 1.8 m/s versus 9.2 ± 1.6 m/s in the subgroup with higher central systolic than brachial BP, $p$ value = 0.064); brachial augmentation index (17.3 ± 15.4% versus −21.1 ± 17.1%, $p < 0.001$) and aortic augmentation index (40.0 ± 5.7% versus 23.7 ± 7.3%, $p < 0.001$) were higher and return time was shorter (106.8 ± 18.7 ms versus 121.8 ± 22.2 ms, $p < 0.001$) in the group with higher central systolic than brachial BP compared to those in the group with lower central systolic than brachial BP, respectively. Of the 55 persons in this subgroup, 44 were female (80%), and they were older,

Table 6: Differences in arterial stiffness and related variables between men and women.

| | Whole group | Males | Females | $p$ value |
|---|---|---|---|---|
| Number of patients ($n$) | 100 | 38 | 62 | |
| PWVao (m/s) | 9.6 ± 1.8 | 9.3 ± 1.9 | 9.7 ± 1.7 | $p = 0.137$ |
| RT (ms) | 113.5 ± 21.6 | 124.1 ± 24.4 | 107.0 ± 16.8 | $p < 0.001$ |
| Aix brachial (%) | 0.04 ± 25.1 | −16.2 ± 24.1 | 10.0 ± 20.0 | $p < 0.001$ |
| Aix aortic (%) | 32.7 ± 10.3 | 25.9 ± 10.5 | 36.8 ± 7.8 | $p < 0.001$ |
| Central systolic BP (mmHg) | 123.2 ± 12.1 | 118.3 ± 10.8 | 126.1 ± 11.9 | $p < 0.001$ |
| Brachial systolic BP (mmHg) | 123.6 ± 10.1 | 122.5 ± 10.7 | 124.2 ± 9.8 | $p = 0.414$ |
| Brachial/central SBP ratio | 1.00 ± 0.05 | 1.04 ± 0.05 | 0.99 ± 0.04 | $p < 0.001$ |
| CSBP > brachial SBP ($n$, %) | 55 (55%) | 11 (29%) | 44 (71%) | $p < 0.001$ |
| Δc-bSBP (mmHg) | −0.41 ± 5.9 | −4.1 ± 6.3 | +1.87 ± 4.4 | $p < 0.001$ |
| Pulse pressure (mmHg) | 48.8 ± 7.3 | 47.2 ± 6.7 | 49.8 ± 7.3 | $p = 0.137$ |
| Heart rate (b/min) | 62.6 ± 8.5 | 62.6 ± 9.0 | 62.6 ± 8.3 | $p = 0.899$ |
| ED (ms) | 324.1 ± 25.4 | 320.7 ± 24.5 | 326.1 ± 25.9 | $p = 0.290$ |
| DRA | 41.2 ± 12 | 46.4 ± 13.6 | 38.0 ± 9.8 | $p < 0.001$ |

PWVao: pulse wave velocity in the aorta; Aix brachial: brachial augmentation index; Aix aortic: aortic augmentation index; ED: duration of ejection from left ventricle; RT: return time; CSBP: central systolic blood pressure = systolic blood pressure in the aorta; Δc-bSBP: difference between central and brachial systolic blood pressure. DRA: diastolic reflection area.

of shorter stature, and with lower BMI; the differences were significant. An overview of arterial stiffness parameters and related variables are provided in Table 7, part C.

Because of the large proportion of women in the group of patients with high CSBP, we statistically evaluated the group based on the sex distribution. The PWVao was nonsignificantly faster in women. However, they had a significantly higher CSBP (126 mmHg versus 118 mmHg), shorter return time (RT), and higher augmentation indexes than men (Table 6).

Antihypertensive therapy was based on a combination of antihypertensive drugs. The mean count of antihypertensive agents per person was 2.6 ± 1.2 (Table 5). We did not find any significant influence of specific drugs on CSBP, the class of drugs, the combinations of drugs, or the number of drugs used. In the laboratory parameters, no important correlations were noted except for a significantly lower GFR in the group with higher CSBP than brachial BP (Table 7, Part C). LVH was significantly more frequent in the group with CSBP ≥ 130 mmHg (Table 7, Part A).

## 4. Discussion

In this study, we evaluated CSBP in treated hypertensive patients. Unexpectedly high was the proportion of patients who had CSBP levels higher than brachial SBP. These findings are different from most published data, which show the brachial systolic BP higher than CSBP because of peripheral pressure wave amplification [13, 27]. For the estimation of central BP, we used the Arteriograph Tensiomed[Ltd]. The Arteriograph was validated based on the finding of a strong correlation between invasively measured and noninvasively estimated CSBP [20]. Rossen et al. [22] found a mean difference of 4.4 mmHg, where the Arteriograph underestimated the central BP against invasively measured values. Several studies that compared the Arteriograph with other noninvasive methods for arterial stiffness estimation have been published, mainly compared to tonometric (Sphygmocor) or piezo-electronic devices (Complior). Good agreement was also achieved for PWVao estimation. The correlations of PWVao assessed with the Arteriograph and with the Sphygmocor ($r = 0.67$, $p < 0.001$) and the Complior ($r = 0.69$, $p < 0.001$) were considerable, but the techniques are not interchangeable and, therefore, for follow-up measurements, it is necessary to use the same device [23–26, 28]. The variability and reproducibility for PWV were best for the Arteriograph followed by Complior and Sphygmocor [25].

In this study, each patient achieved the target brachial BP (<140/90 mmHg). If we accept the suggested cut-off value of greater or equal to 130 mmHg for the definition of central systolic hypertension [16], we can also analogically assume this value as the target for treated CSBP. CSBP below this value (<130 mmHg) was not attained by 62% of our patients, while the target for brachial BP was achieved by all patients. This finding resembles the results published by McEniery (Anglo-Cardiff Collaborative trial II) who described that 78% of men and 72% of women with high-normal brachial BP (systolic BP < 140 mmHg) had similar aortic systolic BP as patients with brachial systolic pressures in stage I hypertension, indicating that they had overlapping values of CSBP [29].

It is known that central haemodynamics depends on aortic stiffness and reflections of pressure waves from the peripheral arterial tree and is influenced by risk factors and cardiovascular diseases [30].

We analysed the interdependencies between PWVao (as an indicator of aortic stiffness) and CSBP. According to all criteria used for central hypertension, hypertensive patients, in comparison to normotensives, had only nonsignificantly higher PWV; however, the return time of the reflected wave into the aortic root was significantly shorter in hypertensive patients. This discordance between the velocity of the aortic pulse wave (which was similar in both groups) and the shorter return time of the reflected wave may be explained

TABLE 7: Aortic stiffness parameters. Division of patients into subgroups according to blood pressure differences. (A) Higher or lower CSBP than the cut-off value of 130 mmHg for central systolic hypertension (equal for women and men). (B) Sex-specific classification: hypertension in women = CSBP ≥ 137 mmHg; hypertension in men = CSBP ≥ 133 mmHg. (C) Lower CSBP than brachial systolic blood pressure or higher CSBP than brachial blood systolic pressure.

| | | (A) Division according to cut-off value 130 mmHg | | | (B) Division according to sex-specific criteria of CSBP | | | (C) Division according to CSBP to brachial BP | | |
|---|---|---|---|---|---|---|---|---|---|---|
| | Whole group | Normotension CSBP < 130 mmHg | Hypertension CSBP ≥ 130 mmHg | $p$ value | Normotension Male CSBP < 133 Female CSBP < 137 | Hypertension Male CSBP ≥ 133 Female CSBP ≥ 137 | $p$ value | Lower CSBP than brachial systolic BP | Higher CSBP than brachial systolic BP | $p$ value |
| Number of patients ($n$) | 100 | 38 | 62 | | 87 | 13 | | 45 | 55 | |
| Males/females ($n$) | 38/62 | 19/19 | 19/43 | $p = 0.060$ | 37/50 | 1/12 | $p = 0.016$ | 27/18 | 11/44 | $p < 0.001$ |
| Age (years) | 64.0 ± 10.7 | 64.2 ± 11.7 | 63.9 ± 10.1 | $p = 0.730$ | 63 ± 11 | 69 ± 9 | $p = 0.082$ | 61.2 ± 12.4 | 66.3 ± 8.5 | $p = 0.017$ |
| Height (cm) | 169.3 ± 9.2 | 171.4 ± 10.0 | 167.9 ± 8.5 | $p = 0.103$ | 170.3 ± 9.1 | 162.2 ± 7.1 | $p = 0.004$ | 173.0 ± 9.3 | 166.2 ± 8.0 | $p < 0.001$ |
| Weight (kg) | 80.2 ± 15.4 | 83.5 ± 16.2 | 78.2 ± 14.7 | $p = 0.081$ | 81.9 ± 15.6 | 68.8 ± 8.1 | $p < 0.001$ | 87.1 ± 17.4 | 74.6 ± 2.4 | $p < 0.001$ |
| BMI (kg/m$^2$) | 27.9 ± 3.9 | 28.3 ± 4.2 | 27.6 ± 3.9 | $p = 0.314$ | 28.1 ± 3.9 | 26.2 ± 3.4 | $p = 0.106$ | 28.9 ± 4.4 | 27.0 ± 3.3 | $p = 0.013$ |
| PWVao (m/s) | 9.6 ± 1.8 | 9.3 ± 1.8 | 9.7 ± 1.7 | $p = 0.064$ | 9.4 ± 1.7 | 10.2 ± 1.7 | $p = 0.099$ | 9.2 ± 1.6 | 9.8 ± 1.8 | $p = 0.064$ |
| RT (ms) | 113.5 ± 21.6 | 119.2 ± 22.3 | 110.1 ± 20.6 | $p = 0.018$ | 115.4 ± 22.1 | 101.2 ± 13.3 | $p = 0.036$ | 121.8 ± 22.2 | 106.8 ± 18.7 | $p < 0.001$ |
| Aix brachial (%) | 0.04 ± 1.80 | −14.8 ± 20.1 | +9.2 ± 23.5 | $p < 0.001$ | −2.7 ± 25.5 | +18.6 ± 9.9 | $p < 0.001$ | −21.1 ± 17.1 | +17.3 ± 15.4 | $p < 0.001$ |
| Aix aortic (%) | 32.7 ± 10.3 | 26.5 ± 8.9 | 36.4 ± 9.4 | $p < 0.001$ | 31.3 ± 10.3 | 41.9 ± 4.2 | $p < 0.001$ | 23.7 ± 7.3 | 40.0 ± 5.7 | $p < 0.001$ |
| CSBP | 123.2 ± 12.1 | 111.0 ± 7.1 | 130.6 ± 7.5 | $p < 0.001$ | 120.2 ± 10.0 | 142.7 ± 2.1 | $p < 0.001$ | 116 ± 10.1 | 129 ± 10.3 | $p < 0.001$ |
| Brachial systolic BP | 123.6 ± 10.1 | 114.9 ± 8.9 | 128.9 ± 6.5 | $p < 0.001$ | 121.6 ± 9.3 | 136.7 ± 1.8 | $p < 0.001$ | 121.9 ± 11.0 | 125.0 ± 9.2 | $p = 0.192$ |
| Δc-bSBP (mmHg) | −0.41 ± 5.9 | −3.9 ± 4.2 | +1.8 ± 5.3 | $p < 0.001$ | −1.4 ± 5.7 | +5.9 ± 1.6 | $p < 0.001$ | −5.8 ± 4.2 | +4.0 ± 2.3 | $p < 0.001$ |
| Brachial/central SBP ratio | 1.01 ± 0.04 | 1.04 ± 0.05 | 0.99 ± 0.04 | $p < 0.001$ | 1.01 ± 0.05 | 0.96 ± 0.01 | $p < 0.001$ | 1.05 ± 0.04 | 0.97 ± 0.02 | $p < 0.001$ |
| Pulse pressure, PP (mmHg) | 48.8 ± 7.3 | 46.7 ± 7.3 | 50.7 ± 6.6 | $p < 0.001$ | 47.4 ± 6.4 | 58.1 ± 5.9 | $p < 0.001$ | 45.1 ± 10.6 | 51.6 ± 9.7 | $p = 0.002$ |
| Heart rate (b/min) | 62.6 ± 8.5 | 64.5 ± 8.3 | 61.4 ± 8.5 | $p = 0.032$ | 62.8 ± 8.7 | 60.8 ± 0.6 | $p = 0.548$ | 65.2 ± 8.5 | 60.4 ± 8.3 | $p = 0.005$ |
| ED (ms) | 324.1 ± 25.4 | 318.3 ± 26.4 | 327.6 ± 24.2 | $p = 0.130$ | 322.8 ± 25.6 | 332.2 ± 23.5 | $p = 0.232$ | 315.7 ± 23.1 | 330.9 ± 25.2 | $p = 0.002$ |
| DRA | 41.2 ± 12.0 | 43.5 ± 11.9 | 39.8 ± 11.0 | $p = 0.109$ | 41.7 ± 11.9 | 37.7 ± 13.1 | $p = 0.469$ | 45.8 ± 13 | 37.4 ± 9.8 | $p < 0.001$ |
| LVH (LVM$_i$), $n$ (%) | 44 (44%) | 10 (26%) | 34 (55%) | $p = 0.007$ | 37 (43%) | 7 (54%) | $p = 0.553$ | 19 (42%) | 25 (46%) | $p = 0.840$ |
| GFR [ml/(min/m$^2$)] | 81.3 ± 23.3 | 85.9 ± 27.1 | 78.4 ± 20.3 | $p = 0.184$ | 82.9 ± 23.5 | 70.6 ± 20.2 | $p = 0.116$ | 87.8 ± 25.9 | 76.2 ± 19.8 | $p = 0.015$ |

PWVao: pulse wave velocity in the aorta; Aix brachial: brachial augmentation index; Aix aortic: aortic augmentation index; ED: duration of ejection from the left ventricle; RT: return time; CSBP: central systolic blood pressure = systolic blood pressure in the aorta; Δc-bSBP: difference between central and brachial systolic blood pressure. DRA: diastolic reflection area.

Table 8: Multivariate analysis. Influence of important parameters on CSBP.

| Independent parameter | Models | | | | | | | |
|---|---|---|---|---|---|---|---|---|
| | All patients | | All patients (model without sex) | | Males | | Females | |
| | Coeff. *B* | *p* value | Coeff. *B* | *p* value | Coeff. *B* | *p* value | Coeff. *B* | *p* value |
| Sex (M = 0, F = 1) | 5.75 | 0.025 | — | — | — | — | — | — |
| Age | −0.15 | 0.239 | −0.165 | 0.186 | −0.341 | 0.046 | −0.008 | 0.960 |
| Height | −0.073 | 0.750 | −0.271 | 0.050 | 0.004 | 0.992 | 0.089 | 0.762 |
| Weight (kg) | 0.049 | 0.656 | −0.069 | 0.522 | −0.041 | 0.782 | −0.095 | 0.559 |
| RT (ms) | −0.119 | 0.039 | −0.12 | 0.044 | 0.104 | 0.640 | −0.507 | 0.007 |
| PWVao (m/s) | −1.499 | 0.370 | −1.594 | 0.337 | 2.764 | 0.008 | −4.17 | 0.026 |

Coeff.: unstandardized regression coefficient.

by a shorter distance (thus, with a shorter return time) of the reflected pulse wave to reach the central aorta [30], as the patients in the subgroup with central systolic hypertension according to sex-specific criteria and in the group of higher CSBP comparing to brachial SBP were significantly shorter (Table 7, parts B and C). This relationship was only borderline in the subgroup with CSBP higher than 130 mmHg (Table 7, part A). These findings are in agreement with the literature, which shows lower cardiovascular mortality in taller individuals and higher cardiovascular risk in shorter persons [31].

The increase of augmentation pressure, pulse pressure, and late systolic pressure due to shorter return time may increase left ventricular load and can predict heart failure [32]. In agreement with this explanation, the ejection duration from the left ventricle has been significantly prolonged in the patients with central systolic BP higher than brachial systolic BP (330.9 ms versus 315.7 ms) (Table 7, part C). We can assume that prolongation of ED concurrently widens the pulse pressure, which leads to ventricular hypertrophy [33].

When we applied the sex-specific scale for CSBP classification (≥133 mmHg for males, ≥137 mmHg for females) presented in EHJ in 2014 [17], which is more specific in comparison to the simpler classification published in JACC in 2013 (cut-off value for hypertension ≥ 130 mmHg for both sexes) [16], the percentage of patients in the hypertensive range dropped from the initial 62% to only 13%. The reclassification to normotension level involved more men than women.

Because females were more frequently among the centrally hypertensive, we also evaluated our patients from a sex-specific aspect. Women had significantly higher CSBP (126 mmHg versus 118 mmHg), lower height (163 cm versus 178 cm), and higher age (66 years versus 61 years) than men (Tables 1 and 6). These results are in agreement with published data that show that central BP increases more with age, compared to peripheral systolic BP, and that this increase is steeper in women than in men [30]. The accuracy of CSBP estimation depends strongly on blood pressure values used for pressure wave calibration. Cheng and coworkers found substantial improvement of accuracy of noninvasively (applanation tonometry) obtained CSBP when invasively measured BP was used for calibration of the peripheral waveform in comparison to results when cuff BP was used for calibration; cuff BP-based calibration underestimated the CSBP by −8.2 mmHg [34]. Costello et al. [35] have tested a new, brachial cuff-based (suprasystolic) technique for estimation of CSBP (a method similar to the Arteriograph) and found an underestimation of central BP by −7 mmHg in comparison to invasive measurements.

To avoid problems with BP calibration, Benetos et al. [36] in their study published in 2010 suggested the use of the ratio of the carotid/brachial pulse pressure to predict cardiovascular mortality, and they found that this ratio is less dependent on BP calibration and may be directly applicable in large population studies. In our study, we found that the ratio of central to brachial systolic BP in our patients had similar statistical significance as the BP differences (Table 7).

Among the basic echocardiographic parameters, we found that LVH significantly occurred more frequently in women than in men (53% versus 29%) (Table 3). LVH also occurred more frequently in patients with CSBP ≥ 130 mmHg than in patients with CSBP < 130 mmHg (55% versus 26%) (Table 7, Part A).

In a large proportion of our patients (55%), CSBP was higher than brachial systolic BP. In the literature, the prevalent opinion is that CSBP is lower compared to brachial BP because of peripheral BP amplification by wave reflections [13, 27, 33]. Safar et al. [37] found a peripheral amplification, which ranged approximately from 7 to 11 mmHg, and amplification was increased with higher brachial BP. Augmentation, which is the increase of central pressure due to the summation of the reflected pressure wave with the primary pressure wave, usually does not exceed the peripheral systolic pressure. The increase of central pressure due to considerable augmentation is usually referred to as the decrease of amplification [37].

Some results have been published suggesting the augmentation of CSBP above the brachial BP values. Munir et al. [38] emphasised the direct relationship between amplification and augmentation based on their findings that the late systolic shoulder of peripheral pressure waveform closely approximates central systolic pressure and that the peripheral augmentation index was related to central systolic pressure. They found a close agreement between the late systolic shoulder of the peripheral pulse and invasively measured values of central systolic pressure, with a mean difference of 0.5 ± 5.2 mmHg, indicating that in some proportion of patients the invasively measured CSBP exceeds peripheral systolic BP even though the mean value of noninvasively measured brachial SBP was higher than CSBP. These results are compatible with the formation of either the type D pressure wave contour in the ascending aorta where the reflected wave arrives early in systole and merges with the incidental pressure wave or the type A configuration where peak systolic pressure occurs in late systole, with augmentation index greater than 12% [39].

This situation is frequently present in clinical states, which increase the degree of aortic stiffness, such as hypertension, diabetes mellitus, or renal failure or due to natural age-dependent changes [40]. In recent studies, CSBP appears to be an important independent risk factor for cardiovascular disease and mortality and, therefore, antihypertensive treatment should be focused not only on the decrease of brachial BP but also on the lowering of CSBP [41–45].

Antihypertensive drugs decrease both brachial BP and CSBP but they differ in the magnitude of decreasing the CSBP, as was shown in a meta-analysis by Manisty and Hughes [27]. They analysed results of several studies and found significant heterogeneity between drug classes used either as monotherapy or in combinations. Combinations of ARBs with CCBs, ARBs with Ds, and ACEIs with CCBs reduced CSBP and brachial SBP to similar extents. Beta-blockers, diuretics, and combinations containing beta-blockers tended to reduce central to brachial amplification, implying that the decrease of brachial SBP is associated with lesser reduction in CSBP. This could explain the differences in clinical outcomes of trials comparing beta-blocker and diuretic-based therapy with other regimens [10, 27]. Beta-blockers with vasodilating properties (such as nebivolol and carvedilol) are reported to have more beneficial effects [14]. In the CAFE study [10] the combination of amlodipine with ACEI achieved better outcomes in comparison to atenobene with diuretic. This difference was explained by a greater decrease of CSBP in the amlodipine + ACEI group (this difference was 4.3 mmHg). In the EXPLOR Study, the combination of amlodipine and valsartan lowered CSBP to a larger extent than amlodipine and atenolol in combination [46]. Among our patients who were mostly on combination therapy, we did not find any significant influence of drugs or their combination on CSBP. Evaluation of the effects of drug therapy on CSBP would require larger studies.

## 5. Limitations

This study was a retrospective analysis of treated hypertensive patients who had achieved the recommended target arm blood pressure values. One limitation of the study was that patients were treated with different antihypertensive drugs. Most frequently, ACE inhibitors or ARBs were used in combination with calcium channel blockers and/or diuretics; beta-blockers were also frequently used. The average number of antihypertensive agents per person was 2.6 ± 1.2. In this study, central systolic hypertension was more frequently detected in women. The women in our analysis were older and shorter than the men; these factors likely contributed to higher CSBP. Due to the combination therapy and relatively small number of patients in our study, we did not find the influence of specific drugs on CSBP. However, the purpose of this study was more focused on comparing central and brachial systolic BP in well-controlled hypertension.

## 6. Conclusions

We found important differences between brachial and CSBPs in our group of patients with well-controlled hypertension, defined as an arm BP below 140/90 mmHg. A significantly large proportion of these patients have high CSBP. While the brachial pressures in the whole group were within the target range, 62% of patients had estimated CSBPs above the proposed cut-off value of 130 mmHg for central systolic hypertension. Using the sex-specific European proposal for CSBP classification, only 13% of patients (mainly women) remained in the hypertensive range. When we used another approach and compared the central systolic and brachial systolic BPs for each individual, we found that the estimated CSBP was higher than the brachial systolic BP in 55% of patients.

Factors that significantly contributed to higher CSBP included shorter height, older age, and female sex. Generally, women are of shorter stature, which significantly influences the timing of pressure wave propagation and reflection. In CSBP classification, factors such as sex, age, and height should be taken into account. However, this approach requires more complex classification scales. Such a different approach can be seen in recently published papers in the Journal of the American College of Cardiology 2013 [16] and European Heart Journal 2014 [17]. CSBP is an important parameter characterising central haemodynamics and is expected to become the therapeutic target in patients with arterial hypertension. The proportion of our patients in whom CSBP exceeded the brachial SBP was unexpectedly high. This phenomenon has not been clearly described in the literature and its clinical significance deserves attention specifically in evaluation of hypertension treatment.

## Abbreviations

| | |
|---|---|
| sBP-brach: | Brachial systolic blood pressure |
| dBP-brach: | Brachial diastolic blood pressure |
| PP: | Pulse pressure |
| MAP: | Mean arterial pressure |
| HR: | Heart rate |
| CSBP: | Central systolic blood pressure (in the ascending aorta) |
| PPao: | Pulse pressure in the ascending aorta |
| Aix aortic: | Aortic augmentation index |
| Aix brachial: | Brachial augmentation index $((P_2 - P_1)/\mathrm{PP})$ |
| PWVao: | Aortic pulse wave velocity, the estimated velocity of the aortic pulse wave |

RT: Return time, the time between the peak of the primary pressure wave ($P_1$) and the peak of secondary (returned) pressure wave ($P_2$); the shorter the return time the higher central systolic pressure augmentation
ED: Duration of ejection from the left ventricle during systole
DRA: Diastolic reflection area, estimated area under the pressure wave which shows the contribution of reflected pressure wave to diastolic coronary perfusion pressure
SAI: Systolic area index expresses the systolic proportion of the heart cycle
DAI: Diastolic area index expresses the diastolic proportion of the heart cycle.

## Competing Interests

The authors declare that there are no competing interests regarding the publication of this paper.

## Acknowledgments

The authors would like to thank Editage (https://www.editage.com/) for English language editing. This research work was supported by a scientific grant VEGA 1/0939/14 of the Slovak Ministry of Education.

## References

[1] G. Mancia, R. Fagard, and K. Narkiewicz, "The Task Force for the management of arterial hypertension of the European Society of Hypertension (ESH) and of the European Society of Cardiology (ESC): 2013 ESH/ESC guidelines for the management of arterial hypertension," *Journal of Hypertension*, vol. 31, no. 7, pp. 1281–1357, 2013.

[2] P. A. James, S. Oparil, B. L. Carter et al., "2014 evidence-based guideline for the management of high blood pressure in adults," *JAMA*, vol. 311, no. 5, pp. 507–520, 2014.

[3] M. F. O'Rourke and J. B. Seward, "Central arterial pressure and arterial pressure pulse: new views entering the second century after Korotkov," *Mayo Clinic Proceedings*, vol. 81, no. 8, pp. 1057–1068, 2006.

[4] S. S. Franklin, "Beyond blood pressure: arterial stiffness as a new biomarker of cardiovascular disease," *Journal of the American Society of Hypertension*, vol. 2, no. 3, pp. 140–151, 2008.

[5] M. F. O'Rourke and A. Adji, "Basis for use of central blood pressure measurement in office clinical practice," *Journal of the American Society of Hypertension*, vol. 2, no. 1, pp. 28–38, 2008.

[6] G. M. London, "Brachial arterial pressure to assess cardiovascular structural damage: an overview and lessons from clinical trials," *Journal of Nephrology*, vol. 21, no. 1, pp. 23–31, 2008.

[7] C. M. McEniery, J. R. Cockcroft, M. J. Roman, S. S. Franklin, and I. B. Wilkinson, "Central blood pressure: current evidence and clinical importance," *European Heart Journal*, vol. 35, no. 26, pp. 1719–1725, 2014.

[8] C. Vlachopoulos, K. Aznaouridis, M. F. O'Rourke, M. E. Safar, K. Baou, and C. Stefanadis, "Prediction of cardiovascular events and all-cause mortality with central haemodynamics: a systematic review and meta-analysis," *European Heart Journal*, vol. 31, no. 15, pp. 1865–1871, 2010.

[9] E. Agabiti-Rosei, G. Mancia, M. F. O'Rourke et al., "Central blood pressure measurements and antihypertensive therapy: a consensus document," *Hypertension*, vol. 50, no. 1, pp. 154–160, 2007.

[10] "The CAFE Investigators, for the Anglo-Scandinavian Cardiac Outcomes Trial (ASCOT) Investigators. Differential impact of blood pressure-lowering drugs on central aortic pressure and clinical outcomes. Principal results of the Conduit Artery Function Evaluation (CAFE) study," *Circulation*, vol. 113, pp. 1213–1225, 2006.

[11] Y. Ben-Shlomo, M. Spears, C. Boustred et al., "Aortic pulse wave velocity improves cardiovascular event prediction. An individual participant meta-analysis of prospective observational data from 17,635 subjects," *Journal of the American College of Cardiology*, vol. 63, no. 7, pp. 636–646, 2014.

[12] S. Laurent, J. Cockcroft, L. Van Bortel et al., "Expert consensus document on arterial stiffness: methodological issues and clinical applications," *European Heart Journal*, vol. 27, no. 21, pp. 2588–2605, 2006.

[13] G. S. Stergiou, G. Parati, C. Vlachopoulos et al., "Methodology and technology for peripheral and central blood pressure and blood pressure variability measurement: current status and future directions—position statement of the European Society of Hypertension Working Group on blood pressure monitoring and cardiovascular variability," *Journal of Hypertension*, vol. 34, no. 9, pp. 1665–1677, 2016.

[14] R. R. Townsend, I. B. Wilkinson, E. L. Schiffrin et al., "Recommendations for improving and standardizing vascular research on arterial stiffness: a scientific statement from the american heart association," *Hypertension*, vol. 66, no. 3, pp. 698–722, 2015.

[15] P. Boutouyrie and S. J. Vermeersch, "Determinants of pulse wave velocity in healthy people and in the presence of cardiovascular risk factors: 'establishing normal and reference values' The Reference Values for Arterial Stiffness' Collaboration," *European Heart Journal*, vol. 31, pp. 2338–2350, 2010.

[16] H.-M. Cheng, S.-Y. Chuang, S.-H. Sung et al., "Derivation and validation of diagnostic thresholds for central blood pressure measurements based on long-term cardiovascular risks," *Journal of the American College of Cardiology*, vol. 62, no. 19, pp. 1780–1787, 2013.

[17] A. Herbert, J. K. Cruickshank, S. Laurent, and P. Boutouyrie, "Establishing reference values for central blood pressure and its amplification in a general healthy population and according to cardiovascular risk factors," *European Heart Journal*, vol. 35, no. 44, pp. 3122–3133, 2014.

[18] I. B. Wilkinson, C. M. McEniery, and J. R. Cockcroft, "Central blood pressure estimation for the masses moves a step closer," *Journal of Human Hypertension*, vol. 24, no. 8, pp. 495–497, 2010.

[19] J. L. Izzo Jr., "Brachial vs. central systolic pressure and pulse wave transmission indicators: a critical analysis," *American Journal of Hypertension*, vol. 27, no. 12, pp. 1433–1442, 2014.

[20] I. G. Horváth, Á. Németh, Z. Lenkey et al., "Invasive validation of a new oscillometric device (arteriograph) for measuring augmentation index, central blood pressure and aortic pulse wave velocity," *Journal of Hypertension*, vol. 28, no. 10, pp. 2068–2075, 2010.

[21] R. B. Devereux, D. R. Alonso, E. M. Lutas et al., "Echocardiographic assessment of left ventricular hypertrophy: comparison

to necropsy findings," *The American Journal of Cardiology*, vol. 57, no. 6, pp. 450–458, 1986.

[22] N. B. Rossen, E. Laugesen, C. D. Peters et al., "Invasive validation of arteriograph estimates of central blood pressure in patients with type 2 diabetes," *American Journal of Hypertension*, vol. 27, no. 5, pp. 674–679, 2014.

[23] M. Ring, M. J. O. Eriksson, J. R. A. Zierath, and K. Caidahl, "Arterial stiffness estimation in healthy subjects: a validation of oscillometric (Arteriograph) and tonometric (SphygmoCor) techniques," *Hypertension research : official journal of the Japanese Society of Hypertension*, vol. 37, no. 11, pp. 999–1007, 2014.

[24] N. A. Jatoi, A. Mahmud, K. Bennett, and J. Feely, "Assessment of arterial stiffness in hypertension: comparison of oscillometric (Arteriograph), piezoelectronic (Complior) and tonometric (SphygmoCor) techniques," *Journal of Hypertension*, vol. 27, no. 11, pp. 2186–2191, 2009.

[25] J. Baulmann, U. Schillings, S. Rickert et al., "A new oscillometric method for assessment of arterial stiffness: comparison with tonometric and piezo-electronic methods," *Journal of Hypertension*, vol. 26, no. 3, pp. 523–528, 2008.

[26] Arteriograph User's Manual, http://www.tensiomed.com/en/product-arteriograph-en.

[27] C. H. Manisty and A. D. Hughes, "Meta-analysis of the comparative effects of different classes of antihypertensive agents on brachial and central systolic blood pressure, and augmentation index," *British Journal of Clinical Pharmacology*, vol. 75, no. 1, pp. 79–92, 2013.

[28] J. M. Davies, M. A. Bailey, K. J. Griffin, and D. J. A. Scott, "Pulse wave velocity and the non-invasive methods used to assess it: complior, sphygmocor, arteriograph and vicorder," *Vascular*, vol. 20, no. 6, pp. 342–349, 2012.

[29] C. M. McEniery, Yasmin, B. McDonnell et al., "Central pressure: variability and impact of cardiovascular risk factors. The Anglo-Cardiff Collaborative Trial II," *Hypertension*, vol. 51, no. 6, pp. 1476–1482, 2008.

[30] A. P. Avolio, M. L. Van Bortel, P. Boutouyrie et al., "Role of pulse pressure amplification in arterial hypertension. Experts' opinion and review of the data," *Hypertension*, vol. 54, pp. 375–383, 2009.

[31] J. C. Reeve, W. P. Abhayaratna, J. E. Davies, and J. E. Sharman, "Central hemodynamics could explain the inverse association between height and cardiovascular mortality," *American Journal of Hypertension*, vol. 27, no. 3, pp. 392–400, 2014.

[32] J. A. Chirinos, P. Segers, D. A. Duprez et al., "Late systolic central hypertension as a predictor of incident heart failure: the multi–ethnic study of atherosclerosis," *Journal of the American Heart Association*, vol. 4, no. 3, Article ID e001335, 2015.

[33] A. Toprak, J. Reddy, W. Chen, S. Srinivasan, and G. Berenson, "Relation of pulse pressure and arterial stiffness to concentric left ventricular hypertrophy in young men (from the Bogalusa Heart Study)," *The American Journal of Cardiology*, vol. 103, no. 7, pp. 978–984, 2009.

[34] H.-M. Cheng, D. Lang, C. Tufanaru, and A. Pearson, "Measurement accuracy of non-invasively obtained central blood pressure by applanation tonometry: a systematic review and meta-analysis," *International Journal of Cardiology*, vol. 167, no. 5, pp. 1867–1876, 2013.

[35] B. T. Costello, M. G. Schultz, J. A. Black, and J. E. Sharman, "Evaluation of a brachial cuff and suprasystolic waveform algorithm method to noninvasively derive central blood pressure," *American Journal of Hypertension*, vol. 28, no. 4, pp. 480–486, 2014.

[36] A. Benetos, F. Thomas, L. Joly et al., "Pulse pressure amplification: a mechanical biomarker of cardiovascular risk," *Journal of the American College of Cardiology*, vol. 55, no. 10, pp. 1032–1037, 2010.

[37] M. E. Safar, J. Blacher, A. Protogerou, and A. Achimastos, "Arterial stiffness and central hemodynamics in treated hypertensive subjects according to brachial blood pressure classification," *Journal of Hypertension*, vol. 26, no. 1, pp. 130–137, 2008.

[38] S. Munir, A. Guilcher, T. Kamalesh et al., "Peripheral augmentation index defines the relationship between central and peripheral pulse pressure," *Hypertension*, vol. 51, no. 1, pp. 112–118, 2008.

[39] W. W. Nichols, M. F. O'Rourke, and C. Vlachopoulous, *McDonald's Blood Flow in Arteries: Theoretical, Experimental and Clinical Principles*, Hodder Arnold, London, UK, 6th edition, 2011.

[40] M. Janić, M. Lunder, and M. Šabovič, "Arterial stiffness and cardiovascular therapy," *BioMed Research International*, vol. 2014, Article ID 621437, 11 pages, 2014.

[41] M. A. Weber and R. R. Townsend, "Building the case for central blood pressure," *Journal of the American College of Cardiology*, vol. 62, no. 19, pp. 1788–1790, 2013.

[42] C.-M. Huang, K.-L. Wang, H.-M. Cheng et al., "Central versus ambulatory blood pressure in the prediction of all-cause and cardiovascular mortalities," *Journal of Hypertension*, vol. 29, no. 3, pp. 454–459, 2011.

[43] L. Trudeau, "Central blood pressure as an index of antihypertensive control: determinants and potential value," *Canadian Journal of Cardiology*, vol. 30, no. 5, supplement, pp. S23–S28, 2014.

[44] P. Palatini, E. Casiglia, J. Gasowski et al., "Arterial stiffness, central hemodynamics, and cardiovascular risk in hypertension," *Vascular Health and Risk Management*, vol. 7, pp. 725–739, 2011.

[45] R. F. Rosenwasser, N. K. Shah, S. M. Smith et al., "Baseline predictors of central aortic blood pressure: a PEAR substudy," *Journal of the American Society of Hypertension*, vol. 8, no. 3, pp. 152–158, 2014.

[46] P. Boutouyrie, A. Achouba, P. Trunet, and S. Laurent, "Amlodipine-valsartan combination decreases central systolic blood pressure more effectively than the amlodipine-atenolol combination: the EXPLOR study," *Hypertension*, vol. 55, no. 6, pp. 1314–1322, 2010.

13

# Effect of MTHFRC677 T Gene Polymorphism on Early Morning Blood Pressure in Elderly Female Patients with H-Type Hypertension

**Chi Zhang, Jun Li, Jian Zhou, Qiaoling Zheng, Ruicong Dong, Enhong Xing, and Zhijie Dou**

*Affiliated Hospital, Chengde Medical College, Chengde 067000, China*

Correspondence should be addressed to Zhijie Dou; 164201134@stu.cuz.edu.cn

Academic Editor: Sandip K Mishra

The distribution characteristics of Methylenetetrahydrofolate Reductase (MTHFR) gene C677 T polymorphism and its influence on early morning blood pressure in elderly female patients with H-type hypertension are investigated. A total of 220 elderly female patients with hypertension who received diagnosis and treatment in our hospital from March to September 2021 are selected. All patients received serum index detection in our hospital and are grouped according to blood homocysteine (Hcy) level. Patients with Hcy>10 $\mu$mol/L are classified as H-type hypertension and included in H-type hypertension group ($n = 166$). Patients with Hcy≤10 $\mu$mol/L are included in the non-H-type hypertension group ($n = 54$). Both groups underwent 24-hour ambulatory blood pressure monitoring. Base frequency and allele distribution of MTHFR gene C677 T locus are compared between the two groups, and the relationship between different bases of MTHFR gene C677 T locus and morning blood pressure and Hcy level is analyzed. The risk factors of morning hypertension in patients with H-type hypertension are analyzed by binary logistic regression. Binary logistic regression analysis shows that smoking history, drinking history, high-salt diet, MTHFR gene C677 T genotype, and abnormal 24 h systolic blood pressure are the risk factors for the occurrence of morning hypertension in H-type hypertension patients. The frequency of TT homozygous mutation at the C677 T site of the MTHFR gene is high in patients with H-type hypertension, and the mutation of the C677 T site of the MTHFR gene had an effect on systolic blood pressure and Hcy level.

## 1. Introduction

Existing studies have shown that the high incidence of various cardiovascular and cerebrovascular diseases in clinical practice is closely related to hypertension symptoms [1]. A study on the classification of hypertensive patients in China pointed out that 75% of hypertensive patients had H-type hypertension [2]. Blood homocysteine (Hcy) levels can be divided into environmental factors and genetic factors. Methylenetetrahydrofolate Reductase (MTHFR) is the key to Hcy metabolic enzymes; their site gene C677 T mutation can make the MTHFR activity decline so that the blood Hcy goes up. More and more studies have shown that H-type hypertension is an independent risk factor in the occurrence and development of stroke, and with the increase in Hcy level, the risk of stroke also increases correspondingly [3,4]. Therefore, exploring the characteristics of MTHFR gene polymorphism in patients with H-type hypertension, analyze its influence on blood pressure, and exploring the influencing factors of early-morning hypertension in patients with H-type hypertension are of important theoretical and application value for elucidating the mechanism of Hcy level increase and preventing related diseases. Due to the influence of age, the estrogen level of elderly female hypertension patients decreases significantly, the body's immunity and resistance are low, and various body functions decline. The occurrence of cardiovascular and cerebrovascular diseases caused by long-term hypertension will seriously affect the quality of life of patients [5].

In this paper, the MTHFR gene C677 T polymorphism, changes in plasma Hcy level and its role in the occurrence of hypertension in elderly female patients with H-type hypertension are studied, aiming to explore the mutation characteristics of MTHFR C677 T in elderly female population, thus, providing reference data for the prevention and treatment of such patients with H-type hypertension and individualized treatment.

The rest of this paper is organized as follows: Section 2 discusses related work, followed by basic information and the proposed methods designed in Section 3. Section 4 shows the experimental results and analysis, and Section 5 briefly summarizes all of standpoints of the whole text, and points out the shortcomings and future research directions.

## 2. Related Work

Existing studies have confirmed that hypertension and blood Hcy synergistically contribute to the aggravation of the risk of cardiovascular and cerebrovascular adverse events [6]. Some scholars clearly pointed out in the expert consensus on diagnosis and treatment of H-type Hypertension in 2016 that hypertension with high Hcy (≥10 $\mu$mol/L) was defined as H-type hypertension, and the guideline for prevention and treatment of hypertension in China (2018 Revision) pointed out that Hc ≥ 10 $\mu$mol/L was an important factor affecting the cardiovascular prognosis of hypertensive patients. Hcy is recommended as one of the laboratory examination items for patients with hypertension [7]. MTHFR is a key rate-limiting enzyme in Hcy methylation metabolism. The MTHFRC677 T genotype can be divided into CC type (wild type), CT type (heterozygous mutant), and TT type (homozygous mutant). The enzyme activity of MTHFR in individuals carrying the TT genotype is reduced by 60%, thus, affecting the normal metabolism of Hcy in vivo. It leads to elevated blood Hcy [8].

Some scholars have found that there are extensive pathological manifestations of arterial thrombosis and atherosclerosis in the systemic circulation of children who died of hereditary homocystinuria at autopsy, thus, proposing the hypothesis that hyperhomocysteinemia can lead to atherosclerotic vascular disease [9]. Hcy is an amino acid containing a sulfhydryl group. Its predecessor is mainly derived from dietary methionine. It is an intermediate metabolite in the metabolism of methionine and cysteine and does not participate in protein synthesis. Methionine and tetrahydrofolic acid are produced by methionine synthetase in about half of Hcy and methyltetrahydrofolic acid in the human body, and methyltetrahydrofolic acid is produced by MTHFR. The remaining half of MTHFR forms cysteine under the action of cysteine $\beta$ synthase through the sulfur-conversion pathway with serine, cysteine forms cysteine under the action of cysteine lyase, and finally pyruvate, sulfuric acid, and water [10]. Metabolic disorders caused by TT homozygous mutations can lead to elevated plasma Hcy. High Hcy can lead to vascular endothelial cell injury, promote vascular smooth muscle cell proliferation, affect the oxidation of LDL, enhance platelet function, and promote thrombosis, but the mechanism of their interaction is not completely clear. This study suggests that TT homozygous mutation at C677 T of the MTHFR gene is one of the causes of increased plasma Hcy level and an independent risk factor for atherosclerosis. Although the exact pathogenic mechanism of Hcy has not been fully understood, clinical data show that the speed and intensity of arterial damage in patients with H-type hypertension are accelerated and the probability of vascular events such as myocardial infarction and stroke is high, and the harm to patient's life and health is multiplied [11, 12].

Previous clinical studies have confirmed that the 677C-T genotype of the MTHFR gene is related to plasma Hcy level, and patients with the 677C-T allele have significantly higher plasma Hcy level, which is an independent risk factor for hypertension, coronary heart disease, and stroke [13, 14]. Morning hypertension with target organ damage is closely related to cardiovascular events, which can lead to a variety of vascular complications, such as coronary heart disease(CHD), asymptomatic cerebral infarction, myocardial hypertrophy, and the happening of cardiovascular events in patients with the highest risk in the morning, and already more and more research evidence in the early morning of hypertension is closely related to the occurrence of cardiovascular events [15, 16]. Studies have shown that hypertension and elevated plasma Hcy have a synergistic effect on cardiovascular and cerebrovascular events, and the risk of cardiovascular and cerebrovascular diseases in patients with elevated Hcy combined with hypertension increases by 11 times, 25–30 times that of normal people [17]. It should be noted that the occurrence of circadian rhythm in blood pressure is closely related to neurohumoral factors, and the activation of sympathetic nervous system and the hyperactivity of the renin-angiotensin-aldosterone system (RAAS) are the main physiological mechanisms [18]. In this study, the occurrence of morning hypertension in patients with H-type hypertension and related factors were analyzed. Smoking history, drinking history, high-salt diet, MTHFR gene C677 T genotype, and abnormal 24 h systolic blood pressure were all risk factors for the occurrence of morning hypertension in elderly women with H-type hypertension. It suggests that the above risk factors will affect the circadian rhythm of patients' blood pressure, leading to the occurrence of morning hypertension, which is basically consistent with previous research results [19–21].

For elderly women with H-type hypertension, it is important for regular physical examination, early detection, and early treatment. The treatment of high blood pressure in H mainly adopts vitamin folic acid treatment. With the continuous improvement of the H blood pressure ratio in my country, people should pay attention to preventive health care to achieve the healthy development of hypertension prevention and treatment.

## 3. Basic Information and the Proposed Methods

*3.1. Basic Information.* A total of 220 elderly female patients with hypertension who received treatment in the Affiliated Hospital of Chengde Medical College from March to December 2021 were selected. All patients are ≥65 years old. All patients receive serum indicators in our hospital, and are grouped according to blood Hcy level. Patients with Hcy>10 μmol/L are classified as H-type hypertension and included in H-type hypertension group ($n = 166$). Patients with Hcy≤10 μmol/L are non-H-type hypertension and are included in the common hypertension group ($n = 54$). The age range of patients in the H-type hypertension group is 65–80 years, with a mean of (71.75 ± 4.40) years and the duration of hypertension is 3–12 years, with a mean of (7.03 ± 3.24) years. In the common hypertension group, the patients' ages are ranged from 66 to 80 years, with a mean of (71.58 ± 4.51) years and the duration of hypertension was ranged from 3 to 13 years, with a mean of (7.23 ± 3.06) years. There is no statistical difference in age, hypertension course, and other general information between the two groups ($P > 0.05$), which proves that the comparison between the two groups is scientific and reasonable.

There are three inclusion criteria as follows: (1) it meets the diagnostic criteria of hypertension in the 2018 Chinese Guidelines for Prevention and Treatment of Hypertension; (2) the patients are between 65 and 80 years old and all are female; (3) patients with good clinical compliance agree to participate in the study and complete relevant investigations until the end of the study.

There are four exclusion criteria as follows: (1) accompanied by cognitive impairment, memory decline, visual spatial impairment and other cognitive impairment; (2) patients with mental diseases; (3) patients with serious organic dysfunction of liver and kidney; (4) patients with acute/chronic infectious diseases or diseases of the blood system.

*3.2. The Proposed Methods*

*3.2.1. MTHFRC677 T Gene Test Method.* In the morning of the second day after admission, 5 mL of fasting venous blood is taken from all patients, digested by membrane solution/ protease K, and genomic DNA is extracted, which is stored at −20°C. Polymerase Chain Reaction(PCR) 50 μL, consisting of 10 x PCR buffer 5 μL, 25 mmol/L magnesium chloride solution, 3 μL, 2 mmol/L dNTP mixture 5 μL, 1.25U AmpliTaq DNA polymerase, 0.5 μmol/L primer and 100 μg genomic DNA. Primer sequence of MTHFRC677 T gene: upstream: 5′-CAGTCCCTGTGGTCTCTTCAT-3′, downstream: 5′- CTCACCTGGATGGGAAagat-3′. PCR cycle conditions: pre-denaturation at 95°C for 10 min, denaturation at 94°C for 30s, renaturation at 60°C for 30s, extension at 72°C for 30s, 37 cycles of reaction, and extension at 72°C for 10 min. The amplified primers are detected by 2% agarose gel electrophoresis and stored at 4°C for testing. PCR products are purified and used as sequencing templates. According to the complete sequence provided by the GenBank database, primer design software is used to design PCR primers and corresponding endonuclease for each site.

*3.2.2. Collection of Clinical Indicators and Measurement of Blood Pressure.* Clinical data are collected after admission, including age, medical history, and Body Mass Index (BMI). 24-hour ambulatory blood pressure monitoring is performed by the German TM2430EX noninvasive portable dynamic sphygmomanometer. The cuff is tied to the subjects' left upper arm at 8 : 00 a.m., and the measurement interval is set at 15 minutes during the day (6 : 00 ~ 22 : 00). At night (22 : 00–6:00), the measurement interval is 30 min, and continuous monitoring is conducted for 24 hours. If effective data >80% and blood pressure data missing from 6 : 00 to 8 : 00 in the morning is less than 2, it is regarded as qualified. Otherwise, retest the next day. The mean 24 h, daytime, and nighttime systolic and diastolic blood pressure levels of these subjects are calculated, respectively, and extreme values are removed during the calculation process. The standard deviations and mean values of SBP and diastolic bp at 24 h, daytime and nighttime are calculated. The diagnostic criteria for morning hypertension are as follows: morning hypertension is defined as blood pressure ≥135/ 85 mmHg within 2 hours after waking up.

*3.2.3. Hcy Detection Method.* All subjects are fasted for ≥10h. 5 mL of elbow venous blood is extracted from all patients with an EDTA anticoagulant tube during specimen collection. The blood samples are centrifuged at 3000r/min with a centrifugation radius of 10 cm and a continuous centrifugation time of 15 min. The blood Hcy is determined by chemiluminescence method.

*3.3. Observation Indicators.* There are four observation indicators as follows:

(1) morning blood pressure indexes of the two groups are compared;
(2) Base frequency and allele distribution of MTHFR gene C677 T locus are compared between the two groups;
(3) The relationship between different bases of MTHFR gene C677 T locus and morning blood pressure and Hcy level is analyzed;
(4) Binary logistic regression analysis of morning hypertension in H-type hypertension patients.

*3.4. Statistical Processing.* SPSS26.0 software is used for statistical analysis. A direct counting method is used to calculate the population distribution frequency of the MTHFR C677 T genotype and allele. A chi-square test is used to compare the distribution frequency of gene polymorphism. The risk factors of morning hypertension in H-type hypertension are analyzed by binary logistic regression. Measurement data are expressed by mean ± standard deviation, and $P < 0.05$ is considered statistically significant.

## 4. Experimental Results

*4.1. Comparison of Morning Blood Pressure Indicators.* Table 1 shows the comparison of morning blood pressure indicators between the two groups. It can be seen from

Table 1: Comparison of morning blood pressure indicators between the two groups.

| Group | Systolic blood pressure(mmHg) | Diastolic blood pressure(mmHg) |
|---|---|---|
| H-type hypertension group ($n = 166$) | 157.62 ± 8.76 | 97.83 ± 4.97 |
| Normal hypertension group ($n = 54$) | 153.35 ± 7.07 | 96.61 ± 4.96 |
| $t$ | 3.988 | 1.822 |
| $P$ | < 0.001 | 0.070 |

Table 2: Comparison of base frequency and allele distribution of C677 T locus of MTHFR gene ($n$,%).

| Group | Genotype | | | Allele frequency (%) | |
|---|---|---|---|---|---|
| | CC | CT | TT | C | T |
| H-type hypertension group ($n = 166$) | 21(12.65) | 61(36.75) | 84(50.60) | 103(31.02) | 229(68.98) |
| Normal hypertension group ($n = 54$) | 12(22.22) | 25(46.30) | 17(31.48) | 49(45.37) | 59(54.63) |
| $\chi 2$ | | 5.596 | | 7.417 | |
| $P$ | | 0.018 | | 0.006 | |

Table 3: Comparison of morning blood pressure and Hcy levels of MTHFR C677 T genotypes.

| Group | Parting | Systolic blood pressure(mmHg) | Diastolic blood pressure(mmHg) | Hcy(μmol/L) |
|---|---|---|---|---|
| *H-type hypertension group (n = 166)* | CC($n = 21$) | 153.96 ± 7.39 | 98.78 ± 5.74 | 17.46 ± 4.83$^{a}$ |
| | CT($n = 61$) | 155.51 ± 9.41 | 97.44 ± 5.18 | 20.98 ± 5.46$^{a}$ |
| | TT($n = 84$) | 160.09 ± 7.85$^{bc}$ | 97.95 ± 4.68 | 24.35 ± 5.21$^{abc}$ |
| *Normal hypertension group (n = 54)* | CC($n = 12$) | 151.21 ± 5.41 | 97.02 ± 4.79 | 7.79 ± 0.81 |
| | CT($n = 25$) | 153.08 ± 7.09 | 96.76 ± 4.86 | 8.04 ± 0.80 |
| | TT($n = 17$) | 156.58 ± 7.90$^{b}$ | 95.78 ± 5.45 | 8.22 ± 0.65$^{b}$ |

Table 1 that there is no significant difference in morning diastolic blood pressure ($P > 0.05$), and the morning systolic blood pressure in the H-type hypertension group increases significantly more than in the common hypertension group (all $P < 0.05$).

*4.2. Comparison of Base Frequency and Allele Distribution of MTHFR Gene C677 T Locus.* Table 2 shows the comparison of base frequency and allele distribution of the C677 T locus of the MTHFR gene. It can be seen from Table 2 that there are significant statistical differences in the correlation data of the CC, CT, TT genotype frequency, and allele frequency of C677 T locus of MTHFR gene (all $P < 0.05$).

*4.3. Analysis of the Relationship between Different Bases of MTHFR Gene C677 T Locus and Morning Blood Pressure and Hcy Level.* Table 3 shows the comparison of morning blood pressure and Hcy levels of MTHFR C677 T genotypes. In Table 3, a is compared with the non-H-type hypertension group, $P < 0.05$; $b$ is compared with CC, $P < 0.05$; $c$ is compared with CT, $P < 0.05$. it can be seen from Table 3 that there are no significant differences in systolic blood pressure between CC, CT, and TT patients in H-type hypertension group and non-H-type hypertension group ($P > 0.05$). The systolic blood pressure level of patients with the TT type is higher than that of patients with the CT type and CC type ($P < 0.05$). The systolic blood pressure of patients with TT type is higher than that of patients with CC type in the non-H-type hypertension group, and there is no significant difference in systolic blood pressure between patients with TT type and patients with CT type ($P > 0.05$), suggesting that patients with TT homozygous mutation at C677 T site of MTHFR gene have higher systolic blood pressure. There are no significant differences in diastolic blood pressure levels between CC, CT, and TT type patients (all $P > 0.05$), suggesting that TT homozygous mutation at the C677 T site of the MTHFR gene have no significant effect on diastolic blood pressure levels of patients. The Hcy level of CC, CT, and TT patients in the H-type hypertension group is significantly higher than that in non-H-type hypertension group ($P < 0.05$). In the H-type hypertension group, the level of Hcy in TT type patients is significantly higher than that in CC type and CT type patients (all $P < 0.05$). In the non-H-type hypertension group, the Hcy level of TT patients increases significantly more than that of CC patients ($P < 0.05$), suggesting that the variation of the C677 T locus of the MTHFR gene has a significant impact on the Hcy level of patients.

*4.4. Binary Logistic Regression Analysis of Factors Related to Morning Hypertension in H-type Hypertension Patients.* Table 4 shows the comparison of clinical data. Table 5 shows the binary logistic regression analysis of risk factors for morning hypertension in H-type hypertension patients.

Figure 1 shows the forest map of factors associated with early morning hypertension in H-type hypertensive patients. It can be seen from the above experimental results that the H-type hypertension group included in this study is subdivided according to the occurrence of morning

Table 4: Comparison of clinical data.

| Factors | Morning hypertension group ($n = 52$) | Nonmorning hypertension group ($n = 114$) | $\chi2$ | $P$ |
|---|---|---|---|---|
| *The history of drinking* | | | 10.280 | <0.001 |
| Yes | 28(53.85) | 32(28.07) | | |
| No | 24(46.15) | 82(71.93) | | |
| *Smoking history* | | | 14.968 | <0.001 |
| Yes | 35(67.31) | 40(35.09) | | |
| No | 17(32.69) | 74(64.91) | | |
| *Eating habits* | | | 18.819 | <0.001 |
| High salt diet | 42(80.77) | 51(44.74) | | |
| A low salt diet | 10(19.23) | 63(55.26) | | |
| *Family history of hypertension* | | | 1.039 | 0.308 |
| Yes | 34(65.38) | 65(57.02) | | |
| No | 18(34.62) | 49(42.98) | | |
| *Course of hypertension* | | | 0.044 | 0.835 |
| > 10 years | 21(40.38) | 48(42.11) | | |
| ≤10 years | 31(59.62) | 66(57.89) | | |
| *24 h systolic blood pressure* | | | 23.682 | <0.001 |
| Normal | 7(13.46) | 61(53.51) | | |
| Elevated | 45(86.54) | 53(46.49) | | |

Table 5: Binary logistic regression analysis of risk factors for morning hypertension in H-type hypertension patients.

| Factors | *B* | *S.E.* | *Wald* | *P* | *OR* | *95% CI* |
|---|---|---|---|---|---|---|
| Smoking history | 1.274 | 0.633 | 4.235 | 0.005 | 0.334 | 0.069~0.594 |
| Smoking history | 1.358 | 0.572 | 5.181 | 0.003 | 0.464 | 0.118~0.846 |
| Family history of hypertension | 1.854 | 0.559 | 6.258 | 0.009 | 0.269 | 0.097~0.662 |
| MTHFR gene C677 T genotype | 1.395 | 0.627 | 4.157 | 0.013 | 0.358 | 0.112~0.526 |
| High Hcy levels | 1.428 | 0.812 | 4.362 | 0.004 | 0.447 | 0.065~0.754 |
| Abnormal systolic blood pressure at 24 hours | 1.428 | 0.812 | 4.362 | 0.004 | 0.447 | 0.065~0.754 |

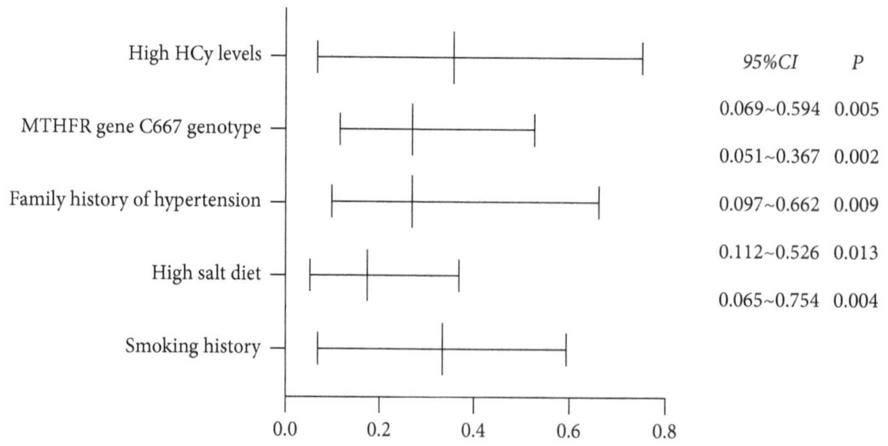


Figure 1: Forest map of factors associated with early morning hypertension in H-type hypertensive patients.

hypertension into two groups: morning hypertension group ($n = 52$) and the nonmorning hypertension group ($n = 114$). The clinical data of the two groups are analyzed by univariate analysis and genotype (CC type: 1; CT type: 2; and TT type: 3) and $P < 0.05$ are included as independent variables. Binary logistic regression analysis shows that smoking history, drinking history, high-salt diet, MTHFR gene C677 T genotype, and 24 h systolic blood pressure elevation are risk factors for the occurrence of morning hypertension in H-type hypertension patients.

## 5. Conclusions

The distribution characteristics of the MTHFR gene C677 T polymorphism and its influence on early morning blood pressure in elderly female patients with H-type hypertension are investigated. Attention should be paid to Hcy and genotype screening for elderly female hypertensive patients. For carriers of TT homozygous mutation at the C677 T site of the MTHFR gene, attention should be paid to early morning blood pressure, prevention, and treatment plans should be adjusted, and targeted antihypertensive drugs should be applied to effectively control early morning hypertension so as to avoid the occurrence of untimely and cerebrovascular events.

## Acknowledgments

This work was supported by the 2022 Medical Science Research Project Plan of Hebei Provincial Health Commission (No. 20220008).

## References

[1] L. Q. Huang, C. X. Wu, H. Q. Wei, and G. Xu, "Clinical characteristics of H-type hypertension and its relationship with the MTHFR C677T polymorphism in a Zhuang population from Guangxi, China," *Journal of Clinical Laboratory Analysis*, vol. 34, no. 11, pp. 1–5, Article ID 234999, 2020.

[2] Y. Wu, Q. Zhang, Y. Hu et al., "Novel binary logistic regression model based on feature transformation of XGBoost for type 2 Diabetes Mellitus prediction in healthcare systems," *Future Generation Computer Systems*, vol. 129, pp. 1–12, 2022.

[3] Z. Wu, M. B. Xia, D. Bertsetseg et al., "Design, synthesis and biological evaluation of novel fluoro-substituted benzimidazole derivatives with anti-hypertension activities," *Bioorganic Chemistry*, vol. 101, pp. 1–11, 2020.

[4] E. Sai, K. Shimada, T. Yokoyama et al., "Myocardial triglyceride content in patients with left ventricular hypertrophy: comparison between hy-pertensive heart disease and hypertrophic cardiomyopathy," *Heart and Vessels*, vol. 32, no. 2, pp. 166–174, 2017.

[5] M. Pasi, G. Boulouis, P. Fotiadis et al., "Distribution of lacunes in cere-bral amyloid angiopathy and hypertensive small vessel disease," *Neurology*, vol. 88, no. 23, pp. 2162–2168, 2017.

[6] J. Wang, "Guidance and suggestions of Chinese experts on clinical management of morning blood pressure," *Chinese journal of cardiovascular disease*, vol. 42, no. 9, pp. 721–725, 2014.

[7] "Chinese Guidelines for prevention and treatment of hypertension 2018 revision, " Prevention and treatment of cardiovascular and cerebrovascular diseases," *Journal of Geriatric Cardiology*, vol. 19, no. 1, pp. 1–44, 2019.

[8] Y. Hasegawa, T. Nakagawa, K. Matsui, and S. Kim-Mitsuyama, "Renal denervation in the acute phase of ischemic stroke provides brain protection in hyperten-sive rats," *Stroke*, vol. 48, no. 4, pp. 1104–1107, 2017.

[9] J. Ni, L. Zhang, T. Zhou et al., "Association between the MTHFR C677T polymorphism, blood folate and vitamin B12 deficiency, and elevated serum total homocysteine in healthy individuals in Yunnan Province, China, Blood folate and vitamin B 12 defi-ciency, and elevated serum total homocysteine in healthy individuals in yunnan province, China," *Journal of the Chinese Medical Association*, vol. 80, no. 3, pp. 147–153, 2017.

[10] M. Hüser, A. Kündig, W. Karlen, V. De Luca, and M. Jaggi, "Forecasting intracranial hypertension using multi-scale waveform metrics," *Physiological Measurement*, vol. 41, no. 1, pp. 014001–014011, 2020.

[11] H. Kayano, S. Koba, T. Hirano et al., "Dapagliflozin influences ventricular hemodynamics and exercise-induced pulmonary hypertension in type 2 diabetes patients - a randomized controlled trial," *Circulation Journal*, vol. 84, no. 10, pp. 1807–1817, 2020.

[12] J. Yao, Y. Bai, and J. Gao, "Research Status and Progress of cerebral apoplexy with H-type hypertension," *Chinese Journal of Practical Internal Medicine*, vol. 37, no. 11, pp. 1034–1036, 2017.

[13] B. Duan, Y. Lian, Z. Dong, and G. Pang, "Research progress on correlation between H-type hypertension and stroke," *Central South Pharmacy*, vol. 15, no. 8, pp. 1088–1092, 2017.

[14] Z. Liu, T. Liu, D. Xie et al., "Relationship between morning peak of blood pressure and early renal impairment in patients with h-type hypertension," *Anhui Medical and Pharmaceutical Journal*, vol. 21, no. 12, pp. 2238–2242, 2017.

[15] J. Zhang, H. Xu, X. Cao, and Y. Jin, "Effects of green aerobic exercise on homocysteine levels and morning blood pressure peaks in Patients with H-type hypertension and ischemic stroke," *Chinese Journal of Practical Nursing*, vol. 35, no. 16, pp. 1214–1218, 2019.

[16] X. Jia, Q. Yang, and J. Ru, "Changes of plasma inflammatory factors and hemodynamics in patients with h-type hypertension," *Journal of Ningxia Medical University*, vol. 39, no. 2, pp. 230–232, 2017.

[17] Z. Zou, H. Zhong, J. Li, and G. Guan, "Prevalence and influencing factors of H-type hypertension in a hospital in Shanghai in 2015," *Anhui Medical Journal*, vol. 38, no. 11, pp. 1440–1444, 2017.

[18] L. Liao, J. Tang, Y. Zhang, and Y. Liu, "Blood pressure variability and circadian rhythm in young and middle-aged patients with H-type hypertension," *Chongqing Medicine*, vol. 47, no. 4, pp. 494–496, 2018.

[19] J. Jiang, W. Miao, S. Tian, and W. Tian, "Blood pressure variability and arteriosclerosis in patients with h-type hypertension:a clinical study," *Chinese Journal of Evidence-based Cardiovascular Medicine*, vol. 10, no. 2, pp. 190–192+195, 2018.

[20] W. Wei, X. Xia, M. Wozniak, X. Fan, R. Damasevicius, and Y. Li, "Multi-sink distributed power control algorithm for Cyber-physical-systems in coal mine tunnels," *Computer Networks*, vol. 161, pp. 210–219, 2019.

[21] Y. Seedat, "Long-term treatment of hypertension with guanfacine alone and in combination therapy," *British Journal of Clinical Pharmacology*, vol. 10, no. S1, pp. 65-66, 2012.

# 14

# Depressive Symptoms and 24-Hour Ambulatory Blood Pressure in Africans: The SABPA Study

**Mark Hamer,[1] Nancy Frasure-Smith,[2,3] François Lespérance,[2,3] Brian H. Harvey,[4] Nico T. Malan,[5] and Leoné Malan[5]**

[1] *Psychobiology Group, Department of Epidemiology and Public Health, University College London, 1-19 Torrington Place, London WC1E 6BT, UK*

[2] *Department of Psychiatry and School of Nursing, McGill University CHUM Research Center, QC, Canada*

[3] *Montreal Heart Institute Research Center, University of Montreal, Montreal, QC, Canada H3C 3J7*

[4] *Unit for Drug Research and Development, Division of Pharmacology, School of Pharmacy, North-West University, Potchefstroom 2520, South Africa*

[5] *Hypertension in Africa Research Team (HART), School for Physiology, Nutrition, and Consumer Sciences, North-West University, Potchefstroom 2520, South Africa*

Correspondence should be addressed to Mark Hamer, m.hamer@ucl.ac.uk

Academic Editor: Tavis S. Campbell

Disturbances in circadian rhythm might play a central role in the neurobiology of depression. We examined the association between depressive symptoms and 24-hour ambulatory BP in a sample of 405 (197 black and 208 Caucasian) urbanized African teachers aged 25 to 60 yrs (mean 44.6 ± 9.6 yrs). Depressive symptoms were assessed using the self-administered 9-item Patient Health Questionnaire (PHQ-9). After adjusting for age, sex, and ethnicity, participants with severe depressive symptoms (PHQ-9 ≥ 15) had higher odds of hypertension defined from ambulatory BP and/or use of antihypertensive medication (odds ratio = 2.19, 95% CI, 1.00–4.90) in comparison to participants with no symptoms. Compared to Caucasians with no depressive symptoms, those with severe symptoms had blunted nocturnal systolic BP drop of 4.7 mmHg (95% CI, −0.5 to 10.0, $P = 0.07$). In summary, depressive symptoms were associated with the circadian BP profile in black and Caucasian Africans.

## 1. Introduction

Studies examining the association between common mood disorder, such as depression and risk of hypertension, have produced mixed findings. Several studies have reported positive associations between depression and risk of incident hypertension [1–4] whereas others have observed null findings [5, 6], or attributed the effects to hypertension labeling [7]. There is even some evidence to suggest lower blood pressure (BP) in participants with depressive symptoms [8, 9]. In the Whitehall II study of British civil servants that examined longitudinal trajectories, the risk of hypertension increased with repeated experience of depressive episodes over time and became evident in later adulthood [10]. Thus, the association between depression and hypertension is complex.

One limitation of this body of work is the reliance on clinic BP readings taken on one occasion. In a recent study of older participants that underwent 24-hour ambulatory BP recordings, those reporting depressive symptoms demonstrated a blunted nocturnal systolic BP fall and were more likely to be nondippers, defined as having nocturnal systolic BP fall of less than 10% [11]. There is increasing recognition that disturbances in circadian rhythm play a central role in the neurobiology of depression, even recognizing its importance as a novel pharmacological target in treating the disorder [12]. Depression is associated with alterations in hormone and catecholamine circadian rhythms [13], which may be the result of poorly regulated neurotransmitter feedback control systems that become erratic when chronically stressed. Melatonin, for example, is an endogenous antihypertensive molecule released by the pineal gland that plays a role in the biological regulation of circadian rhythms and has been associated with depression. In addition, nocturnal melatonin secretion is impaired among nondipper hypertensive patients [14].

Further studies are required to examine the association between depressive symptoms and the circadian BP profile, which might help to further clarify the equivocal nature of existing literature. The aim of this study was therefore to examine the association between depressive symptoms and circadian BP profiles using 24-hour ambulatory monitoring. The study was conducted in a sample of black and Caucasian Africans who were recruited as part of the Sympathetic Activity and Ambulatory Blood Pressure in Africans (SABPA) study—presently the only study in sub-Saharan Africa focusing on the contribution of psychosocial risk factors to cardiovascular health. Thus, a further aim was to assess potential ethnic differences in the association between depression and BP.

## 2. Methods

*2.1. Participants and Procedures.* Participants were recruited as part of the SABPA study conducted between February 2008 and May 2009. The study sample comprised urbanized African teachers working for the Dr. Kenneth Kaunda Education district in the North West Province, South Africa. The reason for this selection was to obtain a homogenous sample from a similar socioeconomic class. All eligible participants between the ages of 25 and 60 years were invited to participate. Exclusion criteria were an oral temperature above 37°C, psychotropic substance dependence or abuse, blood donors, and individuals vaccinated in the past 3 months. Participants were fully informed about the objectives and procedures of the study prior to their recruitment. Assistance was available for any participant who requested conveyance of information in their home language. All participants signed an informed consent form and the study was approved by The Ethics Review Board of the North-West University (Potchefstroom Campus). Participants were transported at 1630 hours to the Metabolic Unit Research Facility of the North-West University and familiarized with the protocol and completed a battery of psychosocial questionnaires. After receiving a standardized dinner participants were encouraged to go to bed at around 2200 hours and were woken at 0545 hours the following morning to undergo a battery of clinical assessments.

*2.2. Depressive Symptoms.* Depressive symptoms were assessed using the self-administered 9-item Patient Health Questionnaire (PHQ-9), which has been extensively validated in various clinical patient groups and different ethnic populations including sub-Saharan Africans [15, 16]. In the present study the PHQ-9 displayed good reliability (Cronbach's alpha = 0.81). The PHQ-9 measures the frequency of depressive symptoms corresponding to the 9 key symptoms of depression used by the *Diagnostic and Statistical Manual of Mental Disorder Fourth Edition* (DSM-IV) criteria to diagnosed major depressive episode. Participants indicated the frequency of experiencing symptoms during the prior two weeks, ranging from "not at all" (scored as zero), "several days" (one point), "more than half the days" (two points), "nearly every day" (three points), thus giving possible scores of 0–27. We used previously described PHQ-9 cut points (15) to derive three categories; no depressive symptoms (score <5), mild-moderate symptoms (score of 5–14), and severe symptoms (score of 15 and above).

*2.3. Blood Pressure Measures.* Semirecumbent clinic BP was measured twice using a mercury Sphygmomanometer with a 5-minute rest between each reading. Participants underwent 24-h ambulatory BP monitoring during the working day prior to the clinic visit. At ~0800 hours, participants were attached with an ambulatory BP monitor (Meditech CE120 CardioTens; Meditech, Budapest, Hungary) on the nondominant arm at their workplace. The apparatus was programmed to measure BP at 30 min intervals during the day (0800–2200 hours) and every hour during nighttime (2200–0600 hours). On average, the cuff successfully inflated 72.6% of the time across all participants. Participants were asked to continue with normal daily activities and record any abnormalities such as headache, nausea, and feeling stressed on their ambulatory diary cards. The data was analyzed using the CardioVisions 1.15 Personal Edition software (Meditech). Hypertension was defined as mean 24-hour BP >125/80 mmHg [17], and nondippers were defined as participants having nocturnal systolic BP fall of less than 10% of their average daytime BP [18].

*2.4. Covariates.* Sodium fluoride, plasma, and serum samples from fasting blood were stored at −80°C for the analysis of biochemical risk markers. Fasting sodium fluoride (glucose) and serum samples for total and high-density lipoprotein (HDL) cholesterol, gamma glutamyl transferase, and high-sensitivity C-reactive protein (CRP) were analyzed using two sequential multiple analyzers (Konelab 20i; Thermo Scientific, Vantaa, Finland; Unicel DXC 800—Beckman and Coulter, Germany). The intra- and intercoefficients of variation for all assays was below 10%.

*2.5. Statistical Analyses.* Differences in the characteristics of participants in relation to depressive symptoms were analysed using ANOVA tests to examine continuous variables and chi-square tests to examine categorical variables. All CRP values were log transformed to normalize the distribution. General linear models were used to examine differences in BP between depressive symptoms categories. Logistic regression was used to examine the associations of depressive symptoms with hypertension and nondipper status. Hypertension was defined from BP readings and/or use of antihypertensive medication. The models were adjusted for covariates, including age, sex, ethnicity, CRP, body mass index, total/HDL cholesterol, and glucose. These covariates were selected on an *a priori* basis, as depressive behavior is accompanied by perturbations in glucose and lipid metabolism, inflammatory, and neural serotonergic system function, all of

Table 1: Characteristics of the study sample ($N = 405$).

| Variable | No depressive symptoms | | Mild- moderate depressive symptoms | | Severe depressive symptoms | |
|---|---|---|---|---|---|---|
| | Black ($n = 42$) | Caucasian ($n = 101$) | Black ($n = 120$) | Caucasian ($n = 95$) | Black ($n = 35$) | Caucasian ($n = 12$) |
| Age (yrs) | 43.8 ± 7.3 | 46.3 ± 10.8 | 44.7 ± 8.3 | 43.8 ± 10.7 | 43.3 ± 7.8 | 43.3 ± 11.3 |
| Sex (% men) | 66.7 | 58.4 | 58.8 | 45.7 | 34.3* | 33.3* |
| Body mass index (kg·m$^2$) | 27.7 ± 6.6 | 27.2 ± 5.4 | 30.7 ± 7.2 | 27.7 ± 6.5 | 31.2 ± 7.1* | 29.8 ± 6.7 |
| Total/HDL cholesterol ratio | 4.41 ± 1.85 | 5.21 ± 1.63 | 4.34 ± 1.58 | 4.71 ± 1.58 | 5.08 ± 3.31 | 5.41 ± 1.69 |
| C-reactive protein (mg/L)† | 3.95 (54.3) | 1.10 (14.1) | 5.05 (53.6) | 1.90 (26.3) | 5.33 (32.5) | 2.90 (25.7)* |
| Glucose (mmol/L) | 5.59 ± 2.23 | 5.80 ± 0.97 | 5.59 ± 1.64 | 5.55 ± 0.62 | 5.92 ± 3.01 | 5.53 ± 0.50 |
| Antihypertensive medication usage (%) | 21.5 | 8.9 | 22.5 | 8.4 | 14.3 | 8.3 |

*$P < 0.05$ for trend across depressive symptom groups compared within own ethnicity; values displayed as mean ± SD unless stated (†non-normally distributed values displayed as median and range).

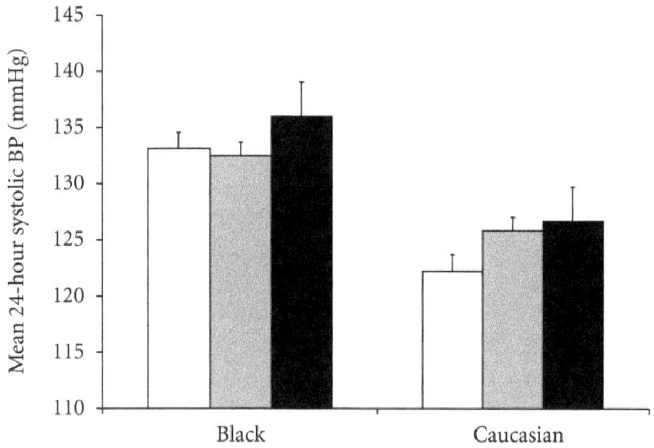


Figure 1: Association between depressive symptoms and mean 24-hour ambulatory systolic blood pressure in black and Caucasian Africans. White, grey, and black bars represent none, mild-moderate, and severe depressive symptoms, respectively. Values for blood pressure are mean ± SEM, adjusted for age, sex, and antihypertensive medication.

which are associated with exacerbated hypertension [19]. We fitted interaction terms in order to assess potential ethnic differences in the association between depression and BP. All analyses were conducted using SPSS version 14.

## 3. Results

The sample comprised 197 black (aged 44.2 ± 8.0 yrs) and 208 Caucasians (aged 45.0 ± 10.8 yrs). Severe depressive symptoms were reported in 11.6% of the sample. Black participants were more likely to report any depressive symptoms compared with Caucasians (age- and sex-adjusted odds ratio = 3.72, 95% CI, 2.35–5.89). Depressive symptoms were associated with several risk factors including higher body mass index and elevated CRP (see Table 1). In addition, black ethnicity was strongly related to other risk factors, including elevated CRP, BMI, and BP.

Hypertension was prevalent in 62.1% of the sample when using the 24-hour ambulatory BP criteria. There was a strong correlation between clinic and ambulatory systolic BP ($r = 0.74$, $P < 0.001$). Black participants recorded higher 24-hour systolic BP (age-, sex-, medication-adjusted $\beta = 7.8$, 95% CI, 5.0–10.6 mmHg) compared to Caucasians. There was an association between depressive symptoms and 24-hour ambulatory BP (see Figure 1). For example, compared to participants with no depressive symptoms, those with severe symptoms had marginally increased 24-hour systolic BP of 4.2 mmHg (95% CI, −0.5 to 8.9, $P = 0.08$) after adjustment for age, sex, ethnicity, and antihypertensive medication. Depressive symptoms were associated with a twofold risk of hypertension defined from 24-hour ambulatory BP monitoring (Table 2), although when hypertension was defined from clinic BP readings (≥140/90 mmHg) there was no associations with depression (odds ratio of hypertension for severe depressive symptoms = 1.36, 95% CI, 0.63–2.96). The associations of depressive symptoms and 24-hour hypertension were slightly attenuated after further adjustments for other risk factors including body mass index, CRP, total/HDL cholesterol, and glucose. We found no evidence for any statistically significant ethnic differences in the association between depression and BP. The removal of four participants who reported use of antidepressant medication did not alter any of the results.

Table 2: The association between depressive symptoms and hypertension defined from 24 hr ambulatory blood pressure readings. ($N = 405$).

| Depressive symptoms | Cases/N | Model 1 OR (95% CI) | Model 2 OR (95% CI) |
|---|---|---|---|
| None | 80/143 | Reference | Reference |
| Mild-moderate | 142/215 | 1.91 (1.15–3.18) | 1.79 (1.02–3.13) |
| Severe | 32/47 | 2.19 (1.00–4.90) | 1.86 (0.76–4.57) |

‡defined as mean 24 hr BP ≥ 125/80 mmHg and/or use of antihypertensive medication.
Model 1; adjustment for age, sex, ethnicity.
Model 2; adjustment for age, sex, ethnicity, + C-reactive protein, body mass index, total/HDL cholesterol, glucose.

Fifty-nine participants (14.5%) recorded experiencing stress on their diary cards during the ambulatory monitoring

TABLE 3: The association between depressive symptoms and nondipper status.

| Depressive symptoms | Cases/N | Model 1 OR (95% CI) | Model 2 OR (95% CI) |
|---|---|---|---|
| None | 45/143 | Reference | Reference |
| Mild-moderate | 75/215 | 1.04 (0.65–1.67) | 1.01 (0.62–1.63) |
| Severe | 23/47 | 1.74 (0.85–3.58) | 1.74 (0.83–3.63) |

Model 1; adjustment for age, sex, ethnicity, antihypertensive medication.
Model 2; adjustment for age, sex, ethnicity, antihypertensive medication + C-reactive protein, BMI, total/HDL cholesterol, glucose.

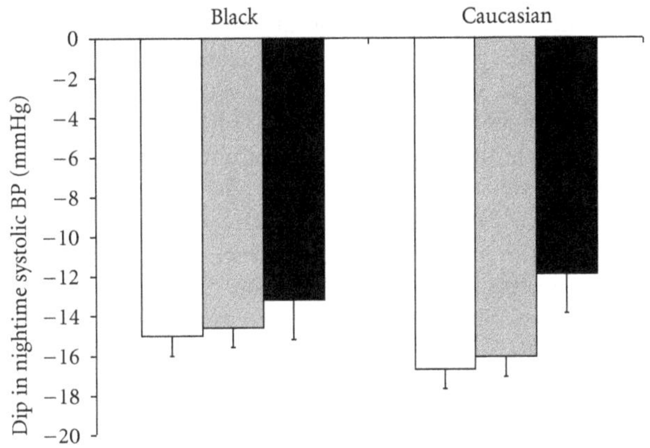


FIGURE 2: Association between depressive symptoms and change in ambulatory systolic blood pressure between daytime and night in black and Caucasian Africans. White, grey, and black bars represent none, mild-moderate, and severe depressive symptoms, respectively. Values for blood pressure are mean ± SEM, adjusted for age, sex, and antihypertensive medication.

day, and those participants had elevated 24-hour systolic BP compared with nonstressed (age-, sex-, ethnicity-adjusted $\beta = 5.5$, 95% CI, 1.7 to 9.3 mmHg, $P = 0.004$). Participants reporting severe depressive symptoms were more likely to report feeling stressed (age-, sex-, ethnicity-adjusted odds ratio = 2.96, 95% CI, 1.16–7.50). When we added stress as a covariate, the difference in 24-hour systolic BP between participants reporting none and severe depressive symptoms was no longer evident ($\beta = 3.3$, 95% CI, −1.4 to 8.0 mmHg, $P = 0.16$), which suggests stress might partly explain the link between depression and the circadian BP profile.

We further examined the association between depressive symptoms and nocturnal BP decline (Table 3 and Figure 2). A nocturnal systolic BP fall of less than 10% (nondipper) was observed in 31.4% of the sample, and black participants were more likely to be nondippers compared with Caucasians (age-, sex-, medication-adjusted odds ratio = 1.62, 95% CI, 1.04–2.51). There was a weak association between depressive symptoms and nocturnal BP decline that was particularly evident in Caucasians. For example, compared to Caucasians with no depressive symptoms, those with severe symptoms had blunted nocturnal systolic BP drop of 4.7 mmHg (95% CI, −0.5 to 10.0, $P = 0.07$) after adjustment for age, sex, and antihypertensive medication (Figure 2). In the whole sample there was evidence of elevated risk of nondipping in participants with severe depressive symptoms although this did not reach statistical significance (Table 3), nor was there any significant interaction by ethnicity.

## 4. Discussion

This is presently the only study in sub-Saharan Africa to examine the association between depressive symptoms and risk of hypertension. Black Africans are known to have elevated BP compared with Caucasians [20], and this was confirmed in the present study. Black participants from the present study also demonstrated a higher prevalence of depressive symptoms. Despite this, the association between depressive symptoms and BP remained independent of ethnicity and there was no evidence for any significant ethnic differences in the association between depression and BP.

Previous studies in this area have been limited by only taking clinic BP readings, but in the present study we also collected data from 24-hour ambulatory BP monitoring. Our main findings show an association between depressive symptoms and 24-hour ambulatory BP. To our knowledge, only one other study examining depression has employed ambulatory BP monitoring [11]. They found an association between depressive symptoms and blunted nocturnal systolic BP fall. Our findings are partly consistent with those results although we did not find strong evidence for an association between depression and risk of nondipping, which might be explained by the older age of participants from the previous study. Several large epidemiological cohort studies have found evidence for an association between depression and elevated risk of incident hypertension at followup [1–3, 10]. However, in other studies depressive disorder was associated with lower systolic BP [8, 9], although use of tricyclic antidepressants was associated with greater risk of hypertension [5, 8]. These inconsistencies might therefore be partially explained by inadequate assessments of BP, antidepressant medication, different measures of symptoms and diagnostic criteria for depression, or other confounding factors.

The associations between depressive symptoms and 24-hour BP were attenuated after further adjustments for other risk factors including body mass index, CRP, cholesterol, and glucose. However, given that these factors might act as intermediate mechanisms on the causal pathway from depression to hypertension, our models may have been overadjusted. For example, depressive symptoms were associated with body mass index and CRP, both of which have been implicated in hypertension risk [21, 22]. Indeed, these mechanisms have also been linked with the association between depression and coronary heart disease [23–25].

From our results we might speculate that daily stress partly explains the link between depression and the circadian BP profile. Participants with severe depressive symptoms were more likely to report feeling stressed on the ambulatory BP monitoring day, which corroborates with observations that depressed individuals are more likely to report events as stressful and to complain and endorse somatic symptoms.

Heightened BP reactivity to laboratory-induced stressors has been prospectively associated with a greater risk of hypertension [26], thus if elicited repeatedly in a person's life these responses might be clinically relevant. Moreover, there is also overlapping biology between the neurohormonal control of BP and the subsequent downstream effects of psychological stress, one in particular being the gaseous transmitter and neuroregulator, nitric oxide [27]. Indeed, naturalistic studies have shown profound effects of acute stressors on BP. For example, the World Trade Centre terrorist attacks in New York on 11th September 2001 produced a substantial and sustained increase in the BP of participants from the local community [28]. There was also a 20% increase in systolic BP following a moderate intensity earth quake that struck central Italy, which was followed by a long lasting period of enhanced BP variability and blunted nocturnal BP fall [29]. Work stress has also been associated with elevated 24-hour ambulatory BP [30] although the findings from prospective cohort studies in relation to work stress and hypertension risk have been generally inconsistent [31–36].

The strengths of this study include the unique sample of participants from sub-Saharan Africa, a well-validated measure of depressive symptoms, and the use of 24-hour ambulatory BP assessments. A limitation is the cross-sectional design, thus we cannot infer causality, identify potential mediators, nor determine the direction of the observed relationship between depression and hypertension. In addition, we did not assess history of major depression and recurrent symptoms, which might be important given the link between persistent depressive symptoms and cardiovascular risk [37]. In summary, we found an association between depressive symptoms and 24-hour ambulatory BP in black and Caucasian Africans. The equivocal nature of the existing work in this area might be explained by reliance on clinic BP readings and failure to capture the circadian BP profile.

## Funding

Funding was provided by HART (North-West University) and National Research Foundation South Africa, Metabolic Syndrome Institute, France. Dr Hamer is supported by the British Heart Foundation, UK. The funding organizations played no role in the design and conduct of the study; collection, management, analysis, and interpretation of the data; preparation, review, or approval of the paper.

## Author's Contributions

M. Hamer had full access to the data and takes responsibility for the integrity of the data and accuracy of the data analyses. M. Hamer performed statistical analyses. L. Malan is the principle investigator and led the study. All authors contributed to the concept and design of study, drafting, and critical revision of the paper.

## Acknowledgments

The authors thank Chrissie Lessing (research nurse) and Szabolcs Péter (MD) for their contribution to data collection and analysis.

## References

[1] S. B. Patten, J. V. A. Williams, D. H. Lavorato, N. R. C. Campbell, M. Eliasziw, and T. S. Campbell, "Major depression as a risk factor for high blood pressure: epidemiologic evidence from a national longitudinal study," *Psychosomatic Medicine*, vol. 71, no. 3, pp. 273–279, 2009.

[2] B. S. Jonas, P. Franks, and D. D. Ingram, "Are symptoms of anxiety and depression risk factors for hypertension? Longitudinal evidence from the National Health and Nutrition Examination Survey I Epidemiologic Follow-up Study," *Archives of Family Medicine*, vol. 6, no. 1, pp. 43–49, 1997.

[3] J. H. Markovitz, K. A. Matthews, W. B. Kannel, J. L. Cobb, and R. B. D'Agostino, "Psychological predictors of hypertension in the Framingham study. Is there tension in hypertension?" *Journal of the American Medical Association*, vol. 270, no. 20, pp. 2439–2443, 1993.

[4] D. Carroll, A. C. Phillips, C. R. Gale, and G. D. Batty, "Generalized anxiety and major depressive disorders, their comorbidity and hypertension in middle-aged men," *Psychosomatic Medicine*, vol. 72, no. 1, pp. 16–19, 2010.

[5] J. A. C. Delaney, B. E. Oddson, H. Kramer, S. Shea, B. M. Psaty, and R. L. McClelland, "Baseline depressive symptoms are not associated with clinically important levels of incident hypertension during two years of follow-up: the multi-ethnic study of atherosclerosis," *Hypertension*, vol. 55, no. 2, pp. 408–414, 2010.

[6] L. L. Yan, K. Liu, K. A. Matthews, M. L. Daviglus, T. F. Ferguson, and C. I. Kiefe, "Psychosocial factors and risk of hypertension: the Coronary Artery Risk Development in Young Adults (CARDIA) study," *Journal of the American Medical Association*, vol. 290, no. 16, pp. 2138–2148, 2003.

[7] M. Hamer, G. D. Batty, E. Stamatakis, and M. Kivimaki, "Hypertension awareness and psychological distress," *Hypertension*, vol. 56, no. 3, pp. 547–550, 2010.

[8] C. M. Licht, E. J. de Geus, A. Seldenrijk et al., "Depression is associated with decreased blood pressure, but antidepressant use increases the risk for hypertension," *Hypertension*, vol. 53, no. 4, pp. 631–638, 2009.

[9] B. Hildrum, A. Mykletun, E. Stordal, I. Bjelland, A. A. Dahl, and J. Holmen, "Association of low blood pressure with anxiety and depression: the Nord-Trøndelag Health Study," *Journal of Epidemiology and Community Health*, vol. 61, no. 1, pp. 53–58, 2007.

[10] H. Nabi, J. F. Chastang, T. Lefèvre et al., "Trajectories of depressive episodes and hypertension over 24 years: the whitehall II prospective cohort study," *Hypertension*, vol. 57, pp. 710–716, 2011.

[11] A. Scuteri, G. Spalletta, M. Cangelosi et al., "Decreased nocturnal systolic blood pressure fall in older subjects with depression," *Aging—Clinical and Experimental Research*, vol. 21, no. 4-5, pp. 292–297, 2009.

[12] C. R. Dolder, M. Nelson, and M. Snider, "Agomelatine treatment of major depressive disorder," *Annals of Pharmacotherapy*, vol. 42, no. 12, pp. 1822–1831, 2008.

[13] H. W. Koenigsberg, M. H. Teicher, V. Mitropoulou et al., "24-h Monitoring of plasma norepinephrine, MHPG, cortisol,

growth hormone and prolactin in depression," *Journal of Psychiatric Research*, vol. 38, no. 5, pp. 503–511, 2004.

[14] M. Jonas, D. Garfinkel, N. Zisapel, M. Laudon, and E. Grossman, "Impaired nocturnal melatonin secretion in non-dipper hypertensive patients," *Blood Pressure*, vol. 12, no. 1, pp. 19–24, 2003.

[15] K. Kroenke, R. L. Spitzer, and J. B. W. Williams, "The PHQ-9: validity of a brief depression severity measure," *Journal of General Internal Medicine*, vol. 16, no. 9, pp. 606–613, 2001.

[16] P. O. Monahan, E. Shacham, M. Reece et al., "Validity/reliability of PHQ-9 and PHQ-2 depression scales among adults living with HIV/AIDS in western Kenya," *Journal of General Internal Medicine*, vol. 24, no. 2, pp. 189–197, 2009.

[17] G. Mancia, G. De Backer, A. Dominiczak et al., "Guidelines for the management of arterial hypertension: the Task Force for the Management of Arterial Hypertension of the European Society of Hypertension (ESH) and of the European Society of Cardiology (ESC)," *Journal of Hypertension*, vol. 25, no. 6, pp. 1105–1187, 2007.

[18] P. Verdecchia, G. Schillaci, M. Guerrieri et al., "Circadian blood pressure changes and left ventricular hypertrophy in essential hypertension," *Circulation*, vol. 81, no. 2, pp. 528–536, 1990.

[19] C. A. Shively, D. L. Musselman, and S. L. Willard, "Stress, depression, and coronary artery disease: modeling comorbidity in female primates," *Neuroscience and Biobehavioral Reviews*, vol. 33, no. 2, pp. 133–144, 2009.

[20] G. Dwivedi and D. G. Beevers, "Hypertension in ethnic groups: epidemiological and clinical perspectives," *Expert Review of Cardiovascular Therapy*, vol. 7, no. 8, pp. 955–963, 2009.

[21] K. Rahmouni, M. L. G. Correia, W. G. Haynes, and A. L. Mark, "Obesity-associated hypertension: new insights into mechanisms," *Hypertension*, vol. 45, no. 1, pp. 9–14, 2005.

[22] P. Mathieu, P. Poirier, P. Pibarot, I. Lemieux, and J. P. Després, "Visceral obesity: the link among inflammation, hypertension, and cardiovascular disease," *Hypertension*, vol. 53, no. 4, pp. 577–584, 2009.

[23] V. Vaccarino, B. D. Johnson, D. S. Sheps et al., "Depression, inflammation, and incident cardiovascular disease in women with suspected coronary ischemia: the National Heart, Lung, and Blood Institute-sponsored WISE study," *Journal of the American College of Cardiology*, vol. 50, no. 21, pp. 2044–2050, 2007.

[24] V. Vaccarino, C. McClure, B. D. Johnson et al., "Depression, the metabolic syndrome and cardiovascular risk," *Psychosomatic Medicine*, vol. 70, no. 1, pp. 40–48, 2008.

[25] W. J. Kop, P. K. Stein, R. P. Tracy, J. I. Barzilay, R. Schulz, and J. S. Gottdiener, "Autonomic nervous system dysfunction and inflammation contribute to the increased cardiovascular mortality risk associated with depression," *Psychosomatic Medicine*, vol. 72, no. 7, pp. 626–635, 2010.

[26] Y. Chida and A. Steptoe, "Greater cardiovascular responses to laboratory mental stress are associated with poor subsequent cardiovascular risk status: a meta-analysis of prospective evidence," *Hypertension*, vol. 55, no. 4, pp. 1026–1032, 2010.

[27] F. Oosthuizen, G. Wegener, and B. H. Harvey, "Nitric oxide as inflammatory mediator in post-traumatic stress disorder (PTSD): evidence from an animal model," *Journal of Neuropsychiatric Disease and Treatment*, vol. 1, pp. 109–123, 2005.

[28] W. Gerin, W. Chaplin, J. E. Schwartz et al., "Sustained blood pressure increase after an acute stressor: the effects of the 11 September 2001 attack on the New York City World Trade Center," *Journal of Hypertension*, vol. 23, no. 2, pp. 279–284, 2005.

[29] G. Parati, R. Antonicelli, F. Guazzarotti, E. Paciaroni, and G. Mancia, "Cardiovascular effects of an earthquake: direct evidence by ambulatory blood pressure monitoring," *Hypertension*, vol. 38, no. 5, pp. 1093–1095, 2001.

[30] T. G. M. Vrijkotte, L. J. P. van Doornen, and E. J. C. De Geus, "Effects of work stress on ambulatory blood pressure, heart rate, and heart rate variability," *Hypertension*, vol. 35, no. 4, pp. 880–886, 2000.

[31] J. H. Markovitz, K. A. Matthews, M. Whooley, C. E. Lewis, and K. J. Greenlund, "Increases in job strain are associated with incident hypertension in the CARDIA Study," *Annals of Behavioral Medicine*, vol. 28, no. 1, pp. 4–9, 2004.

[32] A. Chapman, J. A. Mandryk, M. S. Frommer, B. V. Edye, and D. A. Ferguson, "Chronic perceived work stress and blood pressure among Australian government employees," *Scandinavian Journal of Work, Environment and Health*, vol. 16, no. 4, pp. 258–269, 1990.

[33] C. Guimont, C. Brisson, G. R. Dagenais et al., "Effects of job strain on blood pressure: a prospective study of male and female white-collar workers," *American Journal of Public Health*, vol. 96, no. 8, pp. 1436–1443, 2006.

[34] P. L. Schnall, J. E. Schwartz, P. A. Landsbergis, K. Warren, and T. G. Pickering, "A longitudinal study of job strain and ambulatory blood pressure: results from a three-year follow-up," *Psychosomatic Medicine*, vol. 60, no. 6, pp. 697–706, 1998.

[35] J. P. Fauvel, I. M'Pio, P. Quelin, J. P. Rigaud, M. Laville, and M. Ducher, "Neither perceived job stress nor individual cardiovascular reactivity predict high blood pressure," *Hypertension*, vol. 42, no. 6, pp. 1112–1116, 2003.

[36] B. Öhlin, G. Berglund, M. Rosvall, and P. M. Nilsson, "Job strain in men, but not in women, predicts a significant rise in blood pressure after 6.5 years of follow-up," *Journal of Hypertension*, vol. 25, no. 3, pp. 525–531, 2007.

[37] M. Hamer, M. Kivimaki, A. Lahiri, M. G. Marmot, and A. Steptoe, "Persistent cognitive depressive symptoms are associated with coronary artery calcification," *Atherosclerosis*, vol. 210, no. 1, pp. 209–213, 2010.

15

# Factors Influencing Compliance and Health Seeking Behaviour for Hypertension in Mukono and Buikwe in Uganda

**Geofrey Musinguzi ,[1,2] Sibyl Anthierens,[2] Fred Nuwaha,[1] Jean-Pierre Van Geertruyden,[3] Rhoda K. Wanyenze,[1] and Hilde Bastiaens[2]**

[1]*Department of Disease Control and Environmental Health, School of Public Health, Makerere University, Kampala, Uganda*
[2]*Primary and Interdisciplinary Care, University of Antwerp, Antwerp, Belgium*
[3]*International Health, University of Antwerp, Antwerp, Belgium*

Correspondence should be addressed to Geofrey Musinguzi; mgeof@musph.ac.ug

Academic Editor: Omotayo O. Erejuwa

*Background and Methods.* Hypertension is a global public health challenge and a leading risk factor for cardiovascular morbidity and mortality. Hypertension control rates are low worldwide, and delay in seeking care is associated with increased mortality. *Methods.* In a qualitative study, known hypertensive patients were interviewed to explore factors influencing compliance and health seeking behaviour (HSB). Data was analyzed following a semantic thematic analysis approach. *Results.* Patients sought various channels of care for their hypertension. Self-medication and access to antihypertensive drugs with or without prescription were common as well as use of herbal remedies. Regular monitoring of blood pressure was not a common practice. Factors influencing HSB were related to health systems and the patient socioeconomic and structural environment. The main system issues were related to availability and attitudes of staff and shortage of supplies and medicines. The patient factors were related to awareness, perceived severity, perceived effectiveness of therapy, adverse effects, and perceived fears of lifelong dependence on medicines. The patient socioeconomic status played a role as did the marketing of traditional medicine. *Conclusion.* Patients seek varied channels of care for their hypertension. Strategies to address the multifactorial dimensions that affect HSB are needed to improve hypertension control in this population.

## 1. Introduction

Hypertension is a leading risk factor for cardiovascular morbidity and mortality worldwide [1]. A comparative risk analysis of the burden of disease and injury associated with 67 risk factors revealed that hypertension (also known as high blood pressure) is the leading risk factor for mortality with 7% of deaths attributable to it [1]. It is predicted that, by 2025, the number of adults with hypertension will increase by about 60% to a total of 1.56 billion and most of the cases will occur in low and middle income countries (LMIC) [2]. Urbanization and the epidemiological transition characterised by an aging population, physical inactivity, obesity, increasing alcohol consumption, and high salt intake are contributing to the increasing rates of hypertension in LMIC [3]. Hypertension is a “silent killer” [4] and data suggests that hypertensive heart disease could be the most common form of cardiovascular disease (CVD) in Africa [5]. Unfortunately, most cases of hypertension are asymptomatic and as a result, hypertensive patients often seek medical attention late or when they have developed complications such as strokes, heart attacks, heart failure, and kidney failure [3]. In their publication, Cruickshank et al. on the rule of halves reported that 50% of the hypertensives are known, of the known hypertensives, half are on treatment and of those on treatment, half are controlled [5]. The World Health Organization (WHO) projected that, over the next ten years, Africa will experience the largest increase in death rates from CVDs. Consequently, the negative economic impact of CVDs will be felt more on the African continent [6] and the cost of handling chronic illness will lead many households to poverty [7].

Health seeking behaviour (HSB) has been defined as any activity undertaken by individuals who perceive themselves to have a health problem or to be ill for the purpose of finding an appropriate remedy. The desired HSB is responding to an illness by seeking help from a trained allopathic doctor in a recognized health care center [8]. It is well established that HSB is influenced by manifestation of symptoms [9, 10]. However, many hypertensive individuals may not be aware and may not have any symptoms to compel them to seek care. Even among those presenting with symptoms and those who are aware hypertensive, their HSB is suboptimal [11, 12]. Hypertension control remains very low [13] and attributable reasons revolve around noncompliance due to side effects of the medication, lack of information and support, difficulty obtaining the medication, poverty, low education, and poor access to health care [14–16]. In addition, health system deficiencies such as lack of antihypertensive medication, the physicians' inertia in treating hypertension, and long distance to the health facilities have been implicated in affecting HSBs and control of hypertension [13, 17, 18]. Delays in seeking care for hypertension are associated with increased mortality [19] and the benefits of early treatment and control are also well established [20–22].

Like most of Sub-Saharan Africa, Uganda's health care system was established with a greater orientation towards communicable diseases. It is only in the past 15 years that the NCD agenda started featuring in the national health strategic plan of the Ministry of Health [23]. The current health service delivery system has a number of gaps ranging from lack of preventive services for NCDs to lack of essential supplies for managing NCDs [24].

Over the last 20 years, Uganda has witnessed an increasingly aging population which has ushered in increasing rates of lifestyle-related chronic noncommunicable diseases [25]. Notably, increasing cases of obesity, diabetes mellitus, and hypertension, along with such complications as stroke, and heart diseases are reported [25]. Data from the Health management information system (HMIS) suggests that hypertension is the most reported NCD and community surveys also suggest that one in five of every adult ≥ 18 years have uncontrolled hypertension [26]. The detailed reasons for low levels of hypertension control and inadequate HSB in this setting are not well understood.

We explored compliance and HSBs for hypertension using qualitative approach in order to understand reasons for low levels of hypertension control. Understanding the HSB for hypertension is vitally important in designing programs for hypertension control and enhancing quality standards in healthcare delivery [8].

## 2. Methods

*2.1. Setting and Design.* From August to October 2014, we conducted a community descriptive qualitative study and performed semistructured individual interviews with 48 patients with known hypertension in Mukono and Buikwe districts in Uganda. According to the Uganda population and housing census area specific profiles, 78% and 72% of the population in Buikwe and Mukono, respectively, live in rural areas [27]. The Uganda National Health System is made up of the Public and the Private sectors. Uganda implements a level based healthcare delivery system with a referral framework from a lower facility (Health Center (HC) II, III, IV) through hospitals at the district, regional, or national level. Mukono and Buikwe districts combined have six (6) hospitals, 4 HCIV, 27 HCIIIs, and 57 HCIIs. Moreover, most of these facilities are ill-equipped to provide services for hypertension. For example, essential ingredients including diagnostic equipment, antihypertensive medicines, and personnel are scarce [28]. Secondly, conducting this study in this setting would provide incremental evidence to our previously conducted WHO Stepwise Approach to Chronic Disease Risk Factor Surveillance (STEPS) study [29]. In the STEPS study, we observed an unacceptably high prevalence rate of hypertension and suboptimal treatment and control [29].

*2.2. Sampling.* A purposive sample of patients with known hypertension was identified from the database gathered two years before [29]. The STEPS, conducted in 2012, enrolled 4653 study participants of whom 258 were hypertensive patients and aware of their hypertension. The data set for the 258 patients was organised by gender, residential status, and district to select patients for enrolment into the current study. To generate a wide range of experiences, a fairly big sample size (48) comprising of a varied group of patients (males' and females, urban and rural, Buikwe and Mukono districts) were interviewed. The final sample is comprised of equal number of patients drawn from both districts of Mukono and Buikwe, 17 males, and 24 rural residents. All participants consented except two males.

*2.3. Data Collection.* Data were collected by one of the lead investigators (GM) and three graduate research assistants who underwent a rigorous and extensive 5-day training to standardise data collection procedures. The training entailed a review of the study objectives, conduct of qualitative inquiries, blood pressure measurement using a validated automated digital sphygmomanometer (Omron model M3W) with an appropriate cuff size, interpersonal communication skills, ethics, confidentiality, and informed consent, seminars on one-on-one interviewing techniques, and detailed instructions on using the semistructured interview protocol. The use of semistructured interview guides (Appendix) enabled data gathering on background characteristics of the study patients, compliance, and HSBs for hypertension. Interviews were conducted at the participants' homes. Each interview lasted one hour on average after which the patients' blood pressure was measured thrice one minute apart. Measuring blood pressure after the interview allowed the patient to relax and also prevented any biased responses that would arise if measurements were done before the interviews. All interviews were audio-recorded with consent from each patient and the average of the three readings was used to estimate the patient blood pressure.

*2.4. Ethics Statement.* Ethical approval was granted by Makerere University School of Public Health Higher Degrees-Research and Ethics Committee and the Uganda National Council of Science and technology. Each participant provided written informed consent.

*2.5. Data Management.* All qualitative data were transcribed verbatim and then translated into English from the local language. Each transcript was reviewed by at least two research assistants and one of the investigators (GM) for content and completeness. Final transcripts were stored securely on pass-worded external drives and later exported to ATLAS.ti version 7, qualitative data management software for further management.

*2.6. Data Analysis.* To identify the factors influencing compliance and health seeking behaviours for hypertension, we analysed the data following a semantic approach in thematic analysis [30]. Using free coding options in ATLAS.ti, GM read each transcript and extracted relevant data to generate codes related to compliance and health seeking behaviours. The codes were reviewed to identify patterns within the data [31] and iteratively compared with the original transcripts. Following the review and with use of code families' options in ATLAS.ti, the codes were sorted into groups (to generate subthemes) and where appropriate were split or dropped or renamed if better subthemes were obtained. The subthemes were further reanalysed to generate themes and overarching themes. For quality control, and to ensure that the interpretation was close to the content and to support reflexivity, the process of analysis and output at every stage of the analysis was regularly reviewed and discussed with SA and HB.

## 3. Results

*3.1. Participants and Context.* Table 1 shows study participants' characteristics and their current blood pressure profiles as measured at the time of the interviews.

As shown in Table 1, 48 patients were interviewed between August and October 2014. Of these, 17 were males, 24 were rural residents, 35 were married, and 23 had attained post-primary education. The median age was 54 (males 54, females 51.5). Very few patients, 8, had their hypertension under control (SBP < 140 mmHg and DBP < 90 mmHg). Majority ($n$ = 20) were stage one hypertensive and sizable proportions were stage 2 ($n$ = 11) and stage 3 ($n$ = 9) hypertensive. Self-medication and access to antihypertensive drugs with or without prescription from drug outlets were common as well as use of herbal remedies. Some patients also reported engaging in life style interventions such as cessation of alcohol consumption, increased physical activity, and dietary modifications. Regular monitoring of blood pressure was not a common practice. Modern healthcare for hypertension was sought widely from all levels of health facilities including drug shops, pharmacies, private health clinics, health centers (II, III, and IV) and hospitals. Herbal remedies in use included garlic, ginger, pumpkin leaves *(essunsa)*, herbal mixtures (names unknown), African eggplant *(Katunkuma)*, Moringa, *Mumbwa*, spider plant *(ejjobyo)*, aloe vera *(kigaji)*, dried banana leaves, neem tree, chlorophyll extracts, human urine, Tianshi (Chinese herbal), and African night shade (Nakati).

TABLE 1

| Characteristics | Number |
|---|---|
| Sex | |
| Male | 17 |
| Female | 31 |
| Residential status | |
| Rural | 24 |
| Urban | 24 |
| Education status | |
| Primary or less | 25 |
| Post primary | 23 |
| Marital status | |
| Single | 13 |
| Married | 35 |
| Age | |
| Overall median age | 54 |
| Median age (female) | 51.5 |
| Median age (male) | 54 |
| Measured BP on the interview date | |
| (SBP < 140 mmHg and DBP < 90 mmHg) | 8 |
| Stage 1 (SBP = 140–159/ DBP = 90–99) | 20 |
| Stage 2 (SBP = 160–179/ DBP = 100–109) | 11 |
| Stage 3 (SBP ≥ 180/DBP ≥ 110) | 9 |

*3.2. Factors Influencing Compliance and Health Seeking Behaviour for Hypertension.* The 3 thematic key issues influencing HSB for hypertension were related to the health system, the patient, and the broader socioeconomic and structural environment. Consequently, we organise the key findings (themes and subthemes) under each of these three overarching thematic areas. Figure 1 illustrates the schema of the identified themes and subthemes.

*3.2.1. Health System Factors.* Under the overarching theme of health system factors, five themes influencing compliance and HSBs were identified: (1) availability of medicines, personnel, and diagnostic supplies; (2) high burden of acute care at health facilities; (3) traditional medicines; (4) perceived provider abilities/behaviours and overall quality of care, and (5) patient waiting times at the facilities.

*(1) Availability of Medicine, Personnel, and Diagnostic Supplies*

*Medicines.* Patients noted that availability of or the assumption of [modern] medicines was readily available at health facilities and related costs played a key role in their seeking behaviours for hypertension. In private health facilities and private pharmacies, patients reported that antihypertensive drugs were readily available. However, high costs of these medicines were a deterrent to access. As such, they echoed that only those who had the money accessed the medicines as illustrated by the following patient in a local proverb.

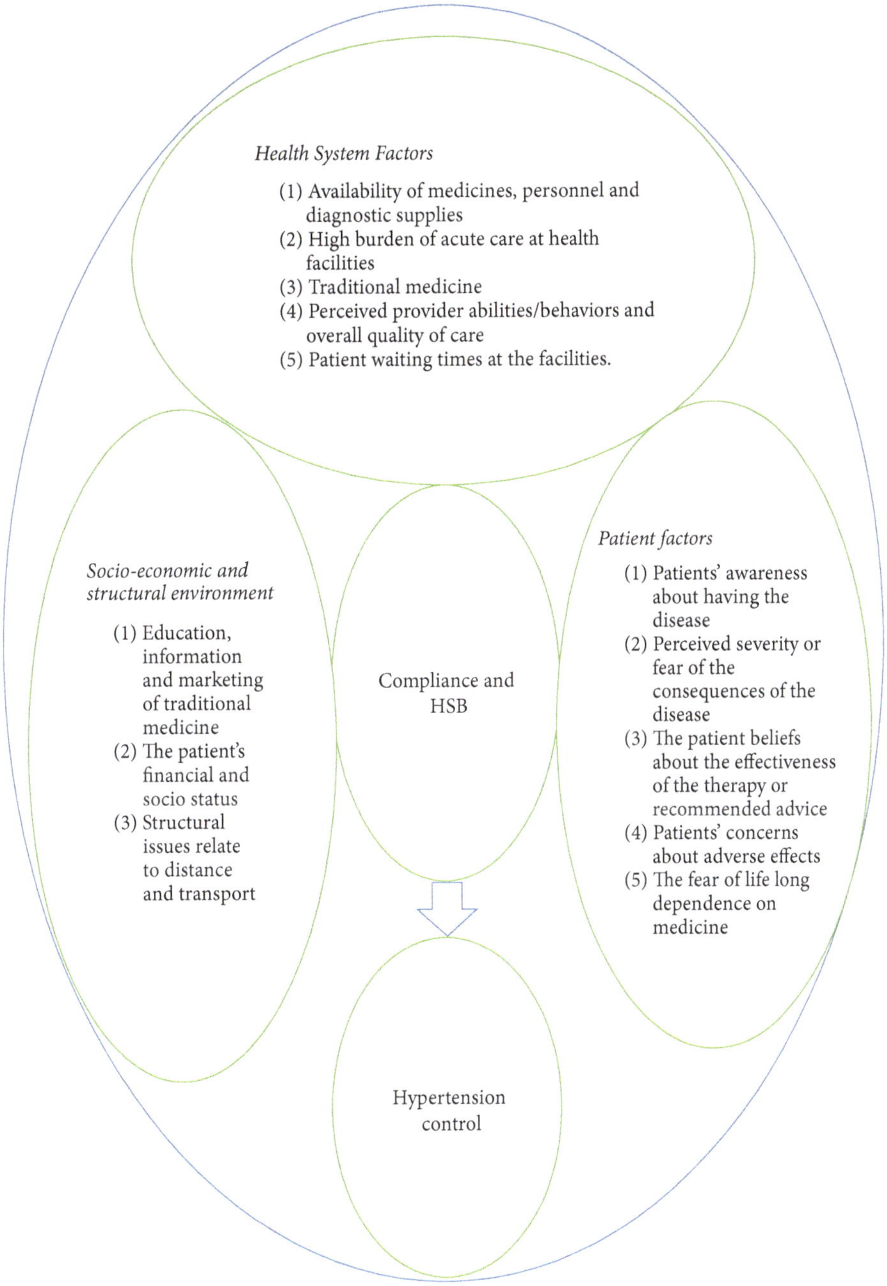


Figure 1: Factors influencing compliance and health seeking behaviours for hypertension among patients in Mukono and Buikwe Districts in Uganda.

> *When you are a poor man, you don't prick a Swahili ban [local bread] or else you get beaten if you prick and don't buy.* (8 Bulamba-Bugungu_Male 1-*Buikwe, Rural*)

As a caveat to turn away from high costs, self-medication was commonly reported from drug outlets, which dispensed medicines with or without prescription and in any quantities depending on the patients' affordability. But even with this option, cost still deterred patients from access as illuminated by the following patient.

> *Apart from the medicine he gave me. I failed to buy the medicine he had prescribed; even the last time I went to him; I failed to buy the medicine because it's expensive. One tablet costs 2,000 shs; and yet I had to swallow one per day for one month. I calculated and it was 60,000 shs; so I only swallowed the medicine he gave me; and then stopped.* (19 Kanyogoga_Male 2-*Buikwe, Urban*)

The costs of antihypertensive medicine were offset when the health facilities provided the medicine free of charge to patients. Indeed, patients attested that finding medicines at the health facilities was a motivation for their health seeking behaviours. However, lack of medicines had a negative implication on their compliance and health seeking behaviours. Patients expressed a sense of disappointment when they visited a health facility in anticipation of getting free medicines only to be given prescriptions to go and buy medicine elsewhere.

> *I went there four times; the first two times I got the medicine; while the other two times I was told that there was no medicine. So I realized that I was wasting time and stopped going there.* (20 Kateete_Female1)

> Another also echoed, "they gave me that medicine that I have told you [valium] and they told me to buy the other drugs since it was out of stock in the hospital. I didn't buy it; the truth is that the medicine was expensive" (12 Geregere Majjani_Female 1-*Buikwe, Urban*).

*Personnel.* Finding a service provider at a health facility was also critical in influencing health seeking behaviour of hypertensive patients. Patients were motivated to go to a health facility where they were sure of finding health workers. Most acknowledged that the situation was improving with establishment of specialised clinics especially at the national referral hospital, which run most days of the week.

> *Previously I only saw a doctor once a month but now, I can see the doctor any day between Monday to Friday.* (1 Anthony_Male 1)

> Some, however, were still hindered by lack of providers at health facilities.

> *Doctors would come once in a month so I didn't have the vigor to go to hospital for care.* (16 Kabumba_female 1-*Mukono, Rural*)

Lack of personnel as a barrier to health seeking behaviour was mainly reported by patients from the rural areas. However, some also stressed that their district hospital operated a one-day clinic in a week for diabetes and hypertension which limited access to specialised health workers for hypertension.

*Diagnostic Supplies.* Supply issues entailed the availability or lack of/or inadequacies in diagnostic equipment. It was common for patients in rural areas to report that they lacked a place where they could have their hypertension routinely monitored.

> *... the clinics here in the village do not have the BP machines ... all they do is to ask you; 'what are you suffering from'? Then they base on what you have told them to give you a few tablets to relieve you from the pain.* (6 Bukamunye B_Female 2-*Buikwe, Urban*)

> Another patient reported, "the biggest challenge we are facing as people with hypertension in this village is lack of somewhere we can go for emergency blood pressure monitoring" (41 Ssaza_female 3- *Mukono, Urban*).

*(2) High Burden of Acute Care at Health Facilities.* It was quite interesting to note that some patients did not seek care because they thought health workers would not attend to them since they [patients] did not have severe symptoms to warrant attention. This was especially in relation to those who desired regular BP monitoring. They said that hospitals were full of the severely ill meaning that a visit to health facilities for routine hypertension monitoring would be an additional burden to an already overwhelmed system. This subtheme was best illuminated by a patient (33 Malongwe Ajjija_male 2-*Buikwe, Urban*) who reported that it was difficult to just walk into a health facility and request a BP measurement. He said that such a daring would be considered luxurious because most of the facilities focus their efforts and resources on the very ill not the healthy looking individuals who walk in for BP measurements. The participant exemplified as follows:

> *One challenge has been the monitoring of blood pressure ... It's hard to just walk up to a health worker and tell them you would like to check your blood pressure ... It's hard for the health worker to really give you attention ... because you would have gone there for luxury and not as a patient. So when I would request for a blood pressure check-up; they would ask what the problem was. They cannot work on a person like me yet there are many patients who need help.* (33 Malongwe Ajjija_male 2-*Buikwe, Urban*)

*(3) Traditional Medicine.* With respect to the challenges surrounding access to modern health services, some patients resorted to using alternative medicines and seeking care from traditional practitioners. Most patients seeking complimentary medicines used herbs and some reported that they consulted traditional healers for their hypertension. Patients considered herbs easily accessible and to a certain extent comparably affordable. Planting them in the back yards enhanced access to herbs. In addition, most of the herbal remedies reported were readily available on the local market. However, it was also noted that some special herbs including those exported from abroad were sometimes difficult to access and expensive and that some traditional healers asked for certain items such as chicken and goats, which deterred patients from consulting them.

> *At first I tried local medicine like mumbwa but when the traditional healers started asking goats from me I couldn't manage that because I didn't have the money to buy these goats so I stopped visiting traditional healers* (47 Vvuluga_female 1-*Buikwe, Urban*). *It was Chinese medicine; ... my brother brought it for me. I drank it ... in fact I improved slightly; the fast heart beats stopped and my head also stopped hurting; only that I failed to use it because of my finances.* (14 Jagary Cable_female 1-*Buikwe, Urban*)

It was also observed that traditional healers do not necessary stay in the same communities where they provide their services. In some cases, patients reported that they abandoned their local treatment remedies because their providers [traditional healers] were out of reach. This patient alluded as follows:

> *From the time I would buy their medicine it would take like two to three months before they [traditional healers] returned to our village, this stopped me from using their medicine.* (16 Kabumba_female 1-*Buikwe, Urban*)

*(4) Perceived Provider Abilities and Behaviours and Overall Quality of Care.* This theme comprises the four subthemes: (1) patients' perceptions about their providers' abilities in terms of skills and knowledge competences; (2) perceived providers' attitudes towards work and the feeling of being treated with or without respect; (3) providers' advising role towards their patients' health seeking behaviours; and (4) perceived quality of care.

*Patients' Perceptions about Their Providers' Abilities in Terms of Skills and Knowledge Competences.* Whereas most patients perceived their providers to have sufficient knowledge and the required skills to manage hypertension, some had reservations. Those who had reservations depicted their providers as not having sufficient competencies. They felt the providers focused on treating symptoms rather than conducting a proper disease diagnosis prior to treatment.

> *... it is better for the health worker to know the disease they are treating by examining the patient, but for them [referring to health workers] they just dish [give] medicine to patients based on whatever disease the patients mentions ... If you tell them [health workers]; 'I have headache due to over sleeping or that I have headache because I have fever', that is it – then he/she [health worker] will give you tablets to treat that.* (6 Bukamunye B_Female 2-*Buikwe, Rural*)

Providers implicated with such incompetence were mainly those operating at the lower level health facilities especially drug outlets, pharmacies, and rural health facilities. On the other hand, most patients had confidence in medical doctors. They also felt that hospitals were better prepared in managing hypertension compared to private and lower health facilities.

*Perceived Provider Attitudes towards Work and the Feeling of Being Treated with or without Respect.* Patients noted that providers exhibited different attitudes towards their work and their patients. They felt very comfortable seeking care from providers who were friendly. Some providers were implicated in having unwelcoming behaviours and negative attitudes towards patients. Examples of negative behaviours reported in this study included barking at patients, treating patients disrespectfully, and being unconcerned. Patients noted that it was common to find such behaviours in the public facilities. Most patients complemented private health facilities for their welcoming and caring attitudes. In fact, one patient stated that, in the private clinics, they are treated as customers which motivates them to seek care from the private clinics although he was also quick to speculate that the warm care was possibly because of the financial incentives [since patients pay for the service] and the strict leadership. Some patients also noted that they did not appreciate the decision making process that their providers followed while helping them to get appropriate remedy for their ailments. They felt that providers exhibited unnecessary delays, which resulted in negative health outcomes. One patient expressed dissatisfaction and wondered why the healthcare workers could not agree on the next course of action and refer her in a timely manner given that they were failing to diagnose and manage her condition.

> *Nurse ... 'her case cannot be handled here' ... 'we have to refer her to Mulago hospital; she will die here.' She would continue to tell the others to allow me go to Mulago stressing that they cannot handle me ... But there was a nurse who would prescribe medicine and tell me, 'These will work for you' so that's how I was. I would always go back to them complaining of not sleeping well; it was like that every time; until I got the doctor from Mulago.* (37 Namengo Female 1- *Buikwe, Urban*)

*Providers' Advising Role towards Their Patients.* In spite of the reported challenges with some modern health care providers, patients were to a greatest extent likely to follow the advice they received from their providers. Certain patients said that they were using herbal remedies because they had been advised to do so by their healthcare providers. However, others said that they were not using herbal remedies because their healthcare providers advised them against arguing that concurrent use of herbal and modern medicine could result in contraindications and that the efficacy and effectiveness of such medicines were not established. On the other hand, some traditional practitioners were also discouraging their patients from using modern medicines arguing that they were not effective.

> *I left Nagalaama [hospital] with some medicine and when I reached the herbalists' place they stopped me from taking modern medicine.* (17 Kabumba_female 2-*Mukono, Rural*)

Health care providers also advised patients on lifestyle modification. Some patients were advised on salt intake, dietary modification, physical activity, alcohol consumption, and smoking. But the patients were also keen on reporting that although they put effort in following their providers' advice, some of the advices were not contextually feasible.

> *... he told me not to eat many things; and yet I cannot stop eating some of those that he mentioned; he told me not to eat 'posho'; sweet potatoes ... and told me not to eat one meal; which is difficult in a village.* (20 Kateete Female 1-*Mukono Rural*)

*Perceived Quality of Care.* This theme generated conflicting reports. Some respondents felt that government hospitals provided high quality services compared to private health facilities in spite of the high patient loads and the long waiting time. On the other hand, patients commended private health providers for being swift in service provision, although they had concerns with regard to provider competencies in private facilities. Meanwhile, the majority felt that modern medicine had an edge over traditional medicine, although some respondents noted that the quality of traditional medicine is improving especially in terms of practice, dosing, and packaging.

*Patient Waiting Time at the Facility.* Patients noted that it was very stressful to spend the whole day at a health facility waiting to be treated. The long waiting time was attributed to (1) high patient volume vis-a-vis the limited number of health workers; (2) sluggishness and being unconcerned on the side of the healthcare workers, and (3) a lack of clear patient flow protocol that was characterised with favouritism and lack of respect.

> *it is because by the time you go to the hospital very early in the morning, you were feeling unwell but in the process of queuing in the hospital, there can come someone who knows the doctor and the person overtakes you – one thing that is annoying because you come to the hospital after you have slept unwell and only to be disappointed – do you see such a thing?* (Njeru_Female 1 *Buikwe, Rural*)

As a consequence, some patients stopped going to certain hospitals because of the long time they spend trying to get a service. Moreover, they reported that they had to cue at every service point (consultation room, laboratory room, and dispensing room). They felt very high workload and long waiting times were most prominent at public health facilities.

*3.2.2. Patient Related Factors.* Another overarching theme influencing compliance and health seeking behaviour for hypertension was "patient related factors." The subthemes building up this theme: (1) awareness about having the disease; (2) perceived severity or fear of the consequences of the disease; (3) beliefs about the effectiveness of the therapy; (4) concerns about adverse effects; and (5) the fear of dependency on long-term medication.

*Patients' Awareness about Having the Disease.* Awareness "the state of being aware or having knowledge that one is hypertensive" played critical role in HSB. Some patients reported presenting with no symptoms at the time of diagnosis, whereas others reported mild or severe symptoms as depicted by the following patients.

> *When I went to the first clinic, they checked me and they said that I was hypertensive – I couldn't believe it. I went to another clinic and they still measured my BP and they told me that I was hypertensive, I still didn't believe it. I went to the third clinic where they measured my BP again and they found me hypertensive and they even started me on the drugs to treat it.* (10 DFI_female 2-*Mukono, Urban*)
>
> Another patient reported, "I did not have any symptom; I was like any other normal person. I did not have rapid heartbeats" (14 Jagary Cable Female 1), and another one also narrated, "I really think that I had been hypertensive for quite a long time though I was unaware" (41 Ssaza_female 3-*Mukono, Urban*).

Respondents felt that creating awareness was dependent on having the patients' blood pressure measurements taken at a health facility or during a community outreach. However, they noted that opportunities to have their blood pressure measurements at the facilities or outreach sites were scarce. Because of the limited opportunities, and the asymptomatic nature of hypertension, most patients got to learn about their hypertension after experiencing severe symptoms or presenting with signs of end organ damage such as stroke.

> *I took long to know that I was hypertensive ... One time in 2000, I was taking my agricultural produce to Kampala for sale, while travelling I got a 'stroke' in the car. I was then taken to a KCC health facility in Kampala. They (health workers) checked and found that I had hypertension, so that's when it started. From that day I knew that I had hypertension. I went on receiving treatment up to this day.* (26 Kyamabale_male 1-*Buikwe, Rural*)

*Perceived Severity or Fear of the Consequences of the Disease.* Patients who had mild symptoms perceived themselves to be at low risk and were likely not to seek care for their hypertension.

> *... here in the village as long as you are still able to walk, there is no need of you monitoring your BP because you have hope that it will subside and you will get back to normal* (6 Bukumunye B_female 2). *I had the disease, but because it was not very serious I kept postponing going to the health facility. (31 Lusozi_male 3-Buikwe, Urban)*

Because of the low risk perceptions, such patients mainly depended on self-medication to treat symptoms or embraced a do nothing scenario. On the other hand, patients who perceived their disease to be severe especially after experiencing life-threatening symptoms were more likely to seek care promptly from bigger hospitals and avoid self-medication

> *... after surviving death, I no longer self-treat or cover up an illness [delay diagnosis]. (41 Ssaza_female 3-Mukono, Urban)*

*The Patient Beliefs about the Effectiveness of the Therapy or Recommended Advice.* Some patients' HSB and compliance were dependent on their perceptions about the effectiveness of the treatment or recommended provider advice. Effective remedies encouraged patients to return to their providers for refills, whereas patients who reported otherwise commonly reported trying out alternatives in search for better therapies.

> *I have managed to treat this disease (Hypertension) for the many years I have lived with*

*it. I have used various treatment methods. I first started with the modern method then later traditional medicine until now. However the traditional (medicine) has helped me more than the modern medicine.* (8 Bulamba_Bugungu_male 1-*Buikwe, Rural*)

Compliance based on perceived effectiveness of therapy applied both to modern as well as herbal medicine. Those who perceived herbal medicines to be effective in relieving their symptoms were likely to report usage of such remedies.

*I use the onions and the small egg plants – they help me a lot because whenever they bring them for me, I tend to feel better after using them* (34 Mayugwe Ssi_female 1-*Buikwe, Rural*). *It's very bitter and I know that hypertension can be controlled with bitter substances. When you take aloe vera, you feel well.* (6 Bulamba_Bugungu_male 1-*Buikwe, Rural*)

Similarly, those who perceived modern medicines to be effective were likely to report modern medicine usage.

*Well I went to the hospital and they diagnosed me with hypertension and they started me on the drugs and later in the process of seeking care from the modern health facility, there was someone who advised me to also use the traditional herbal medicine which I used for a short time and later realized that it was useless. So I returned to the modern health facility and they gave me the drugs to take.* (P 16: Ngogwe_Kikoota_ female 1-*Buikwe, Rural*)

A third category reported using both. This category perceived that using both modern and herbal remedies had complimentary effectiveness and resulted in better health outcomes.

*For the modern medicine, they can tell you to take one tablet a day (1 × 1) of which I have already taken it in the morning at around 8.00 AM. So by evening when I feel my BP raised due to the constant movements, that is when I take that Aloe Vera - it normalizes it and I finally sleep. (2 Bugga female 1-Buikwe, Rural)*

*Patients' Concerns about Adverse Effects.* Patients reported that some therapies were not tolerable. They were associated with unpleasant outcomes. Some noted that adverse effects of some medicines were worse off than their hypertension. On the other hand, if the remedy was tolerable, usage was more likely. These concerns were reported for modern medicines as well as herbal medicines.

*In the beginning they introduced me to start using herbal medicine; but when I started using it I realized that it had bad side effects; my hands and legs were swelling. So I stopped and remained on the modern medicine (14 Jagary_cable_female 1-Buikwe, Urban). I do not like the [modern] medicine they provide; the medicine is bitter; others are tiny others are big. It makes 'you' weak, and dizzy; even if 'you' have a baby crying next to 'you'; it's hard to carry the baby because 'you' get weak.* (29 Lusozi_female 2-*Buikwe, Urban*)

*The Fear of Life Long Dependence on Medicine.* Lifelong dependence on antihypertensive was perceived as a burden and some patients could not believe that they were ready for such a course of action. As a result, some patients reported that they swallowed drugs occasionally to try and avoid over dependency on medicine in controlling their hypertension.

*3.2.3. The Socioeconomic and Structural and Cultural Environment.* Besides, the healthcare and the patient related factors and several other issues were reported that influenced HSBs. We have summarized these factors under the socioeconomic and structural/cultural environment issues. More specifically, three topics were discussed: (1) education, information, and marketing of traditional medicine, (2) the patients' financial and social status, and (3) distance and transport.

*(1) Education, Information, and Marketing of Traditional Medicine.* Education, information, and marketing greatly influenced the use of alternative medicine for hypertension in this population. Patients reported that traditional practitioners, distributors, and proponents of herbal medicines embraced the power of sociomarketing, education, and active information sharing about their products. The most popular avenues of communication and promotion of herbal remedies included media houses such as radios and television, door-to-door information and drug distribution, and use of public address system in populated areas such as markets and assembly places.

*They give us the herbal medicine that is packed in the bottles and sold on the cars that pass by advertising the herbal medicine for the people to buy. They say that their medicines heal every sickness. So I buy those Rwenzori bottles with herbal medicine and take.* (23 Kikoota_female 1 *– Buikwe Rural*)

Another patient stated, "I would listen to him (traditional health practitioner) over the radio – that was before he went to the television; because up to date he is still on the radio and on the television. I listened to him and then I got his telephone contact and first I rang him and then I went there to see him" (11 DFI_male 1-*Mukono, Urban*).

On the other hand, no data was generated about efforts to use education, information, and marketing strategies to promote modern health care for hypertension.

*(2) The Patient's Financial and Social Status.* Financial and socioeconomic status of the patients was critical in influencing compliance and HSBs of patients with hypertension. Specifically, financial and social aspects included the ability of the patients to meet their healthcare needs, family support,

and advice from significant others. Most patients reported that hypertension was a lifetime disease that in the long run was too expensive. In fact some of them said they were already struggling with more pressing basic needs of life such as food and children school fees, which took precedence over their hypertension problems. For example, this patient narrated her story:

> *... its money; because you may have the money and think you will go [to the hospital] at the end of the week and then there comes a person who needs the money more than you do, for example your child calls saying mammy send me money; there is this problem; so you decide to send the money to them; so you postpone and say I will go next week. So it gets to that; you later realize you spent two months without treatment.* (20 Kateete_female 1-*Mukono, Rural*)

On the other hand, those who had better financial standing were more likely to seek care for their hypertension.

> *I don't have money problem to buy medicine. I have my work which earns me money that I use to buy medicine.* (1 Anthony male 1-*Mukono, Urban*)

In addition, patients with family members [children or other relatives] with better financial standing were reportedly supported to enhance their HSBs for hypertension.

> *In fact my children and my brothers' money have been spent big time – most especially my son's money has been spent so much because he wishes me to get better but all in vain.* (Mayugwe_Female 2-*Buikwe, Rural*)

Family members also provided patients with psychosocial and moral support as well as reminding them about their scheduled appointments, drug refills, and taking the medicines. Moreover, acquaintances such as friends, community members with similar challenges, or community resource persons such as religious leaders were also reported. These particularly played a key role in providing guidance to patient on whether to use modern or traditional medicine.

*(3) Distance and Transport.* The study shows that transport, distance, and related costs influenced health seeking behaviour of patients for hypertension. Patients from far-off areas (mainly rural) incurred higher costs of transport compared to their counterparts from urban neighbourhoods and those near the health facilities. Moreover, means of transport were not always reliably available in some settings. Consequently, rural residents commonly reported transport as a key barrier to seeking care, including adhering to scheduled hospital appointments.

> *The only challenge I faced was lack of transport; the place was really far so it was hard to go there on foot.* (P 8: 16 Kabumba_female 1-*Mukono Rural*)

On the other hand, urban resident either did not mention transport as a barrier or they reported ease of access to health facilities as a motivator to seek care for their hypertension.

> *It's because I am near the hospital so I don't spend on transport to go to Kawolo hospital. I just walk to the hospital.* (P 6: 14 Jagary_cable_ female 1-*Mukono, Rural*)

## 4. Discussion

The study shows that most patients in this setting utilise varied channels of care for their hypertension. In spite of the varied health seeking behaviours (HSBs), 8 in 10 patients interviewed in this qualitative study had uncontrolled hypertension. Insufficient hypertension control is prevalent in most of Sub-Saharan Africa [13] and data suggest that these high levels of uncontrolled hypertension are attributed to non-compliance, difficulty in obtaining medication, poverty, and poor access to health care [14–16]. In addition, health system deficiencies such as lack of antihypertensive medication and long distance to facilities have been implicated in affecting HSBs and control of hypertension [13, 17, 18]. Similarly, our study found that a range of health system challenges such as inadequate services, high cost of services and medicines, frequent drug stock outs, and quality concerns were strongly attributed to noncompliance and poor HSB patterns for hypertension.

In addition, HSBs were influenced by awareness, perceived severity, perceived effectiveness of recommended intervention/therapy, concerns about adverse effects, and fear of long-term dependence on medication. The influence of awareness on HSBs for hypertension is well established [11, 32]. Being aware of one's hypertension status is critical in initiation of care and impacts on self-care management practices [32] and is associated with reduced hypertension related complications and mortalities. However, availability and access to BP monitors were reported as a challenge in this study. However, perceived disease severity was critical in determining treatment compliance and HSB. In fact some of the patients reported that it was not necessary for them to continue with treatment or go to hospital if they felt well. On the other hand, manifestation of symptoms enhanced their compliance and HSBs. With mild symptoms, they mostly self-treated with herbal or modern medicines or consulted with providers at lower level health facilities including drug shops and pharmacies, whereas patients with severe symptoms reportedly sought care from hospitals or higher level health centers. The behaviours of these patients are consistent with those of the Koreans in the stroke study whose choice of care depended on their perceived severity of symptoms. For those who perceived themselves to have mild symptoms, they used over-the-counter drugs and folk remedies or visited health care facilities such as drugstores, public health agency, herbal clinic, or hospital [33]. These findings confirm the assertion that signs and symptoms influence people to seek diagnosis and treatment. The patients contemplate about the symptoms and then decide to take appropriate actions according to their perceived degree of disease severity [33]. When they perceive that the disease is very severe, they seek more specialised care but if they feel that the disease is less severe, they embark on self-care to try and resolve the discomfort.

HSBs were also influenced by the perceived effectiveness of the recommended treatment advice and this factor applied to modern as well as herbal alternative usage. Similar findings have been reported before [34–36]. In our previous study, use of traditional medicine was associated with the perception that herbal medicines were effective [34] and in Nigeria, patients strongly considered herbal medicines as viable alternative for a cure for their hypertension [37].

Another key factor was experiencing adverse reactions. Some patients reported that they experienced terrible side effects which were regarded worse off than their hypertension. Likewise, patients in Nigeria stopped medication as a result of experienced side effects [36]. Additional studies in Nigeria [11, 36], Democratic Republic of Congo [14], and Vietnam [3] have reported similar findings.

Health seeking behaviour was to a greater extent also influenced by the socioeconomic status of patients and structural and cultural factors. Patients with better socioeconomic standing had better compliance and better health seeking behaviour. The former were more likely to afford both the direct and indirect costs of health care, whereas the later, even basic amenities of life such as food, was sometimes a problem. Osamor argued that when people are hungry, nothing else matters to them except food [36]. Similar findings related to socioeconomic status and its influence on compliance and health seeking behaviour have been reported in other settings [38, 39]. In South Africa, authors reported that patients with greater economic resources were more likely to seek treatment from private doctors and spend considerably more for all types of health services compared to their counterparts in the low socioeconomic index [39]. Likewise in Nigeria, poor socioeconomic status, low level of education, unemployment, lack of effective social support networks, unstable living conditions, long distance from treatment center, and high cost of transport negatively influenced treatment compliance and health seeking behaviours for hypertension [38].

## 5. Implications for Policy and Practice

These findings have significant policy and practical implications on the delivery of services for hypertension. These revolve around the need for educating both the patients and the general population on hypertension, conducting routine screening, ensuring continuity of care, adherence to treatment, patient provider relations, organisation of services to minimize multiple movements across service points, availing services, and enhancing competences of staff.

Although the multiple channels of care for hypertension increase the reach of the services, the channels make it difficult for providers to monitor treatment success rates. Nonetheless, it is unlikely that the patients' behaviour of seeking care from various channels will stop in the near future as long as the comparative advantages of the different care pathways remain. For example, self-medication is comparatively cheaper and saves a lot of patients' time. Yet, it denies the patient the opportunity to receive professional management of the disease which may result in disease complication due to poor management. Therefore, empowering lower level facilities including private drug outlets through training, support supervision, and regulations may be harnessed to reduce risks of self-medication and enhance screening and monitoring, drug refills, and referral compliance. This empowerment would also reduce the challenges related to distance and access especially among the rural folks. On the other hand, higher level facilities should progressively be exempted from routine screening and monitoring which contributes to high patient volumes but instead be equipped and motivated to deal with referral cases in a timely manner. Meanwhile, it is also desirable to enhance the integration of traditional health practice with modern practice to bridge the gaps. Such integration would reduce bickering and situations where traditional health practitioners advice patients not to use prescribed modern medicines. Moreover, increased integration would increase interest in understanding traditional medicine and exploring its efficacy and effectiveness. With the increasing burden of chronic disease, a more sustainable financing mechanism is also warranted. A life time disease like hypertension in the long run becomes unaffordable even to the middle income category in this population. Hence, noncompliance and poor seeking behaviour and related negative health outcomes are inevitable. Exploring feasibility of instituting insurance schemes for chronic disease is recommended.

The patient related barriers have also significant implications. Jin and colleagues recommend that therapy related concerns should be addressed to contribute positively in improving patient's compliance. Prescribing medication with noninvasive route of administration and simple dosing regimens might motivate patients to be compliant [40]. Long duration of treatment period and medication side effects might compromise patient's beliefs about medication effectiveness. Therefore, healthcare providers should consider therapy related problems when designing the therapy plan and involve the patients in the process to minimize the possible therapeutic barriers [40].

## 6. Strengths and Limitations

This qualitative study highlights the factors influencing compliance and health seeking behaviour for hypertension among aware hypertensive patients in Mukono and Buikwe Districts in Uganda. The strength of the study lies in accruing the patients in their natural environment and learning from their experiences by using interviews in the community at the patients' homes. The patients were purposively selected to obtain a varied sample comprising of different gender, residential status, and district of residence. Limited transferability can be claimed given the small scale sized nature of the study which was conducted in only two districts in Uganda. Despite these limitations, the findings are insightful and of practical importance for programs and intervention trials aimed at feasible strategies to lower hypertension in this population.

## 7. Conclusions

Hypertension control among aware hypertensive patients in this setting is very low with eight in ten of patients aware of their hypertension not controlled. These control levels are attributable to poor compliance and health seeking behaviours which in turn are influenced by a number of factors which are closely related to the health system, the patient, and the socioeconomic circumstances and the culture of using traditional medicines. Strategies are needed to improve hypertension control in this population. Such strategies should leverage the opportunities at the various levels and traditions of care and address the barriers to health seeking behaviours.

## Appendix

### Factors Influencing Health Seeking Behaviours of Hypertensive Patients in Mukono and Buikwe in Uganda

*Qualitative Interview Guide*

(1) For how long have you had (known that you have) hypertension?

(2) What are you're own thoughts about the cause of your hypertension?

(3) How did you get to know that you had hypertension?

  (a) Probe for symptoms and diagnosis.

  (b) How did you deal with those symptoms before you got diagnosed?

    (i) Probe for things the patient did before he/she got actually diagnosed with hypertension (selftreatment, traditional healers, ...)

  (c) How and when did you decide to seek treatment, what changed?

    (i) Probe for change in symptoms, or things that might have encouraged them to actually go and seek help

    (ii) How did they actually seek help, who helped them in making that decision where to go

    (iii) how was the process of seeking help (meaning did you see many different people before actually seeing a doctor, how did you become diagnosed with hypertension)

(4) Can you explain the care and treatment process from the time you discovered that you are hypertensive?

  (a) Probe for access to treatment and care (traditional healers, drug shops, self medication with herbs or modern medicine, health care facilities)

    (i) Probe for barriers and facilitators

  (b) frequency of blood pressure monitoring and who monitors this?

  (c) Who helps you deal with your hypertension (family, neighbours, Village health team member (VHT))

  (d) What do they help you with?

  (e) Adherance to treatment and defaults.

(5) Since you became hypertensive, have you used any other methods to treat your hypertension?

  (a) Probe for herbs or other things that they might have tried

    (i) If yes, where do you get them from?

    (ii) Does that interfere with your other medication (if used)

    (iii) Why do you use herbs for your hypertension?

    (iv) Can you explain how you came to use these products (who introduced you to these methods)

(6) Since you became hypertensive, have you visited or consulted a traditional healer for your hypertension?

  (a) Probe for advice and treatment received, experience with the treatment or advice

  (b) What influenced your decision to go to the traditional healer for your hypertension?

  (c) How were you treated?

(7) Since you became hypertensive, have you been to a modern healthcare facility (health center, hospital or private clinic) for your hypertension? If yes:

  (a) Probe for treatment and advice recieved, level of satisfaction

  (b) What influcend your decision to go to a modern healthcare facility for your hypertension?

  (c) How where you treated?

(8) What is your preferred healthcare service provider (modern or traditional)? Explain your preference, why do you choose one over the other or both and why?

(9) What recommendations would you make that can help hypetensive patients to seek care from modern healthcarefacility?

We are now at the end of the interview and the questions I wanted to ask you. Are there any other issues you find important regarding this topic that we did not talk about? What?

Thank you for your valuable time and accepting to participate in this study.

## Disclosure

The funders had no role in study design, data collection and analysis, decision to publish, or preparation of the manuscript.

## Authors' Contributions

Geofrey Musinguzi contributed to the study design and conception, study implementation, data analysis, and interpretation of results, wrote the initial draft of the manuscript, and edited the final submitted version. Sibyl Anthierens contributed to conceptualisation, development of study tools, and interpretation of results, conducted data analysis, and participated in peer writing. Fred Nuwaha contributed to study design, conceptualisation, and training research assistants, reviewed the draft manuscript, and provided useful comments. Jean-Pierre Van Geertruyden contributed to data analysis, interpretation, and manuscript writing. Rhoda K. Wanyenze contributed to interpretation of results, manuscript writing, and critical review of the manuscript. Hilde Bastiaens contributed to conceptualisation, development of study tools, data analysis, and interpretation of results and participated in peer writing. All authors have read and approved the final manuscript.

## Acknowledgments

The authors would like to acknowledge the research assistants, the mobilisers, the study participants, and district health officers of Mukono and Buikwe. This study has received funding from the European Union's Horizon 2020 Research and Innovation Programme under Grant agreement no. 733356 (SPICES project) and the Flemish Interuniversity Council (VlIR-UOS) through the HEFS Platform Harvest Call (ZIUS2013VOA0902).

## References

[1] S. S. Lim, T. Vos, A. D. Flaxman, G. Danaei, K. Shibuya et al., "comparative risk assessment of burden of disease and injury attributable to 67 risk factors and risk factor clusters in 21 regions, 1990–2010: a systematic analysis for the Global Burden of Disease Study 2010," *The Lancet*, vol. 380, no. 9859, pp. 2224–2260, 2012.

[2] P. M. Kearney, M. Whelton, K. Reynolds, P. Muntner, P. K. Whelton, and J. He, "Global burden of hypertension: analysis of worldwide data," *The Lancet*, vol. 365, no. 9455, pp. 217–223, 2005.

[3] PT. Son, *Hypertension in Vietnam from Community-Based Studies to A National Targeted Programme*, 2012.

[4] D. Hoel, "Hypertension Stacking the silent killer," *Postgraduate Medical Journal*, vol. 101, no. 2, pp. 116–121, 1997.

[5] J. K. Cruickshank, J. C. Mbanya, R. Wilks et al., "Hypertension in four African-origin populations: Current 'Rule of Halves', quality of blood pressure control and attributable risk of cardiovascular disease," *Journal of Hypertension*, vol. 19, no. 1, pp. 41–46, 2001.

[6] WHO, *Global Status Report on Noncommunicable Diseases 2010*, World Health Organization, Geneva, 2011.

[7] WHO, *Impact of out-of-pocket payments for treatment of non-communicable diseases in developing countries: A review of literature WHO Discussion Paper*, World Health Organization, Geneva, 2011.

[8] Conner M. N. P., "The theory of planned behaviour and health behaviours," in *Predicting Health Behaviours: Research and Practice with Social Cognition Models*, M. Conner and P. Norman, Eds., pp. 121–162, Open University Press, Buckingham, 1996.

[9] K. Hjelm and F. Atwine, "Health-care seeking behaviour among persons with diabetes in Uganda: an interview study," *BMC International Health and Human Rights*, vol. 11, no. 1, article 11, 2011.

[10] M. Ali and A. de Muynck, "Illness incidence and health seeking behaviour among street children in Rawalpindi and Islamabad, Pakistan - A qualitative study," *Child: Care, Health and Development*, vol. 31, no. 5, pp. 525–532, 2005.

[11] B. S. Godfrey and S. I. I. Iyalomhe, "Hypertension-related knowledge, attitudes and life-style practices among hypertensive patients in a sub-urban Nigerian community," *Journal of Public Health and Epidemiology*, vol. 2, no. 4, pp. 71–77, 2010.

[12] J. Benson and N. Britten, "What effects do patients feel from their antihypertensive tablets and how do they react to them? Qualitative analysis of interviews with patients," *Journal of Family Practice*, vol. 23, no. 6, pp. 80–87, 2006.

[13] J. Kayima, R. K. Wanyenze, A. Katamba, E. Leontsini, and F. Nuwaha, "Hypertension awareness, treatment and control in Africa: a systematic review," *BMC Cardiovascular Disorders*, vol. 13, article 54, 2013.

[14] J.-P. F. Lubaki, L. Mabuza, N. Malete, P. Maduna, and J. V. Ndimande, "Reasons for non-compliance among patients with hypertension at Vanga hospital, Bandundu Province, Democratic Republic of Congo: A qualitative study," *African Journal of Primary Health Care and Family Medicine*, vol. 1, no. 1, pp. 107–111, 2009.

[15] P. A. Bourne, "Impact of poverty, not seeking medical care, unemployment, inflation, self-reported illness, and health insurance on mortality in Jamaica," *North American Journal of Medical Science*, pp. 99–109, 2009.

[16] P. Bourne, "Health literacy and health seeking behavior among older men in a middle-income nation," *Patient Related Outcome Measures*, p. 39.

[17] J. E. Pires, Y. V. Sebastião, A. J. Langa, and S. V. Nery, "Hypertension in Northern Angola: Prevalence, associated factors, awareness, treatment and control," *BMC Public Health*, vol. 13, no. 1, article no. 90, 2013.

[18] I. I. Ulasi, C. K. Ijoma, B. J. C. Onwubere, E. Arodiwe, O. Onodugo, and C. Okafor, "High prevalence and low awareness of hypertension in a market population in Enugu, Nigeria," *International Journal of Hypertension*, vol. 2011, Article ID 869675, 5 pages, 2011.

[19] J. Moodley, "Maternal deaths associated with hypertension in South Africa : lessons to learn from the Saving Mothers report, 2005-2007," *Cardiovascular Journal of Africa*, pp. 31–35, 2011.

[20] C. Lenfant, A. V. Chobanian, D. W. Jones, and E. J. Roccella, "Seventh report of the Joint National Committee on the prevention, detection, evaluation, and treatment of high blood pressure (JNC 7): resetting the hypertension sails," *Hypertension*, vol. 41, no. 6, pp. 1178-1179, 2003.

[21] P. Isaakidis, M.-E. Raguenaud, C. Say et al., "Treatment of hypertension in rural Cambodia: Results from a 6-year programme," *Journal of Human Hypertension*, vol. 25, no. 4, pp. 241–249, 2011.

[22] R. Beaglehole, J. Epping-Jordan, V. Patel et al., "Improving the prevention and management of chronic disease in low-income and middle-income countries: a priority for primary health care," *The Lancet*, vol. 372, no. 9642, pp. 940–949, 2008.

[23] MoH, *Health Sector Strategic and Investment Plan 2010/11–2014/15*, Ministry of Health, Kampala, Uganda, 2010.

[24] R. W. Mayega, S. Etajak, E. Rutebemberwa, G. Tomson, and J. Kiguli, "'Change means sacrificing a good life': Perceptions about severity of type 2 diabetes and preventive lifestyles among people afflicted or at high risk of type 2 diabetes in Iganga Uganda," *BMC Public Health*, vol. 14, no. 1, article no. 864, 2014.

[25] D. Maher, L. Smeeth, and J. Sekajugo, "Health transition in Africa: Practical policy proposals for primary care," *Bulletin of the World Health Organization*, vol. 88, no. 12, pp. 943–948, 2010.

[26] G. Musinguzi, J.-P. Van Geertruyden, H. Bastiaens, and F. Nuwaha, "Uncontrolled hypertension in Uganda: A comparative cross-sectional study," *The Journal of Clinical Hypertension*, vol. 17, no. 1, pp. 63–69, 2015.

[27] UBOS, *National Population and Housing Census 2014 Area Specific Profiles Uganda Bureau of Statistics*, 2014.

[28] G. Musinguzi, H. Bastiaens, R. K. Wanyenze, A. Mukose, J.-P. Van Geertruyden, and F. Nuwaha, "Capacity of health facilities to manage hypertension in Mukono and Buikwe districts in Uganda: Challenges and recommendations," *PLoS ONE*, vol. 10, no. 11, Article ID e0142312, 2015.

[29] G. Musinguzi, F. Nuwaha, and N. Ashton, "Prevalence, awareness and control of hypertension in Uganda," *PLoS ONE*, vol. 8, no. 4, Article ID e62236, 2013.

[30] V. Braun and V. Clarke, "Using thematic analysis in psychology," *Qualitative Research in Psychology*, vol. 3, no. 2, pp. 77–101, 2006.

[31] H. F. Hsieh and S. E. Shannon, "Three approaches to qualitative content analysis," *Qualitative Health Research*, vol. 15, no. 9, pp. 1277–1288, 2005.

[32] T. S. Ferguson, M. K. Tulloch-Reid, N. O. Younger, S. R. McFarlane, D. K. Francis, and R. J. Wilks, "Prehypertension in Jamaica: A review of data from recent studies," *West Indian Medical Journal*, vol. 60, no. 4, pp. 429–433, 2011.

[33] H.-S. Oh and H.-A. Park, "Decision-tree model of treatment-seeking behaviors after detecting symptoms by Korean stroke patients.," *Taehan Kanho Hakhoe chi*, vol. 36, no. 4, pp. 662–670, 2006.

[34] F. Nuwaha and G. Musinguzi, "Use of alternative medicine for hypertension in Buikwe and Mukono districts of Uganda: A cross sectional study," *BMC Complementary and Alternative Medicine*, vol. 13, article no. 301, 2013.

[35] D. A. Oke and E. O. Bandele, "Misconceptions of hypertension," *Journal of the National Medical Association*, vol. 96, no. 9, pp. 1221–1224, 2004.

[36] P. E. Osamor, *Health Care Seeking For Hypertension In South West Nigeria*, Medical Sociology Online, 2011.

[37] D. A. Oke and E. O. Bandele, "Misconceptions of hypertension," *J Natl Med Assoc*, vol. 96, pp. 1221–1224, 2004.

[38] M. R. Akpa, D. I. Agomuoh, and O. J. Odia, "Drug compliance among hypertensive patients in Port Harcourt, Nigeria," *Nigerian Journal of Medicine*, vol. 14, no. 1, pp. 55–57, 2005.

[39] R. J. Petrella, E. P. Merikle, and J. Jones, "Prevalence, treatment, and control of hypertension in primary care: gaps, trends, and opportunities.," *Journal of clinical hypertension (Greenwich, Conn.)*, vol. 9, no. 1, pp. 28–35, 2007.

[40] J. Jin, G. E. Sklar, O. V. Min Sen, and L. S. Chuen, "Factors affecting therapeutic compliance: a review from the patient's perspective," *Therapeutics and Clinical Risk Management*, vol. 4, no. 1, pp. 269–286, 2008.

16

# Epidemiology of Hypertension Stages in Two Countries in Sub-Sahara Africa: Factors Associated with Hypertension Stages

**Kirubel Zemedkun Gebreselassie[1] and Mojgan Padyab[2]**

[1]*Epidemiology and Global Health, Department of Public Health and Clinical Medicine, Umeå University, 901 85 Umeå, Sweden*
[2]*Centre for Population Studies, Ageing and Living Conditions Programme, Umeå University, Umeå, Sweden*

Correspondence should be addressed to Kirubel Zemedkun Gebreselassie; kirubelgebresilassie@yahoo.com

Academic Editor: Olugbenga Ogedegbe

Studies using the revised hypertension classification are needed to better understand epidemiology of hypertension across full distribution. The sociodemographic, biological, and health behavior characteristics associated with different stages of hypertension in Ghana and South Africa (SA) were studied using global ageing and adult health (SAGE), WAVE 1 dataset. Blood pressure was assessed for a total of 7545 respondents, 2980 from SA and 4565 from Ghana. Hypertension was defined using JNC7 blood pressure classification considering previous diagnosis and treatment. Multivariate multinomial logistic regression analysis using Stata version 12 statistical software was done to identify independent predictors. The weighted prevalence of prehypertension and hypertension in Ghana was 30.7% and 42.4%, respectively, and that of SA was 29.4% and 46%, respectively, showing high burden. After adjusting for the independent variables, only age (OR = 1.32, 95% CI: 1.14–1.53), income (OR = 1.9, 95% CI: 1.04–3.47), and BMI (OR = 1.16, 95% CI: 1.1–1.22) remained independent predictors for stage 1 hypertension in Ghana, while, for SA, age (OR = 2.27, 95% CI: 1.53–3.36), sex (OR = 0.28, 95% CI: 0.08–1), and BMI (OR = 1.15, 95% CI: 1.07–1.25) were found to be independent predictors of stage 1 hypertension. Healthy lifestyle changes and policy measures are needed to promptly address these predictors.

## 1. Introduction

Worldwide prevalence estimates for hypertension may be as much as 1 billion individuals, and approximately 7.1 million deaths per year may be attributable to hypertension. The World Health Organization reports that suboptimal systolic blood pressure (SBP) >115 mmHg is responsible for 62 percent of cerebrovascular disease and 49 percent of ischemic heart disease (IHD), with little variation by sex [1]. Hypertension has been identified as the leading risk factor for developing congestive heart failure [2], stroke [3], chronic kidney disease, and end stage renal disease [4] and is ranked third as a cause of disability-adjusted life-years [5].

The risk of developing these complications depends on the level of elevated blood pressure and has been seen in all age groups starting from blood pressure as low as SBP 115 and DBP of 75 [6]. Data from observational studies involving more than 1 million individuals have also indicated that death from both IHD and stroke increases progressively and linearly from levels as low as 115 mmHg SBP and 75 mmHg DBP upward especially in individuals ranging from 40 to 89 years of age, indicating need for new blood pressure classification [6]. The risk of coronary heart disease increased significantly in the high range prehypertension individuals (SBP 130–139 or DBP 85–89 mmHg) but not in the low range prehypertensive population (SBP from 120 to 129 or DBP 80 to 84 mmHg) [7].

Because of the new data on lifetime risk of hypertension and the highly increased risk of cardiovascular morbidity associated with levels of BP previously considered to be normal, the JNC 7 report has introduced a new classification that includes the term "prehypertension" for those with BPs ranging from 120 to 139 mmHg systolic and/or 80 to 89 mmHg diastolic. This new designation is intended to identify those individuals in whom early intervention by adoption of healthy lifestyles could reduce BP, decrease the rate of progression of BP to hypertensive levels with age, or prevent hypertension entirely [8]. Robust population-based data using these recent blood pressure categories are still needed to confirm prior estimates and inform policy decision makers in Sub-Saharan Africa.

Increasing urbanization has fueled social and economic changes in Sub-Saharan Africa, which have contributed to a surge in noncommunicable disease (NCD), including hypertension [9]. Epidemiological studies on hypertension in this region have been conducted over the years in an attempt to estimate the burden of hypertension, and these have reported variable rates within and between different population groups. In the first national Demographic and Health Survey, of 12,952 randomly selected South Africans aged 15 years, a high risk of hypertension was associated with less than tertiary education, older age groups, overweight and obese people, excess alcohol use, and a family history of stroke and hypertension [10]. Prehypertension was also more common in those aged 35 years compared with those aged <35 years and in overweight and obese people compared with people of normal weight [11]. Hypertension was defined in these studies as individuals with self-reported treated hypertension or with an average of 2 blood pressure measurements of at least 140/90 mmHg [9, 12, 13].

Prior studies on hypertension mainly focused on these dichotomous definitions of hypertension and did not examine the sociodemographic characteristics and risk factors for hypertension across full distribution of blood pressure. The current study follows the work of Basu and Millet on social epidemiology of hypertension in low- and middle-income countries from World Health Organization's Study on global AGEing and adult health (SAGE) [13]. Their work further showed additional variation in hypertension prevalence and social determinants of awareness when categorical definitions of hypertension were used compared to dichotomous definitions. Men had significantly lower probability of hypertension awareness than women at stage 1, but not at stage 2 [14]. This empirical study with an objective of studying social determinants and risk factors of different stages of hypertension tries to address this question. It determines the prevalence and independent predictors of different stages of hypertension in two countries in Sub-Saharan Africa, Ghana and South Africa.

## 2. Methods

*2.1. Study Design and Population.* We conducted a cross-sectional analysis of the Study on global AGEing and adult health (SAGE), WAVE 1 dataset which is a part of longitudinal survey program in WHO's multicountries study unit. The main SAGE surveys compile comparable longitudinal information on the health and well-being of adult populations and the ageing process from nationally representative samples in six middle- and low-income countries. We used the dataset of two Sub-Saharan countries, Ghana and South Africa. The SAGE study included nationally representative sample of persons aged 50 years and sample from younger adults aged 18–49 years as comparison which were also selected from both countries. Multistage cluster sampling was used [15]. The sampling design entailed two-stage probabilistic sample that yielded national and subnational estimates. In the first stage, a total sample of 600 enumeration areas (EA) in South Africa and 300 (EA) in Ghana were drawn from the master sample and used as the primary selection units (PSU). The second stage of the sample design was the selection of households from the EA's which formed the secondary sampling units. This stage of the process involved georeferenced aerial photograph maps of urbanized areas on which the locations of households were plotted. The total sample size of individuals was targeted to be 1000 people in the age group 18–49 years and 5000 people aged 50 years or older in each country.

*2.2. Questionnaire.* We recorded information about the household members from household and individual questionnaires; living place variable from the household questionnaire and sociodemographic characteristics, work history, blood pressure measurements, and risk factors including preventive health behaviors were taken from the individual questionnaire. Both the household and individual questionnaires were translated into six local South African and three local languages of Ghana. The respondents were interviewed face to face.

*2.3. Blood Pressure Measurements and Classification.* Blood pressure was measured three times while the respondent seated using automated OMRON R6 Wrist Blood Pressure Monitor, HEM-6000-E, Health Care Europe, B.V., Hoofddorp, The Netherlands. Such digital monitors have been shown to have high degree of agreement with mercury sphygmomanometers for systolic blood pressure [16, 17]. Average blood pressure was calculated arithmetically for the 3 measurements of each systolic and diastolic blood pressure. Missing values were excluded from being included in the study. Blood pressure classification was done using JNC 7 algorithm [1]. Prehypertension was defined as systolic blood pressure (SBP) measurement of 120–139 mmHg or diastolic blood pressure (DBP) of 80–89 mmHg. Stage 1 hypertension was defined as SBP of 140–159 mmHg or DBP of 90–99 mmHg and stage 2 as SBP of greater than or equal to 160 mmHg or DBP of greater than or equal to 100 mmHg. Accordingly normal pressure was defined as SBP of less than 120 mmHg and DBP of less than 80 mmHg.

All respondents were initially asked if they have ever been diagnosed with hypertension and if they did, whether or not they have been taking any kind of drugs or other treatment for the last 2 weeks and last 12 months. Normal blood pressure was defined as SBP <120 and DBP <80 mmHg and either no previous history of diagnosis or not taking antihypertensive medication. Those with SBP of 120 or more and DBP of 80 or more who did not have prior diagnosis nor treatment were designed as to have hypertension. They were subsequently stratified into three mutually exclusive different stages of hypertension. Those who reported as either having a diagnosis of hypertension previously or taking antihypertensive medication were excluded from analysis due to overlapping.

*2.4. Sociodemographic Characteristics.* All participants older than 18 years, of both sexes, were included in the study and classified as living in urban or rural area. Current marital status (married or single that included unmarried, widowed, or separated) was asked about using the individual questionnaire. Educational level was assessed by first asking whether respondents have been in any school, and those who answered yes were asked for the highest educational level completed according to the international standard classification of education [18]. Respondents were asked whether they had ever worked for pay, type of work, and employer. Occupation responses were written verbatim by the interviewer, then coded, and mapped to the International Standard Classifications of Occupations (ISCO) scheme [19]. Classification of income quintiles was based on permanent income estimates derived from household assets and characteristics of the dwelling upon which The 2001 WHO World Health Survey/SAGE WAVE 0 relied [15]. Recent alcohol intake was asked for by asking whether the respondents have consumed alcohol in the past 30 days. Response was documented as yes and no. Current smoking (yes or no), with provision for the collection of information on other forms of smoking apart from cigarettes, such as cigars, pipes, snuff, or chewing smokeless tobacco, was asked about. Question was formulated based on guidelines for controlling and monitoring the tobacco epidemic [20]. Work related and sport or leisure time physical activities were separately asked in a typical week. Vigorous or moderate physical activities required hard or moderate physical effort and caused an increase in breathing or heart rate for at least 10 minutes [21]. Fruit and vegetable servings in typical 24 hours were asked about. Inadequate intake was defined based on WHO recommendations and labeled as less than 5 servings (80 g per serving) on a typical day [22].

*2.5. Anthropometric Measurements.* Height was measured in centimeters after the respondents took off their shoes, put their feet and heels close together, stood straight, and stood forward with their back, head, and heels touching the wall. Next body weight was measured in kilograms. Body composition and fatness were assessed using WHO body mass index (BMI) derived from measured weight in kilograms and normalized by dividing by height in meters squared. It was categorized as underweight <18.5, normal weight 18.5–24.9, overweight 25 to 29.9, and obese greater than or equal to 30. Since abdominal obesity is highly correlated with atherosclerotic cardiovascular morbidity and mortality than BMI indices [23], waist circumference was also used to measure central obesity. The interviewer identified the top of the hip bone and after making sure the tape measure is parallel to the floor all the way around the body measured waist circumference (WC). The National Cholesterol and Education Program: Adult Treatment Panel III (NCEP: ATP III) guideline was used to designate central obesity: accordingly men with WC measurements greater than or equal to 102 cm and women with greater than or equal to 88 cm were considered to have one [24].

*2.6. Statistical Analysis.* Stata version 12 statistical software was used to analyze data after being cleaned. The individual and household data were merged together. Living place variable was taken from the household data while all the others were included from the individual dataset. To make sure the results of the individual country dataset represent the respective country population, weighting at the country level was done which was available in the SAGE dataset. Individual weights were poststratified according to the 2009 projected population estimates in Ghana and to the 2009 medium midyear population estimates in South Africa [25]. Weighted estimates of different stages of hypertension prevalence were reported as proportions of the actual sample size. Invalid blood pressure measurements such as values of diastolic blood pressure greater than systolic and those in the outliers were considered missing and excluded from analysis.

The associations between sociodemographic, biological, and health behavior variables and stages of hypertension (prehypertension, stage 1, and stage 2) were assessed in a two-step procedure where individuals with the different stages of hypertension were compared separately with those having normal blood pressure. In the first step, each variable was evaluated independently in a bivariate multinomial logistic regression analysis with different stages of hypertension as dependent variable to generate unadjusted OR with respondents' characteristics in each country separately. Those variables with $P$ values less than 0.2 were retained and entered into multinomial logistic regression model in ascending stepwise manner to determine variables that were independently associated with the stages of hypertension. A probability level of $P < 0.05$ was considered significant. Age and BMI variables were entered in the multivariable multinomial models as continuous due to fewer numbers of people in the most upper and lower categories. All other variables were retained as categorical.

*2.7. Ethical Approval.* Informed consent was obtained from each respondent for interviews and measurements of anthropometrics. SAGE study received ethical clearance from WHO ethical review committee [26].

## 3. Results

The total sample size of the study was 8939, 3974 from South Africa and 4965 from Ghana. Participants who have been diagnosed previously with high blood pressure or who were already taking treatment were excluded from analysis due to overlap and difficulty to stratify them into mutually exclusive hypertension stages. Those with previous diagnosis of hypertension were 587 (12%) in Ghana and 1,111 (28%) in South Africa. Individuals taking antihypertensive medications were 396 (8%) in Ghana and 981 (25%) in South Africa. Completed interview response in South Africa was 2853 (96%) and 5057 (99%) in Ghana. Of these blood pressure was assessed for a total of 7545, 2980 (75%) respondents from South Africa and 4565 (92%) from Ghana which was included for analysis (Table 1). A higher number of study participants in Ghana were males (50.2%) compared to 48.5% in South Africa. More people lived in Urban areas in South Africa (69.7%) compared to only 44.4% in Ghana. In South Africa,

Table 1: Sociodemographic, health behavior, and biological characteristics (%) of study subjects, by country and hypertension stages.

| $N$ = 7545 | Ghana ($n$ = 4565) | | | | | South Africa ($n$ = 2980) | | | | |
|---|---|---|---|---|---|---|---|---|---|---|
| | Normal | Pre-HTN | Stage 1 HTN | Stage 2 HTN | Total (%) | Normal | Pre-HTN | Stage 1 HTN | Stage 2 HTN | Total (%) |
| **Sociodemographic variables** | | | | | | | | | | |
| Age groups (years) | ** | | | | | ** | | | | |
| 18–49 | 28.1 | 32.6 | 20.5 | 18.8 | 762 (76.9) | 28.2 | 31.7 | 16.2 | 23.9 | 334 (79.7) |
| 50–59 | 20.1 | 23.2 | 28.3 | 28.4 | 1532 (9.4) | 9.1 | 20.9 | 24.9 | 45.1 | 1242 (11.1) |
| 60–69 | 18.5 | 24.7 | 23.1 | 33.7 | 1055 (6.3) | 6.9 | 20.6 | 28.5 | 44.1 | 803 (5.7) |
| 70–74 | 18.4 | 26.7 | 23.9 | 30.9 | 837 (5.1) | 9.5 | 15 | 33.1 | 42.4 | 424 (2.5) |
| 80+ | 19.0 | 27.6 | 24.5 | 29 | 374 (2.3) | 5.8 | 20.4 | 29.6 | 44.2 | 171 (1.1) |
| Sex | | | | | | * | | | | |
| Male | 26.2 | 29.3 | 20.7 | 23.8 | 2466 (50.2) | 16.4 | 33.9 | 18.5 | 31.2 | 1361 (48.5) |
| Female | 25.9 | 32.1 | 22.6 | 19.4 | 2099 (49.8) | 31.3 | 25.1 | 18.4 | 25.3 | 1617 (51.5) |
| Living place | | | | | | * | | | | |
| Urban | 23.6 | 30.3 | 24 | 22.2 | 1747 (44.4) | 28.3 | 28.6 | 18.3 | 24.9 | 1890 (69.7) |
| Rural | 28 | 31.1 | 19.8 | 21.1 | 2818 (55.6) | 14.7 | 31.4 | 18.2 | 35.7 | 1084 (30.3) |
| Marital status | | | | | | | | | | |
| Married | 25.6 | 28.1 | 23.8 | 22.5 | 1758 (26.6) | 28.9 | 29.1 | 19.5 | 22.6 | 1346 (46.5) |
| Single | 26.3 | 31.8 | 20.8 | 21.1 | 2782 (73.4) | 20 | 29.4 | 17.8 | 32.8 | 1578 (53.6) |
| Educational level | * | | | | | ** | | | | |
| No school | 21.9 | 27.6 | 22.1 | 28.4 | 2337 (31.1) | 7.7 | 20.8 | 22.4 | 49.1 | 647 (7.3) |
| <6 yrs | 29.3 | 30.3 | 23.5 | 17 | 498 (12.8) | 5.5 | 23.4 | 22.2 | 48.9 | 556 (13.9) |
| Primary | 26.4 | 29.3 | 24.8 | 19.6 | 567 (20.1) | 10.4 | 28.9 | 22 | 38.7 | 557 (13.9) |
| Secondary | 21.8 | 41.3 | 21 | 15.8 | 244 (10.9) | 35.2 | 26.2 | 17.4 | 21.3 | 391 (27.7) |
| High school | 29.5 | 32.3 | 18.2 | 20.1 | 737 (20.7) | 40.3 | 19.2 | 18.4 | 22.1 | 221 (29.1) |
| University | 36.8 | 28.8 | 18.2 | 16.3 | 154 (4.4) | 41.7 | 27.1 | 11.6 | 19.6 | 143 (8.1) |
| Occupation | * | | | | | | | | | |
| Public sector | 23.6 | 34.1 | 21.8 | 20.6 | 380 (7.2) | 26.9 | 30.1 | 10.7 | 32.4 | 395 (19.8) |
| Private | 26.7 | 20.1 | 24.1 | 29.1 | 180 (5.2) | 13.4 | 32.7 | 23 | 31 | 1421 (53.1 |
| Self-employed | 25 | 32.3 | 22 | 20.7 | 3564 (80.8) | 44 | 31.8 | 10.5 | 13.8 | 106 (4) |
| Informal | 25.2 | 24.0 | 15 | 35.8 | 332 (6.8) | 33.9 | 16.9 | 18.9 | 30.3 | 592 (23.1) |
| Income | ** | | | | | | | | | |
| Quintile 1 (poorest) | 33.4 | 28.3 | 21.5 | 16.9 | 939 (15.6) | 20 | 30 | 21.2 | 28.8 | 640 (19.6) |
| Quintile 2 | 33 | 29 | 16.9 | 21.1 | 932 (18) | 28.3 | 23.6 | 22.8 | 25.3 | 631 (20) |
| Quintile 3 | 19.3 | 31 | 20.8 | 28.8 | 922 (19.4) | 27.4 | 19.6 | 17.3 | 35.6 | 545 (20.2) |
| Quintile 4 | 18.8 | 34.8 | 24.6 | 21.8 | 921 (22.2) | 21.1 | 35.6 | 13 | 30.4 | 551 (19.5) |
| Quintile 5 (richest) | 28.2 | 29.6 | 23.2 | 19.1 | 845 (24.9) | 23.7 | 37.7 | 17.7 | 20.9 | 595 (20.8) |
| **Biological variables** | | | | | | | | | | |
| BMI (kg/m$^2$) | ** | | | | | ** | | | | |
| Underweight | 31 | 33 | 14.4 | 21.5 | 670 (9.3) | 21.1 | 35.7 | 8.2 | 35 | 130 (3.5) |
| Normal | 30.6 | 29.4 | 19.8 | 20.2 | 2543 (54.4) | 35.9 | 35.6 | 12.2 | 16.4 | 777 (36.1) |
| Overweight | 21.4 | 32.8 | 22.2 | 23.6 | 889 (24.2) | 32.4 | 21.2 | 21.4 | 25 | 849 (30) |
| Obese | 10.8 | 30.4 | 33.4 | 25.3 | 444 (12.1) | 5.7 | 23.2 | 25.7 | 45.4 | 1148 (30.5) |
| Waist circumference | * | | | | | | | | | |
| Normal | 27.9 | 29.9 | 20.2 | 22 | 3608 (76.7) | 24.5 | 32 | 18.4 | 25.1 | 1574 (63.2) |
| Abnormal | 20.2 | 32.8 | 26.2 | 20.9 | 930 (23.3) | 20 | 25.2 | 20.8 | 34 | 1180 (36.9) |
| **Health related behaviors** | | | | | | | | | | |
| Smoking | * | | | | | | | | | |
| No | 25.9 | 31.4 | 22.2 | 20.5 | 3416 (84.1) | 26.5 | 32.3 | 16.9 | 24.4 | 1819 (67.6) |

TABLE 1: Continued.

| N = 7545 | Ghana (n = 4565) Normal | Pre-HTN | Stage 1 HTN | Stage 2 HTN | Total (%) | South Africa (n = 2980) Normal | Pre-HTN | Stage 1 HTN | Stage 2 HTN | Total (%) |
|---|---|---|---|---|---|---|---|---|---|---|
| Yes | 26.2 | 27.6 | 18.8 | 27.5 | 1143 (15.9) | 19.1 | 23.2 | 22.2 | 35.6 | 1077 (32.4) |
| Current alcohol use | | | | | | | | | | |
| No | 25.9 | 31.7 | 20.7 | 21.7 | 1181 (44.3) | 25.4 | 21.2 | 31.2 | 22.2 | 347 (33.5) |
| Yes | 28.2 | 27.2 | 22.7 | 22 | 1492 (55.7) | 14.9 | 27.8 | 18.5 | 38.8 | 489 (66.5) |
| Work related physical activity | * | | | | | * | | | | |
| High | 25.5 | 33.5 | 19.9 | 21.2 | 1868 (44.7) | 30.7 | 15.6 | 27 | 26.7 | 306 (12.4) |
| Moderate | 29 | 28.7 | 22.5 | 19.7 | 1400 (27.5) | 33.3 | 28.1 | 14.5 | 24.1 | 852 (36.3) |
| Low | 23.5 | 28.5 | 23.7 | 24.3 | 1289 (27.8) | 16 | 33.6 | 19.3 | 31.1 | 1734 (51.4) |
| Fruit intake/day | * | | | | | ** | | | | |
| 0-1 | 25.7 | 27.9 | 23.9 | 22.5 | 1726 (32.3) | 17.6 | 24.9 | 21.1 | 36.4 | 1476 (46.3) |
| 2–4 | 28 | 31.9 | 19.8 | 20.3 | 2374 (57.8) | 29.8 | 34.2 | 17.4 | 18.6 | 1305 (50.2) |
| >=5 | 13.7 | 32.7 | 24.7 | 29 | 402 (9.9) | 37.8 | 9.2 | 7 | 46 | 79 (3.5) |
| Vegetable intake/day | * | | | | | ** | | | | |
| 0-1 | 29.9 | 24.1 | 24.5 | 21.5 | 1112 (24.9) | 14.9 | 24.8 | 24.4 | 35.9 | 1160 (35.7) |
| 2–4 | 24.1 | 32.4 | 21.2 | 22.3 | 3269 (74.3) | 30.8 | 32.7 | 15.3 | 21.2 | 1592 (60.6) |
| >=5 | 21.8 | 36.2 | 29.8 | 12.2 | 57 (0.9) | 5.4 | 10.1 | 21.7 | 62.9 | 116 (3.7) |
| Blood pressure number | 957 | 1205 | 1108 | 1295 | 4565 | 301 | 647 | 738 | 1294 | 2980 |
| Weighted prevalence (%) | 26.1 | 30.7 | 21.6 | 21.6 | | 24.1 | 29.4 | 18.5 | 28.1 | |

*$P < 0.2$, **$P < 0.05$.
$n$ = number of observations in the sample.
All percentages (%) are put as weighted estimates of the sample to represent population.

the proportion of obesity was 30.5% as compared to 12.1% in Ghana. Income quintile distribution was similar in both countries. Only 26.1% of the respondents in Ghana and 24.1% in South Africa fulfilled the definition of normal blood pressure. Prehypertension was more prevalent in Ghana (30.7%) than South Africa (29.4%). The weighted prevalence of hypertension (both stages 1 and 2) was 42.4% in Ghana and 46% in South Africa. The age group distribution across stages of hypertension was similar in both countries, the majority of prehypertensive individuals being in the age group of 18 to 49. Obese individuals constituted 45.4% of stage 2 hypertension in South Africa while they constituted only 25.3% of stage 2 hypertension in Ghana.

Prehypertension was significantly associated in Ghana with income distribution (OR = 1.9, 95% CI: 1.11–3.23) and BMI category (OR = 2.64, 95% CI: 1.11–6.3) in the bivariate multinomial analysis when compared with normal blood pressure measurement while in South Africa age (OR = 2.66, 95% CI: 1.34–5.28) and educational level (OR = 0.18, 95% CI: 0.05–0.63) only had a significant association (Table 2). Income and BMI remained to have a significant association with stage 1 hypertension. In addition age emerged as a new variable with significant correlation with stage 1 hypertension in Ghana in the bivariate analysis (OR = 1.71, 95% CI: 1.25–2.33). In South Africa stage 1 hypertension was significantly associated with age of the study participants (OR = 6.02, 95% CI: 2.61–13.88), educational level (OR = 0.09, 95% CI: 0.02–0.49), type of occupation (OR = 4.32, 95% CI: 1.06–17.55), BMI category (OR = 11.72, 95% CI: 2.35–58.43), and number of vegetable servings per day in the bivariate multinomial analysis (OR = 0.3, 95% CI: 0.11–0.82). Age, income, and BMI remained to be significantly associated with stage 2 hypertension in the bivariate multinomial analysis in Ghana. In addition educational level (OR = 0.07, 95% CI: 0.02–0.35) became a significant correlate with stage 2 hypertension. In South Africa factors significantly associated with stage 2 hypertension were age, living place, educational level, and fruit and vegetable intake.

## 4. Multinomial Logistic Regression Model with Pooled Multivariable Analysis

*4.1. Ghana.* For the multinomial logistic regression analysis, 10 independent variables which were associated with hypertension stages at level of $P$ value < 0.2 in the bivariate analysis were retained in the model. These were age, educational level, type of occupation, income quintile, smoking status, BMI category, abdominal waist circumference, work related physical activity, and fruit and vegetable intake per day. Those with $P$ values <0.05 in the multivariable model were considered statistically significant and were considered independent predictors of hypertension stages (Figure 1). At prehypertension level BMI (OR = 1.08, 95% CI: 1.03–1.14), income (OR = 2,24, 95% CI: 1.27–3.97), and number of vegetable intakes per day were found to be independent predictors after being adjusted for the other variables in the model. Income and BMI remained independent predictors

Table 2: Association between sociodemographic, health behavior, and biological variables with stages of hypertension (pre-HTN, stage 1, and stage 2) compared to normal blood pressure: bivariate multinomial analysis.

| $N$ = 7545 | Ghana ($n$ = 4565) Pre-HTN OR (95% CI) | Stage 1 OR (95% CI) | Stage 2 OR (95% CI) | South Africa ($n$ = 2980) Pre-HTN OR (95% CI) | Stage 1 OR (95% CI) | Stage 2 OR (95% CI) |
|---|---|---|---|---|---|---|
| Age groups (years) | | | | | | |
| 18–49 | 1 | 1 | 1 | 1 | 1 | 1 |
| 50–59 | 1 (0.78–1.29) | 1.93 (1.47–2.54)* | 2.12 (1.59–2.83) | 2.06 (1.04–4.09) | 4.77 (2.13–10.67) | 5.88 (3.01–11.48) |
| 60–69 | 1.15 (0.86–1.54) | 1.71 (1.25–2.33)* | 2.72 (2.02–3.67) | 2.66 (1.34–5.28) | 7.19 (3.38–15.28) | 7.57 (3.87–14.82) |
| 70–74 | 1.25 (0.94–1.66) | 1.78 (1.26–2.51)* | 2.51 (1.8–3.51) | 1.4 (0.57–3.44) | 6.02 (2.61–13.88*) | 5.25 (2.39–11.5)* |
| 80+ | 1.25 (0.8–1.97) | 1.77 (1.1–2.84)* | 2.29 (1.47–3.57)* | 3.17 (1.19–8.43)* | 8.95 (3.5–22.89) | 9.09 (3.77–21.93) |
| Sex | | | | | | |
| Male | 1 | 1 | 1 | 1 | 1 | 1 |
| Female | 1.11 (0.78–0.58) | 1.1 (0.75–1.61) | 0.82 (0.56–1.21) | 0.39 (0.14–1.09) | 0.52 (0.19–0.44) | 0.43 (0.17–1.06) |
| Living place | | | | | | |
| Urban | 1 | 1 | 1 | 1 | 1 | 1 |
| Rural | 0.86 (0.6–1.24) | 0.69 (0.47–1.03) | 0.8 (0.51–1.25) | 2.12 (0.82–5.49) | 1.92 (0.75–4.88) | 2.76 (1.14–6.68)* |
| Marital status | | | | | | |
| Married | 1 | 1 | 1 | 1 | 1 | 1 |
| Single | 1.1 (0.71–1.72) | 0.85 (0.55–1.3) | 0.91 (0.59–1.4) | 1.46 (0.49–4.34) | 1.32 (0.46–3.77) | 2.1 (0.8–5.52) |
| Educational level | | | | | | |
| No school | 1 | 1 | 1 | 1 | 1 | 1 |
| <6 yrs | 0.82 (0.45–1.49) | 0.8 (0.44–1.44) | 0.45 (0.25–0.8) | 1.58 (0.38–6.53) | 1.39 (0.44–4.34) | 1.4 (0.47–4.15) |
| Primary | 0.88 (0.52–1.49) | 0.93 (0.53–1.64) | 0.57 (0.33–0.98)* | 1.03 (0.28–3.84) | 0.73 (0.2–2.66) | 0.58 (0.17–1.95) |
| Secondary | 1.5 (0.77–2.9) | 0.95 (0.48–1.92) | 0.56 (0.26–1.2) | 0.27 (0.07–1.05) | 0.17 (0.05–0.61) | 0.09 (0.03–0.3) |
| High school | 0.87 (0.52–1.45) | 0.61 (0.35–1.07) | 0.53 (0.3–0.92) | 0.18 (0.05–0.63)* | 0.16 (0.04–0.7) | 0.09 (0.02–0.33) |
| University | 0.62 (0.25–1.56) | 0.49 (0.18–1.34) | 0.34 (0.11–1.06) | 0.24 (0.05–1.13) | 0.09 (0.02–0.49)* | 0.07 (0.02–0.35)* |
| Occupation | | | | | | |
| Public sector | 1 | 1 | 1 | 1 | 1 | 1 |
| Private | 0.52 (0.17–1.57) | 0.97 (0.29–3.23) | 1.25 (0.38–4.09) | 2.18 (0.4–12.03) | 4.32 (1.06–17.55)* | 1.93 (0.49–7.64) |
| Self-employed | 0.89 (0.47–1.72) | 0.95 (0.49–1.85) | 0.95 (0.46–1.97) | 0.65 (0.06–7.18) | 0.6 (0.07–5.23)) | 0.26 (0.03–2.33) |
| Informal | 0.66 (0.27–1.62) | 0.64 (0.27–1.55) | 1.63 (0.6–4.39) | 0.45 (0.07–2.99) | 1.4 (0.22–8.72) | 0.74 (0.16–3.51) |
| Income | | | | | | |
| Quintile 1 (poorest) | 1 | 1 | 1 | 1 | 1 | 1 |
| Quintile 2 | 1.04 (0.6–1.79) | 0.79 (0.44–1.41) | 1.26 (0.74–2.14) | 0.56 (0.14–2.26) | 0.76 (0.17–3.43) | 0.62 (0.18–2.14) |
| Quintile 3 | 1.9 (1.11–3.23)* | 1.67 (0.94–2.96) | 2.95 (1.76–4.95) | 0.48 (0.1–2.37) | 0.6 (0.11–3.15) | 0.9 (0.2–4.12) |
| Quintile 4 | 2.19 (1.3–3.68) | 2.03 (1.14–3.64)* | 2.29 (1.32–3.97)* | 1.13 (0.28–4.6) | 0.58 (0.15–2.29) | 1 (0.27–3.73) |
| Quintile 5 (richest) | 1.24 (0.72–2.12) | 1.27 (0.74–2.21) | 1.33 (0.73–2.42) | 1.06 (0.25–4.43) | 0.7 (0.2–2.42) | 0.61 (0.18–2.06) |
| **Biological variables** | | | | | | |
| BMI (kg/m$^2$) | | | | | | |
| Underweight | 1 | 1 | 1 | 1 | 1 | 1 |
| Normal | 0.9 (0.51–1.6) | 1.39 (0.76–2.55) | 0.95 (0.53–1.71) | 0.59 (0.12–2.87) | 0.88 (0.16–4.68) | 0.27 (0.05–1.38) |
| Overweight | 1.44 (0.76–2.74) | 2.23 (1.09–4.56)* | 1.58 (0.77–3.26) | 0.39 (0.07–2.06) | 1.71 (0.28–10.53) | 0.47 (0.08–2.77) |
| Obese | 2.64 (1.11–6.3)* | 6.62 (2.79–15.69) | 3.37 (1.37–8.26)* | 2.42 (0.53–11.03) | 11.72 (2.35–58.43)* | 4.81 (0.98–23.54) |
| Waist circumference | | | | | | |
| Normal | 1 | 1 | 1 | 1 | 1 | 1 |
| Abnormal | 1.52 (0.97–2.38) | 1.79 (1.12–2.87)* | 1.31 (0.8–2.13) | 0.96 (0.25–3.75) | 1.38 (0.38–5.04) | 1.66 (0.49–5.56) |
| **Health related behaviors** | | | | | | |
| Smoking | | | | | | |
| No | 1 | 1 | 1 | 1 | 1 | 1 |
| Yes | 0.87 (0.56–1.34) | 0.83 (0.51–1.36) | 1.33 (0.85–2.07) | 1 (0.33–3.04) | 1.83 (0.57–5.84) | 2.02 (0.69–5.95) |

Table 2: Continued.

| $N$ = 7545 | Ghana ($n$ = 4565) Pre-HTN OR (95% CI) | Stage 1 OR (95% CI) | Stage 2 OR (95% CI) | South Africa ($n$ = 2980) Pre-HTN OR (95% CI) | Stage 1 OR (95% CI) | Stage 2 OR (95% CI) |
|---|---|---|---|---|---|---|
| Current alcohol use | | | | | | |
| No | 1 | 1 | 1 | 1 | 1 | 1 |
| Yes | 1.27 (0.77–2.1) | 0.99 (0.6–1.65) | 1.08 (0.66–1.76) | 0.44 (0.1–1.93) | 0.98 (0.15–6.56) | 0.33 (0.08–1.42) |
| Work related physical activity | | | | | | |
| High | 1 | 1 | 1 | 1 | 1 | 1 |
| Moderate | 0.75 (0.49–1.15) | 1 (0.63–1.58) | 0.82 (0.5–1.33) | 1.66 (0.35–7.95) | 0.5 (0.08–2.93) | 0.83 (0.19–3.62) |
| Low | 0.92 (0.57–1.5) | 1.29 (0.75–2.23) | 1.24 (0.72–2.16) | 4.14 (0.9–19.13) | 1.38 (0.26–7.42) | 2.24 (0.56–8.98) |
| Fruit intake/day | | | | | | |
| 0-1 | 1 | 1 | 1 | 1 | 1 | 1 |
| 2–4 | 1.05 (0.72–1.53) | 0.76 (0.5–1.16) | 0.83 (0.55–1.25) | 0.81 (0.28–2.32) | 0.49 (0.17–1.38) | 0.3 (0.11–0.81)* |
| >=5 | 2.2 (1.06–4.56) | 1.94 (0.91–4.14) | 2.42 (1.29–4.54) | 0.17 (0.02–1.34) | 0.15 (0.02–1.03) | 0.59 (0.07–4.65) |
| Vegetable intake/day | | | | | | |
| 0-1 | 1 | 1 | 1 | 1 | 1 | 1 |
| 2–4 | 1.67 (1.09–2.57) | 1.07 (0.69–1.68) | 1.28 (0.78–2.12) | 0.64 (0.24–1.68) | 0.3 (0.11–0.82)* | 0.29 (0.11–0.72)* |
| >=5 | 2.07 (0.58–7.43) | 1.67 (0.36–7.63) | 0.78 (0.22–2.7) | 1.13 (0.19–6.74) | 2.46 (0.29–20.65) | 4.86 (0.66–35.82) |

*$P < 0.05$.

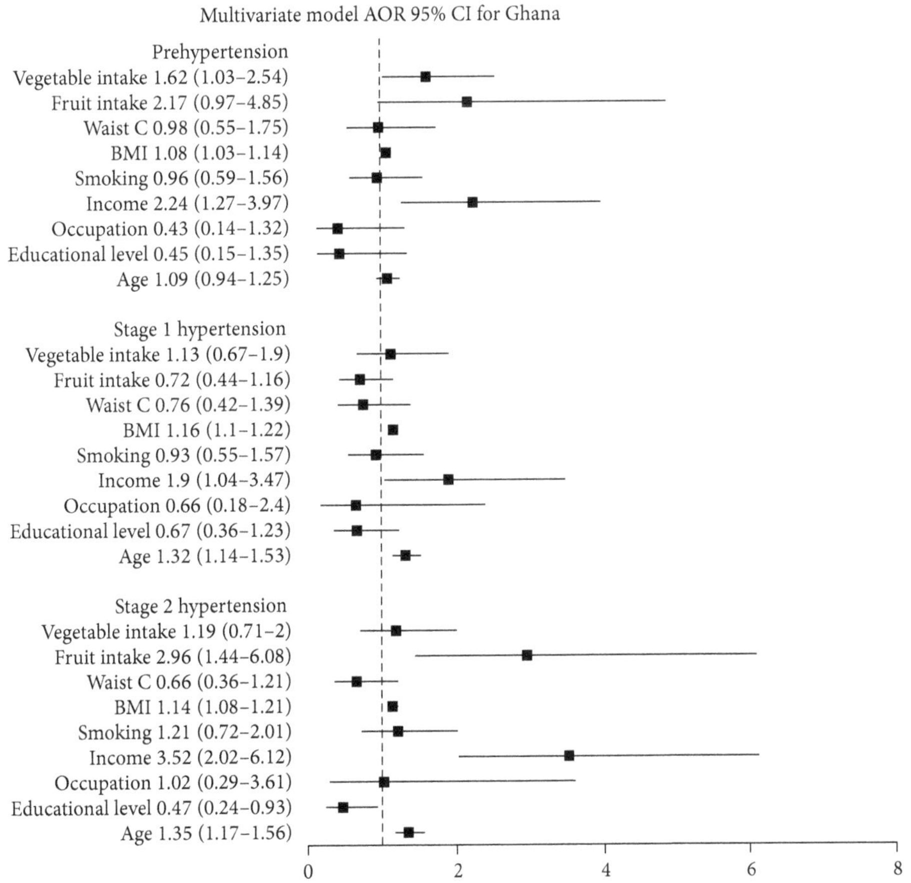


Figure 1: Adjusted odds ratios and 95% confidence intervals for stages of hypertension, Ghana.

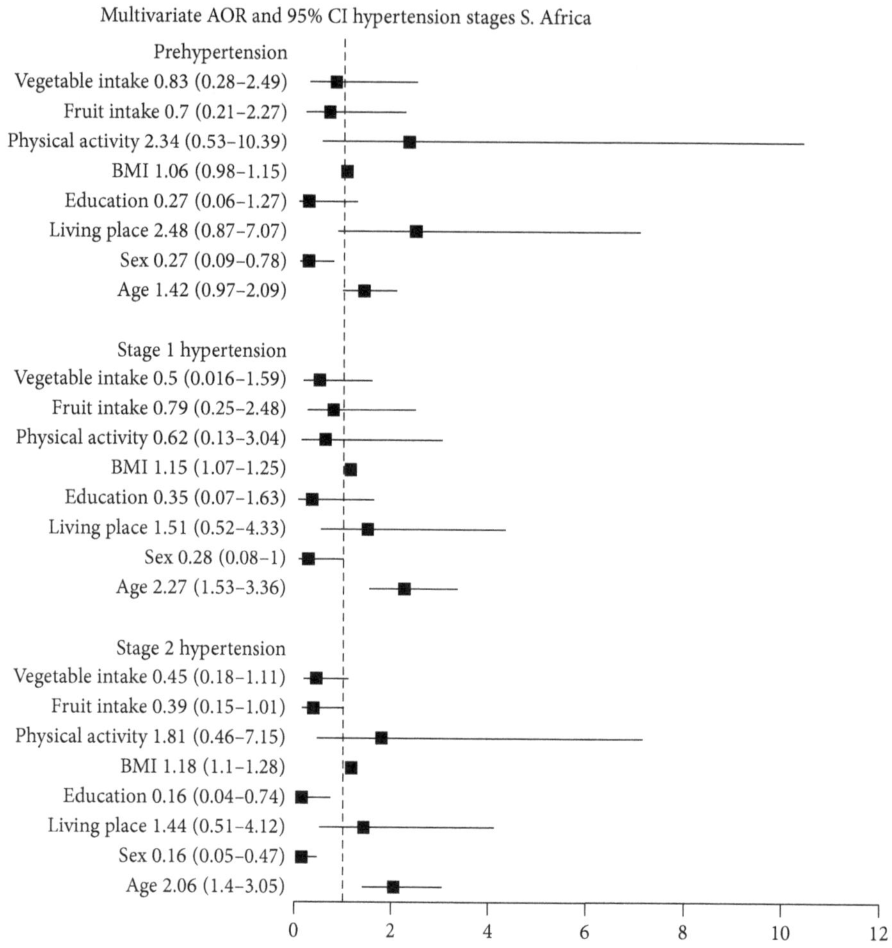


FIGURE 2: Adjusted odds ratios and 95% confidence intervals for stages of hypertension, South Africa.

for stage 1 hypertension as well. There was 32% increased risk of having stage 1 hypertension for every age increase by one year (OR = 1.32, 95% CI: 1.14–1.53). Age (OR = 1.35, 95% CI: 1.17–1.56), income (OR = 3.52, 95% CI: 2.02–6.12), and BMI (OR = 1.14, 95% CI: 1.08–1.21) remained as independent predictors for stage 2 hypertension as well. In addition higher educational level emerged as a protective variable against stage 2 hypertension in the model (OR = 0.47, 95% CI: 0.24–0.93).

*4.2. South Africa.* Eight variables which were associated with stages of hypertension in the bivariate analysis at probability level of $P < 0.2$ were retained in the multinomial logistic regression model. These were age, sex, living place, educational level, BMI category, work related physical activity, and fruit and vegetable servings per day (Figure 2). Only sex (OR = 0.27, 95% CI: 0.09–0.78) remained independent predictor of prehypertension in the multivariate logistic regression model after being adjusted for the other variables. Age and BMI emerged as independent predictors of stage 1 hypertension (OR = 2.27, 95% CI: 1.53–3.36 and OR = 1.15, 95% CI: 1.07–1.25). Sex remained as an independent predictor of stage 1 hypertension (OR = 0.28, 95% CI: 0.08–1). Being female resulted in 72% lower risk of having stage 1 hypertension than being male (OR = 0.28, 95% CI: 0.08–1). Age (OR = 2.06, 95% CI: 1.4–8.7), sex (OR = 0.16, 95% CI: 0.05–0.47), and BMI (OR = 1.18, 95% CI: 1.1–1.28) remained independent predictors of stage 2 hypertension in the final model. Educational level emerged as an independent predictor of stage 2 hypertension. Those with high school education tended to have 84% lower odds of stage 2 hypertension compared to those with no education (OR = 0.16, 95% CI: 0.04–0.74).

## 5. Discussion

The study has showed high burden of prehypertension and hypertension stages in the Sub-Saharan African countries, Ghana and South Africa. The weighted prevalence of hypertension (including both stages 1 and 2) was higher in South Africa (46%) compared to Ghana (42.4%). The high prevalence of hypertension in the current study is mostly due to higher age distribution of participants. More than 85% of respondents in Ghana and around 90% South Africans were in the age group more than 50, as part of the WHO SAGE study. The probability that a middle-aged or elderly individual will develop hypertension in his or her lifetime is 90% [27], explaining the higher prevalence in this study. Higher prevalence of hypertension (77.3%) than the current study was also reported in hypertension and associated factors in older adults study in South Africa [28]. Comparing the two countries South Africa had higher prevalence of hypertension that could be explained by higher proportion of people living in urban area (69.7% in South Africa and 44.4% in Ghana) and increased number of obese people (30.5% in South Africa and 12.1% Ghana). In addition lower rate of physical activity and fruit intake per day was reported in South Africa.

The weighted prevalence of prehypertension was higher in Ghana (30.7%) than South Africa (29.4%). Higher reports were made from the PURE hypertension trial done on 153,996 adults aged 35 to 70 years, from 628 communities in 3 high-income, 10 upper-middle and low-middle-income, and 4 low-income countries of 36.8% [12]. These are groups of people with increased cardiovascular risk but who do not need pharmacologic treatment unless there is another compelling medical indication such as diabetes or chronic kidney disease [29]. They have higher likelihood of progression to overt hypertension and need lifestyle changes as a treatment such as weight reduction, physical activity, and decreased salt intake [30]. Progression from prehypertension to stage 1 hypertension was positively related to male gender, higher waist circumference, and having parents with hypertension in population-based study Keelung, Taiwan [31]. Identifying these individuals has high public health importance as such measures taken could delay or prevent progression or development of hypertension.

The weighted prevalence of stage 1 hypertension in Ghana was higher (21.6%) than in South Africa (18.5%) and the weighted estimate of stage 2 hypertension was higher in South Africa (28.1%) and Ghana (21.6%). Prior studies on these two countries were mainly done on dichotomized blood pressure classification using SBP of 140 mmHg or DBP of 90 mmHg and more. According to hypertension in South African adults, results from the Demographic and Health Survey, 1998, the prevalence rate of hypertension was 11% in males and 14% in females when blood pressure cut-off point (160/95 mmHg) was used [32]. In the current study BMI was an independent predictor for prehypertension in both Ghana and South Africa which was a similar finding in the study done in the Ashanti region of Ghana which showed age (OR = 1.56, 95% CI: 1.12–2.18; $P < 0.01$), obesity (OR = 2.71; 95% CI: 1.40–5.24; $P < 0.001$), and sex (OR = 2.36, 95% CI: 1.77–3.15; $P < 0.001$) being independent predictors of prehypertension on multivariable logistic regression [11]. In addition income became one of the strongest predictors for prehypertension in Ghana in our study, with higher income quintiles associated with higher levels of prehypertension. This was similar with household characteristics for older adults and study background from SAGE Ghana WAVE 1, which showed people with the higher income quintiles generally reported more hypertension (income quintile 5, wealthiest = 26.7%, versus quintile 1, poorest = 5.5%) and received more current and chronic therapy [15]. Other studies in US and Canada have shown the opposite effect; inverse linear relationship between household income and hypertension prevalence in the United States, but no evidence of such a relationship in Canada, was seen due to similar burden of hypertension across different socioeconomic classes [33]. Middle-income was a high correlate in another study in urban India [34]. Getting income data reliably was difficult as income was generated from ho usehold assets and converted later to quintiles, hence requiring cautious interpretation of result. The proportion of both overweight and obese was higher in the 4th and 5th income quintiles than the lower ones (23% and 30%, resp.) which could explain the high prevalence of prehypertension in the group.

Being in the higher BMI category contributed significantly to having prehypertension and could be related to the low physical activity of the current study participants [35]. Those with the lowest work related physical activity had the highest rates of prehypertension. South Africa has one of the lowest rates of insufficient physical activity (49% in adult women and 43% in adult men) compared to global figure of 17% and Africa's coverage of about 10% [36]. Some of the explanations were high rate of urbanization, increased mechanized labour, and television watching [37]. The very low report of physical activity contributing to both obesity and prehypertension needs to be addressed in South Africa by clinicians, public health specialists, patients, and policy makers at the government level.

We have tried to see the social determinant and risk factors for different hypertension stages (1 and 2) separately and whether they differ in the two countries and across different hypertension stages in the same country. The study has showed only age, income, and BMI remaining as independent predictors of stage 1 hypertension in Ghana. We found educational level and number of fruit intakes per day having an inverse relationship to stage 1 hypertension in South Africa in the bivariate multinomial analysis. This is similar with the first demographic and health survey study: determinants and treatment of hypertension in South Africa which showed higher risk of having hypertension with less than tertiary education [10]. Adults with no education or less than primary school were more than 50%, and the highest report of stage 1 hypertension was seen in this group in the current study. Curriculum reforms and models to increase opportunity of education in the postapartheid education system are undergoing [38] and should be further strengthened.

Increasing fruit and vegetable intake was seen to have significant blood pressure lowering effect in stage 1 and stage 2 hypertension. This effect was not seen in the final model. The finding is consistent with other trials that demonstrated the greatest benefit of dietary changes at lower stages of hypertension [30]. The DASH (Dietary Approaches to Stop Hypertension) trials introduced the DASH diet which is comprised of four-five servings of fruit, four-five servings of vegetables, two-three servings of low-fat dairy per day, and <25 percent fat [39]. Drop in average systolic blood pressure by 11.4 mmHg and diastolic blood pressure by 5.5 mmHg in hypertensive individuals has been seen as early as two weeks, with the DASH diet. Increasing fruit intake is thus highly recommended in individuals especially with lower stages of hypertension to prevent progression of disease. Countries should be working on ways to make availability of fruits accessible and affordable. The weighted estimate of people taking the recommended fruit intake was very low (9.9%) in Ghana and (3.5%) South Africa. Vegetable intake was even much worse (0.9%) in Ghana and (3.5%) in South Africa. The wide confidence interval and attenuated beneficial effects of fruits and vegetables could be attributed to the very little proportion of people in these categories making the expected statistical association loose.

Though smoking cigarette was one of the most important risk factors for cardiovascular disorders and acute myocardial infarction in the INTERHEART Africa study [40], it was associated only in the bivariate analysis when studied individually. The effect was lost when multiple variables were retained in the regression model in both countries at every stage of hypertension. The incidence of hypertension increases in those who smoke 15 or more cigarettes per day [41] and could be the reason why strong association was not seen as only less than 2% individuals (Ghana) and around 7% (South Africa) smoked more than 15 cigarettes per day. Other studies have also documented "lower blood pressure measurements in those habitual smokers than nonsmokers due to weight loss and some vasodilatory effect of cotinine a metabolite of nicotine" [42, 43].

Only increasing age, income, BMI, and educational level were found to be independent risk factors for stage 2 hypertension in the final model in Ghana. There was no significant variation of stage 2 hypertension between sexes in Ghana, although it is known that men had higher systolic blood pressure measurements in early adulthood, while older women have steeper age-related rate of rise [27]. This could be in part due to the higher proportion of women who are overweight and obese in both countries.

This particular study has assessed the burden of hypertension in Sub-Saharan African countries. It focused mainly on risk factors and social determinants across different stages of hypertension among the two countries. This helps to identify newly emerging associated risk factors at different stages of hypertension and helps to be able to recommend measures accordingly. As it is always said "Prevention is better than Cure," we also recommend identifying individuals and treating accordingly at pre- and early hypertension stages, where the maximum benefit of lifestyle changes can be seen. These include having regular and intense physical exercise, reduction of body weight which can decrease average SBP by 5–20 mmHg for every 10 kg weight loss [1], increasing the opportunity to have basic education for all, and educating people with higher income in Ghana who are at high risk of prehypertension and subsequent overt hypertension due to probable acculturation to change their lifestyle. Government bodies at policy level and health specialists need to design methods to improve diagnosis and treatment of hypertension at earlier stages in respective countries.

## 6. Limitation

One of the major limitations of the current study was high number of missing and some invalid values in the original dataset. Missing and invalid blood pressure measurements accounted for 8% in Ghana and 25% in South Africa. They were excluded during the data cleaning period and not included in analysis. Alcohol consumption was an independent variable with the highest missing values (63%) in Ghana and (35%) in South Africa. This could be the reason for not seeing the expected protection from moderate dose of alcohol against hypertension and increased risk from excess dose [44]. The other components of therapeutic lifestyle changes that include intake of salt, saturated fat, and amount of calories [45] were not included in the SAGE questionnaire and their association with hypertension was not studied. The current study as any other cross-sectional studies determines only associations that are statistically significant without inferring causality. Further cohort studies that examine risk and causality are recommended. And finally using the JNC 7 blood pressure classification that was originally designed for US population and using its blood pressure cut-off points for Sub-Saharan population could impose risk of overgeneralization. Blood pressure cut-off points at which cardiovascular morbidity starts should be looked for in Sub-Saharan Africa context and guidelines should develop in the future.

## Abbreviations

AOR: Adjusted odds ratio
BP: Blood pressure
BMI: Body mass index
CVD: Cardiovascular disorder
CI: Confidence interval
DASH: Dietary approaches to stop hypertension
DBP: Diastolic blood pressure
EA: Enumeration area
HTN: Hypertension
IHD: Ischemic heart disease
ISCO: International standard classification of occupation
JNC 7: Joint national committee 7 for hypertension
NCD: Noncommunicable disease
NCEP: ATP III: National Cholesterol Education Program: Adult Treatment Panel III
OR: Odds ratio
PSU: Primary selection unit
SA: South Africa
SAGE: Study on global AGEing and adult health
SBP: Systolic blood pressure
WC: Waist circumference
WHO: World Health Organization.

## Acknowledgments

The authors wish to thank the WHO SAGE study group, Umeå International School of Public Health (UISPH), particularly Kjerstin Dahlblom, Nawi Ng, and Jennifer Stewart Williams, and Swedish Institute (SI) scholarships.

## References


[1] A. V. Chobanian, G. L. Bakris, H. R. Black et al., "The seventh report of the joint national committee on prevention, detection, evaluation, and treatment of high blood pressure: the JNC 7 report," *Journal of the American Medical Association*, vol. 289, no. 19, pp. 2560–2572, 2003.

[2] F. Palano, F. Paneni, S. Sciarretta, G. Tocci, and M. Volpe, "The progression from hypertension to congestive heart failure," *Recenti Progressi in Medicina*, vol. 102, no. 12, pp. 461–467, 2011.

[3] J. A. Staessen, R. Fagard, L. Thijs et al., "Randomised double-blind comparison of placebo and active treatment for older patients with isolated systolic hypertension," *The Lancet*, vol. 350, no. 9080, pp. 757–764, 1997.

[4] J. Coresh, G. L. Wei, G. McQuillan et al., "Prevalence of high blood pressure and elevated serum creatinine level in the United States: findings from the third national health and nutrition examination survey (1988–1994)," *Archives of Internal Medicine*, vol. 161, no. 9, pp. 1207–1216, 2001.

[5] M. E. Hendriks, F. W. N. M. Wit, M. T. L. Roos et al., "Hypertension in Sub-Saharan Africa: cross-sectional surveys in four rural and urban communities," *PLoS ONE*, vol. 7, no. 3, Article ID e32638, 2012.

[6] S. Lewington, R. Clarke, N. Qizilbash, R. Peto, and R. Collins, "Age-specific relevance of usual blood pressure to vascular mortality: a meta-analysis of individual data for one million adults in 61 prospective studies," *The Lancet*, vol. 360, no. 9349, pp. 1903–1913, 2002.

[7] L. Shen, H. Ma, M.-X. Xiang, and J.-A. Wang, "Meta-analysis of cohort studies of baseline prehypertension and risk of coronary heart disease," *American Journal of Cardiology*, vol. 112, no. 2, pp. 266–271, 2013.

[8] C. Lenfant, A. V. Chobanian, D. W. Jones, and E. J. Roccella, "Seventh report of the Joint National Committee on the prevention, detection, evaluation, and treatment of high blood pressure (JNC 7): resetting the hypertension sails," *Hypertension*, vol. 41, no. 6, pp. 1178–1179, 2003.

[9] P. Kotwani, D. Kwarisiima, T. D. Clark et al., "Epidemiology and awareness of hypertension in a rural Ugandan community: a cross-sectional study," *BMC Public Health*, vol. 13, no. 1, article 1151, 2013.

[10] K. Steyn, D. Bradshaw, R. Norman, and R. Laubscher, "Determinants and treatment of hypertension in South Africans: the first demographic and health survey," *South African Medical Journal*, vol. 98, no. 5, pp. 376–380, 2008.

[11] C. Agyemang and E. Owusu-Dabo, "Prehypertension in the Ashanti region of Ghana, West Africa: an opportunity for early prevention of clinical hypertension," *Public Health*, vol. 122, no. 1, pp. 19–24, 2008.

[12] C. K. Chow, K. K. Teo, S. Rangarajan et al., "Prevalence, awareness, treatment, and control of hypertension in rural and urban communities in high-, middle-, and low-income countries," *Journal of the American Medical Association*, vol. 310, no. 9, pp. 959–968, 2013.

[13] W. K. Bosu, "Epidemic of hypertension in Ghana: a systematic review," *BMC Public Health*, vol. 10, article 418, 2010.

[14] B. D. Capistrant and P. Kowal, "Social epidemiology of hypertension stages," *Hypertension*, vol. 62, no. 6, article e41, 2013.

[15] R. B. Biritwum, G. Mensah, N. Minicuci et al., "Household characteristics for older adults and study background from SAGE Ghana Wave 1," *Global Health Action*, vol. 6, no. 1, Article ID 20096, 2013.

[16] A. M. B. Menezes, S. C. Dumith, R. B. Noal et al., "Validity of a wrist digital monitor for blood pressure measurement in comparison to a mercury sphygmomanometer," *Arquivos Brasileiros de Cardiologia*, vol. 94, no. 3, pp. 345–370, 2010.

[17] H. Takahashi, M. Yoshika, and T. Yokoi, "Validation of Omron RS8, RS6, and RS3 home blood pressure monitoring devices, in accordance with the European Society of Hypertension International Protocol revision 2010," *Vascular Health and Risk Management*, vol. 9, pp. 265–272, 2013.

[18] S. L. Schneider and I. Kogan, "The International Standard Classification of Education 1997: challenges in the application to national data and the implementation in cross-national surveys," in *The International Standard Classification of Education (ISCED-97): An Evaluation of Content and Criterion Validity for 15 European Countries*, pp. 13–46, MZES, 2008.

[19] L. Wirth, Copyright International Labour Organization 2001 First published 2001 Second impression 2001 Publications of the International Labour Office enjoy copyright under Protocol 2 of the Universal Copyright Convention, Nevertheless, short excerpts from them may be reproduced without authorization, 2001.

[20] World Health Organization, *Guidelines for Controlling and Monitoring the Tobacco Epidemic*, World Health Organization, 1998.

[21] T. Armstrong and F. Bull, "Development of the World Health Organization Global Physical Activity Questionnaire (GPAQ)," *Journal of Public Health*, vol. 14, no. 2, pp. 66–70, 2006.

[22] World Health Organization, *Global Health Risks: Mortality and Burden of Disease Attributable to Selected Major Risks*, World Health Organization, 2009.

[23] J. I. Recio-Rodriguez, M. A. Gomez-Marcos, M. C. Patino-Alonso, C. Agudo-Conde, E. Rodriguez-Sanchez, and L. Garcia-Ortiz, "Abdominal obesity vs general obesity for identifying arterial stiffness, subclinical atherosclerosis and wave reflection in healthy, diabetics and hypertensive," *BMC Cardiovascular Disorders*, vol. 12, article 3, 2012.

[24] A. M. Gotto, "NCEP ATP III guidelines incorporate global risk assessment," *The American Journal of Managed Care*, supplement, pp. 1–3, 2003.

[25] W. He, M. N. Muenchrath, and P. R. Kowal, *Shades of Gray: A Cross-Country Study of Health and Well-Being of the Older Populations in SAGE Countries, 2007–2010*, Economics and Statistics Administration, US Census Bureau, 2012.

[26] N. Naidoo, S. Abdullah, A. Bawah et al., *Ageing and Adult Health Status in Eight Lower-Income Countries: the INDEPTH WHO-SAGE Collaboration*, Global Health Action, 2010.

[27] A. S. Fauci, *Harrison's Principles of Internal Medicine*, McGraw-Hill Medical, New York, NY, USA, 2008.

[28] K. Peltzer and N. Phaswana-Mafuya, "Hypertension and associated factors in older adults in South Africa," *Cardiovascular Journal of Africa*, vol. 24, no. 3, pp. 67–71, 2013.

[29] S. Chaturvedi, "The seventh report of the joint national committee on prevention, detection, evaluation, and treatment of high blood pressure (JNC 7): is it really practical?" *National Medical Journal of India*, vol. 17, no. 4, p. 227, 2004.

[30] L. J. Appel, M. W. Brands, S. R. Daniels, N. Karanja, P. J. Elmer, and F. M. Sacks, "Dietary approaches to prevent and treat hyper-

tension: a scientific statement from the American Heart Association," *Hypertension*, vol. 47, no. 2, pp. 296–308, 2006.

[31] Y.-H. Chiu, S.-C. Wu, C.-D. Tseng, M.-F. Yen, and T. H.-H. Chen, "Progression of pre-hypertension, stage 1 and 2 hypertension (JNC 7): a population-based study in Keelung, Taiwan (Keelung Community-based Integrated Screening No. 9)," *Journal of Hypertension*, vol. 24, no. 5, pp. 821–828, 2006.

[32] K. Steyn, T. A. Gaziano, D. Bradshaw, R. Laubscher, and J. Fourie, "Hypertension in South African adults: results from the demographic and health survey, 1998," *Journal of Hypertension*, vol. 19, no. 10, pp. 1717–1725, 2001.

[33] M. S. Kaplan, N. Huguet, D. H. Feeny, and B. H. McFarland, "Self-reported hypertension prevalence and income among older adults in Canada and the United States," *Social Science and Medicine*, vol. 70, no. 6, pp. 844–849, 2010.

[34] S. Yadav, R. Boddula, G. Genitta et al., "Prevalence & risk factors of pre-hypertension & hypertension in an affluent North Indian population," *Indian Journal of Medical Research*, vol. 128, no. 6, pp. 712–720, 2008.

[35] S. Mora, I.-M. Lee, J. E. Buring, and P. M. Ridker, "Association of physical activity and body mass index with novel and traditional cardiovascular biomarkers in women," *The Journal of the American Medical Association*, vol. 295, no. 12, pp. 1412–1419, 2006.

[36] J. Joubert, R. Norman, E. V. Lambert et al., "Estimating the burden of disease attributable to physical inactivity in South Africa in 2000," *South African Medical Journal*, vol. 97, no. 8, pp. 725–731, 2007.

[37] E. V. Lambert, M. I. Lambert, K. Hudson et al., "Role of physical activity for health in communities undergoing epidemiological transition," *World Review of Nutrition and Dietetics*, vol. 90, pp. 110–126, 2001.

[38] J. D. Jansen, "Curriculum Reform in South Africa: a critical analysis of outcomes-based education," *Cambridge Journal of Education*, vol. 28, no. 3, pp. 321–331, 1998.

[39] L. J. Appel, T. J. Moore, E. Obarzanek et al., "A clinical trial of the effects of dietary patterns on blood pressure," *Journal of Materials Science: Materials in Medicine*, vol. 8, no. 4, pp. 1117–1124, 1997.

[40] K. Steyn, K. Sliwa, S. Hawken et al., "Risk factors associated with myocardial infarction in Africa: the INTERHEART Africa Study," *Circulation*, vol. 112, no. 23, pp. 3554–3561, 2005.

[41] T. S. Bowman, J. M. Gaziano, J. E. Buring, and H. D. Sesso, "A prospective study of cigarette smoking and risk of incident hypertension in women," *Journal of the American College of Cardiology*, vol. 50, no. 21, pp. 2085–2092, 2007.

[42] K. A. Perkins, L. H. Epstein, B. L. Marks, R. L. Stiller, and R. G. Jacob, "The effect of nicotine on energy expenditure during light physical activity," *The New England Journal of Medicine*, vol. 320, no. 14, pp. 898–903, 1989.

[43] N. L. Benowitz and D. S. Sharp, "Inverse relation between serum cotinine concentration and blood pressure in cigarette smokers," *Circulation*, vol. 80, no. 5, pp. 1309–1312, 1989.

[44] H. C. Bucher, L. Bujanda, J. M. Marimon et al., "Mortality and light to moderate alcohol consumption after myocardial infarction," *Lancet*, vol. 353, no. 9160, pp. 1272–1273, 1999.

[45] J. A. Iestra, D. Kromhout, Y. T. van der Schouw, D. E. Grobbee, H. C. Boshuizen, and W. A. van Staveren, "Effect size estimates of lifestyle and dietary changes on all-cause mortality in coronary artery disease patients: a systematic review," *Circulation*, vol. 112, no. 6, pp. 924–934, 2005.

# 17

# Characteristics of Inpatient Hypertension Cases and Factors Associated with Admission Outcomes in Ashanti Region, Ghana

**Kenneth Nuamah,[1] Harriet Affran Bonful,[2] Joseph Danso Yeboah,[3] Ebenezer Antwi Amankwaah,[1] Daniel Boakye,[1] Samuel Kwame Owusu,[1] Adwoa Aduako Owusu,[4] Freddie Amponsah,[5] Fred Adomako-Boateng,[1] Alexis Nang-Beifubah,[1] Margaret Gyapong,[6,7] Anthony Ofosu,[5] Bertha Garshong,[6] and Evelyn K. Ansah[6,7]**

[1]*Ashanti Regional Health Directorate, P.O. Box 1908, Kumasi, Ghana*
[2]*Department of Epidemiology and Disease Control, School of Public Health, University of Ghana, P.O. Box LG 13, Legon, Accra, Ghana*
[3]*Sekyere Central District Health Directorate, P.O. Box 36, Nsuta, Ashanti, Ghana*
[4]*Suntreso Government Hospital, P.O. Box 14775, Kumasi, Ghana*
[5]*Policy Planning Monitoring and Evaluation Division, Ghana Health Service, PMB Ministries, Accra, Ghana*
[6]*Research Development Division, Ghana Health Service, P.O. Box MB-190, Accra, Ghana*
[7]*Institute of Health Research, University of Health & Allied Science, PMB 31, Ho, Ghana*

Correspondence should be addressed to Kenneth Nuamah; kenneth.nuamah@ghsmail.org

Academic Editor: Tomohiro Katsuya

*Background*. Hypertension remains a cause of morbidity and mortality in the Ashanti Region of Ghana. It has been featured in the top ten causes of OPD attendance, admissions, and deaths since 2012. We investigated the sociodemographic characteristics and spatial distribution of inpatient hypertensives and factors associated with their admission outcomes. *Methods*. A 2014 line list of 1715 inpatient HPT cases aged ≥25 years was used for the cross-sectional analytic study. Accounting for clustering, all analyses were performed using the *"svy"* command in Stata. Frequencies, Chi-square test, and logistic regression analysis were used in the analysis. Arc view Geographic Information System (ArcGIS) was used to map the density of cases by place of residence and reporting hospital. *Results*. Mean age of cases was 58 (S.D 0.0068). Females constituted 67.6% of the cases. Age, gender, and NHIS status were significantly associated with admission outcomes. Cases were clustered in the regional capital and bordering districts. However, low case densities were recorded in the latter. *Conclusion*. Increasing NHIS access can potentially impact positively on hypertension admission outcomes. Health educational campaigns targeting men are recommended to address hypertension-related issues.

## 1. Introduction

The World Health Organization (WHO) defines hypertension as a systolic blood pressure equal to or above 140 mm Hg and/or diastolic blood pressure equal to or above 90 mm Hg [1]. Overall health and wellbeing of human rely on efficient functioning of vital organs such as the heart, brain, and kidneys [1]. This largely depends on both systolic and diastolic blood pressure being normal. If hypertension is left uncontrolled, it can lead to several cardiovascular complications including a heart attack, an enlargement of the heart, and eventually heart failure [1]. Kidney failure, blindness, rupture of blood vessels, and cognitive impairment can be attributed to hypertension [1].

The prevalence of hypertension rose from 600 million in 1980 to about 1 billion in 2013 [1]. Worldwide, there are over

17 million deaths attributed to cardiovascular diseases, which is nearly one-third of total deaths in a year [2]. Complications due to hypertension account for 9.4 million deaths every year [3]. Hypertension accounts for at least 5% of deaths from heart disease and 51% of deaths due to stroke [3].

The African region has the highest prevalence of hypertension, affecting 46% of all adult aged 25 years and above [4]. The prevalence (35%) in high-income countries is lower compared to 40% in low-income countries. The greatest health challenge facing the African region after HIV/AIDS is hypertension [4].

In sub-Saharan Africa, Noncommunicable Diseases (NCDs) have become important causes of morbidity and mortality, contributing 22% of total deaths [4]. It has been forecasted that, by 2025, the hypertensive population in developing countries will be 125.5 million people, which will correspond to an increase of 68% from 2008 to 2025 [5, 6].

Hypertension disease risk factors include age, race, family history, being overweight or obese, physical inactivity, tobacco use, high-salt diet, too little vitamin D and potassium in diet, excessive alcohol use, stress, and certain chronic conditions [3]. The prevalence of hypertension increases with increasing age. Sidhu and colleagues noted that the highest prevalence is found in ages equal to or above sixty (60 years) followed by ages between fifty and fifty-nine (50–59 years) [7] whilst Opie and Seedat also noted that, at age 65 in rural West Africa, there is a 30%–40% chance of being hypertensive as compared to 50% chance in semiurban areas in West Africa [4].

Others have identified level of education and occupation as factors associated with hypertension [8]. The risk of hypertension can vary in geographical areas depending on environmental conditions and socioeconomic position [9]

Ghana like other middle-income countries is no exception as hypertension is the number three killer today [10]. The prevalence of high blood pressure in Ghana is estimated at 12.9% and 15% for women and men, respectively [10]. The 2014 Demographic Health Survey puts the prevalence of hypertension in Ashanti at 15.3% for women and 18.1% for men, which is higher than the national average [10]. Prevalence of hypertension for Ashanti is highest among males in Ghana and second highest for females [10].

Earlier studies in the Ashanti Region have shown that there is a long-standing perception that hypertension disease is associated with affluence and that it is a disease of the rich and wealthy in society [11]. This perception has led to many people in low-income communities failing to report for medical check-ups and undertake routine exercises and not fully participate in health education programmes [11].

Over the years, some of the steps taken to control the increasing burden of hypertension in the country by the Ghana Health Service (GHS) have included the introduction of the Regenerative Health and Nutrition Program as well as the institutionalization of hypertension clinics in health facilities. In a systematic review by Tagoe and Dake in 2011, it was concluded strongly that more females exhibited healthier life style compared with males after the introduction of the Regenerative Health Policy [12]. Despite these interventions, morbidity and mortality due to hypertension continue to rise in the region. The proportion of hypertension to total OPD attendance increased from 3.8% in 2012 to 5.4% in 2014 [13]. More importantly, the proportion of admissions attributed to hypertension increased from 1.1% in 2010 to 2.4% in 2014. In 2014, hypertension was ranked sixth, third, and fifth, for top ten causes of OPD attendance, cause of admissions and deaths, respectively [13]. A review of literature suggests that there is little knowledge on the local factors driving the increasing burden of the disease and hospitalization. This study describes the characteristics of inpatient hypertension cases; establishes the factors associated with the outcomes of hypertension admissions; and also determines the geospatial distribution of these admissions in the Ashanti Region for the year 2014.

## 2. Materials and Methods

Data collected was used purposely for a cross-sectional analytic study. The study was conducted in Ashanti Region, which is one of the ten administrative regions of Ghana located in the middle belt of the country and covers about 10.2% of the total land surface area. It has an estimated 2014 mid-year population of 5,461,933, constituting 19.8% of the national population (projection from 2010 population and housing census, Ghana Statistical Service). The Komfo Anokye Teaching Hospital (KATH) is the teaching hospital for the region. Health services are delivered in public, private, quasi-, and mission facilities totaling 548. These facilities are comprised of 121 hospitals, 103 health centres, 282 clinics, and 133 CHPS compounds. Inpatient services are rendered in the 121 hospitals for hypertensive patients. Population to health facility ratio is 1 : 9967. Most facilities report on health indicators into the District Health Information Management System (DHIMS2) software; however, the only teaching hospital which also serves as the main referral hospital in the region does not.

This study used secondary data extracted from *DHIMS 2* for the Ashanti Region. DHIMS 2 is a developed software that operates on *DHIS2 (District Health Information Software)* application platform. DHIMS 2 is used by GHS to collect and collate data on health care service provision. DHIMS 2 helps to generate routine data, analyse reports using maps, and graphs and health profiles for indicators across facilities over a period.

The study population included records of all hypertension patients on admission aged between 25 years and above, diagnosed by clinicians within the Ashanti Region and reported in the DHIMS platform.

Diagnosis made in this study was done by prescribers in accordance with the standard Treatment Guidelines of Ghana [14]. Recruitment of study participants was based on diagnosis of hypertension by clinicians providing care in the health facility. Clinician practice is in accordance with the Standard Treatment Guidelines of Ghana and WHO. There is a system of regular supervision by different levels of health managers to ensure that the guidelines and protocols are adhered to. According to the treatment guideline, prescribers are expected to take an average of two or more properly measured blood pressure readings of a patient before diagnosing them of being hypertensive. At the point of call, the patient to be diagnosed is made to assume a relaxed and comfortable position for at least thirty (30) minutes [14]. Blood pressure (BP) of patients is checked with the use of manual mercury sphygmomanometer and a stethoscope. The arm (preferably left arm) is positioned to face the prescriber and a cuff is wrapped around the upper arm with the cuff lower edge about one inch above the antecubital fossa of the patient [14]. The average of the second and third or more outcomes of systolic blood pressure (SBP) and Diastolic Blood Pressure (DBP) within constant time intervals is recorded as the actual BP of the Patient. An adult with persistent SBP equal to or higher than 140 mm Hg and DBP equal to or higher than 90 mm Hg in nondiabetic or SBP equal to or higher than 130 mm Hg and DBP equal to or higher than 80 mm Hg in diabetics is diagnosed as being hypertensive.

Majority (>95%) of the sphygmomanometer used in the health facilities involved in this study are manufactured by Accoson from England; 3M Littmann stethoscopes from USA are also the commonly used stethoscopes in the Ashanti Region. According to the clinical engineering department, apart from the mandatory conformance to standard specifications checks made on the equipment, other factors including availability and accessibility to spare parts from manufacturers and user friendliness of the equipment, influences the choice of the equipment. Health facilities in Ghana procure clinical equipment including the manual mercury sphygmomanometer and the stethoscope with prior approval and in consultation with the clinical engineering department at the regional headquarters of the Ghana Health Service. The regional clinical engineer's approval and recommendation are paramount in the decision-making process to procure clinical equipment according to standard specifications at all levels of health care delivery (i.e., district hospitals, health centres, and polyclinics).

Hypertension-related conditions excluded in the *ICD-10-CM* (International Classification and Coding of Diseases) tabular list of diseases and injuries codes *(I10–I15)* were excluded in this study. Due to incomplete data for previous years, only data for the year 2014 was used. This study employed a cross-sectional analytic design approach.

The data was "svyset" to account for clustering in facilities and all analyses were conducted using the "svy:" command in Stata version 13 S.E (Stata Corporation, College Station, Texas). The data extracted was checked for internal consistency and completeness using simple summary statistics of the selected variables. Patient folder numbers were used as unique identifiers instead of patient names. All duplicate numbers were deleted before analysis. Frequencies were used to describe the characteristics of cases. Where there was evidence of skewness in the data, means were estimated for continuous variables after log transformation.

The independent variables were age, sex, educational level, occupation, place of residence, length of stay, facility ownership type, and District and National Health Insurance status. Educational level was recategorized from 7 levels (none, primary, JHS/middle school, SHS, technical/vocation, tertiary, and unspecified) to 4 levels (no formal education, primary, secondary, and tertiary) by merging primary and JHS, SHS, and technical vocation. Occupation was recoded from 13 to 6 groups by merging occupational status with similar characteristics as follows: *formal employment* (professional), clerical worker; *self-employed,* business person, farmer, hairdresser, and trader; *unemployed,* housewife, retiree, unemployed, and unskilled laborer; *others; student; and unspecified.* Age and length of stay were also recoded into categorical variables with uniform intervals, that is, age (5 groups with 10-year interval from 25 years to 65 and above.) and length of stay in days (5 groups from 1 day to 5 days and above).

The dependent variable, hypertension admission outcome, and a categorical ordinal variable with three categories *(died, discharged, and referred)* were used to perform Chi-square tests of associations with the independent variables. This variable was then recoded into a binary variable *(died and did not die)* by merging the referred and discharged cases. To identify the predictors of inpatient hypertension admission outcomes, univariable and multivariable logistic regression analyses were performed to determine the predictors of inpatient hypertension admission at 95% confidence level and a $p$ value of 0.05.

*2.1. Geospatial Distribution.* To generate the spatial distribution of the cases, the data in Ms Excel format was imported into Arc GIS Version 10.2. The shape files for all the districts in the region adopted from the Ghana Survey Department were used to draw thematic maps for the study since the shape files for the actual communities were not available. The communities of residence (addresses) of the cases were aligned with their respective districts for the analysis of the geographical distribution. Ninety-five (95) individual records were deleted from the list because their addresses could not be linked to any district in the region.

## 3. Results and Discussion

The total sample size obtained after data validation was 1,715. However, there were missing data in some variables in the dataset; therefore the sample size varied for the analysis conducted on these variables. The cases reported were seen in 30 hospitals comprising 17 public (government), 10 quasi-/mission facilities, and 3 private health facilities. Majority of the cases (59.3%) were seen in public hospitals.

Females constituted 67.5%. The mean age of these patients was 58.2 (S.D 0.00685) years, ranging from 25 years to 106 years. More than half (57.7%) of the hypertensive patients on admission had no formal education with the rest having been in some form of academic training as shown in Table 1. A proportion of 85.2% ($n$ = 1695) accessed health care with the National Health Insurance Scheme (NHIS) card. The mean length of stay on admission was 2 days, ranging from one to ninety-one (1–91) days. 90% of hypertensive patients on admission were engaged in one form of employment or the other. Less than ten percent (7.5%) were not engaged in any form of occupation.

Table 1: Sociodemographic characteristics of inpatient hypertension clients in Ashanti Region, 2014.

| | Female | | Male | | Total | |
|---|---|---|---|---|---|---|
| | Freq | % (95% CI) | Freq | % (95% CI) | Freq | % (95% CI) |
| Age group | | | | $N$ = 1714 | | |
| 25–34 | 61 | 35.60 (2.79–4.52) | 30 | 1.75 (1.01–3.03) | 91 | 5.31 (3.98–7.05) |
| 35–44 | 158 | 9.22 (7.04–11.99) | 74 | 4.32 (3.29–5.64) | 232 | 13.54 (11.55–15.80) |
| 45–54 | 249 | 14.53 (12.80–16.44) | 132 | 22.23 (6.03–9.78) | 381 | 22.23 (20.34–24.24) |
| 55–64 | 229 | 13.36 (11.73–15.17) | 119 | 6.94 (5.71–8.42) | 348 | 20.3 (18.58–22.14) |
| 65+ | 460 | 26.84 (24.51–29.31) | 202 | 11.79 (8.99–15.30) | 662 | 38.62 (36.26–41.05) |
| Total | 1157 | 67.5 (61.56–72.93) | 557 | 32.50 (27.07–38.44) | 1714 | 100 |
| Sex | | | | $N$ = 1714 | | |
| Female | 1157 | 67.5 (61.56–72.93) | 0 | — | 1157 | 67.5 (61.56–72.93) |
| Male | 0 | — | 557 | 32.5 (27.07–38.44) | 557 | 32.5 (27.07–38.44) |
| Total | 1157 | 67.5 (61.56–72.93) | 557 | 32.50 (27.07–38.44) | 1714 | 100 |
| Educational level | | | | $N$ = 1713 | | |
| No education | 706 | 41.21 (31.31–51.88) | 282 | 16.46 (12.53–21.32) | 988 | 57.68 (45.38–69.09) |
| Primary | 393 | 22.94 (16.96–30.26) | 212 | 12.38 (8.37–17.92) | 605 | 35.32 (25.92–46.01) |
| Secondary | 33 | 1.93 (0.73–4.99) | 37 | 2.16 (1.00–4.59) | 70 | 4.09 (1.86–8.74) |
| Tertiary | 24 | 1.4 (0.67–2.89) | 26 | 1.52 (0.70–3.26) | 50 | 2.92 (1.46–5.75) |
| Total | 1156 | 67.48 (61.55–72.91) | 557 | 32.52 (27.09–38.45) | 1713 | 100 |
| NHIS status | | | | $N$ = 1694 | | |
| Not having NHIS | 148 | 8.74 (5.06–14.68) | 103 | 6.08 (3.57–10.17) | 251 | 14.82 (8.82–23.83) |
| Have NHIS | 993 | 58.62 (50.21–66.55) | 450 | 26.56 (22.69–30.83) | 1443 | 85.18 (76.17–91.18) |
| Total | 1141 | 67.36 (61.49–72.72) | 553 | 32.64 (27.28–38.51) | 1694 | 100 |
| Occupation | | | | $N$ = 1711 | | |
| Unemployed | 88 | 5.14 (1.84–13.54) | 41 | 2.40 (12.09–5.20) | 129 | 7.54 (3.02–17.60) |
| Formal employment | 16 | 0.94 (14.38–43.87) | 23 | 1.34 (0.66–2.73) | 39 | 2.28 (1.23–4.18) |
| Self-employed | 455 | 26.59 (14.38–43.87) | 227 | 13.27 (7.22–23.13) | 682 | 39.86 (20.67–62.77) |
| Student | 1 | 5.8$e$ − 02 (6.7$e$ − 03–0.51) | 2 | 0.12 (2.5$e$ − 02–0.54) | 3 | 0.18 (4.8$e$ − 02–0.64) |
| Unspecified | 470 | 27.47 (10.07–56.15) | 161 | 9.41 (3.4–23.48) | 631 | 36.88 (12.52–70.46) |
| Others | 125 | 7.31 (3.18–15.89) | 102 | 5.96 (2.88–11.93) | 227 | 13.27 (6.41–25.47) |
| Total | 1155 | 67.50 (61.53–72.96) | 556 | 32.50 (27.04–38.47) | 1711 | 100 |
| Facility ownership | | | | $N$ = 1714 | | |
| Quasi-/mission | 403 | 23.51 (7.12–55.23) | 201 | 11.73 (4.97–25.22) | 604 | 35.24 (10.8–70.97) |
| Public | 700 | 40.84 (21.03–64.16) | 317 | 18.49 (9.60–32.66) | 1017 | 59.33 (27.20–85.07) |
| Private | 54 | 3.15 (0.63–14.29) | 39 | 2.28 (0.56–8.79) | 93 | 5.43 (1.27–20.40) |
| Total | 1157 | 67.50 (61.56–72.93) | 557 | 32.50 (27.07–38.44) | 1714 | 100 |
| District status | | | | $N$ = 1714 | | |
| Rural | 337 | 19.66 (8.29–39.84) | 200 | 11.67 (4.87–25.43) | 537 | 31.33 (12.48–59.34) |
| Urban | 820 | 47.84 (30.18–66.06) | 357 | 20.83 (13.86–30.08) | 1177 | 68.67 (40.66–87.52) |
| Total | 1157 | 67.5 (61.56–72.93) | 557 | 32.50 (27.07–38.44) | 1714 | 100 |

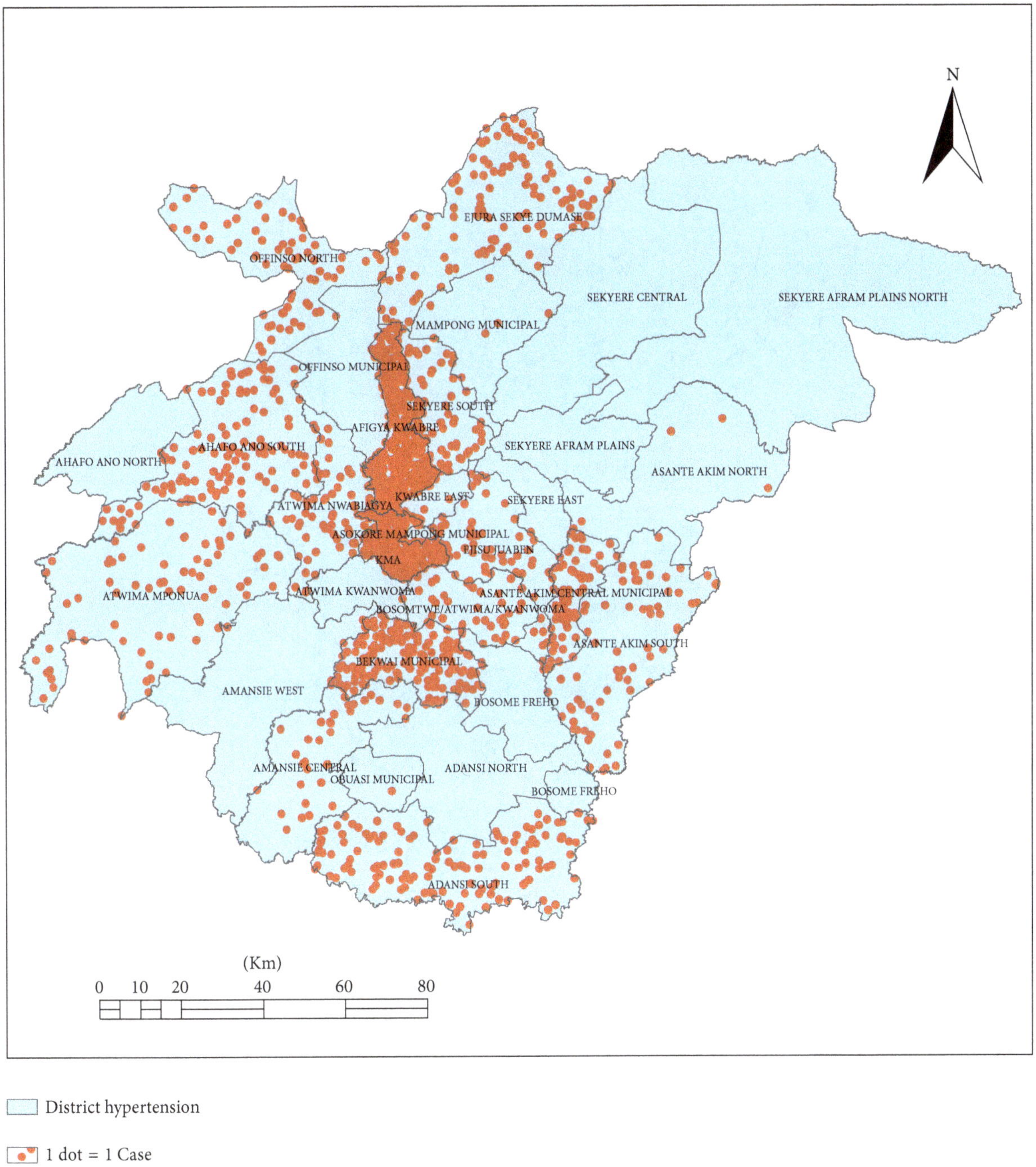


Figure 1: Case density of the hypertension admissions by clients place of residents, Ashanti Region, 2014.

Figure 1 shows the spatial pattern of cases by place of residence (address) across the study area. Most cases were clustered around the regional capital, Kumasi, and adjoining districts, whereas 9 districts including Sekyere Afram plains, Sekyere Central, Sekyere Kumawu, Obuasi Municipal, Ahafo Ano North, Asokore Mampong, and Sekyere East recorded admissions below 5 cases. Four out of these 9 districts do not have district hospitals.

Figure 2 is a spatial distribution of hypertension admission case density per hospital. Four (4) hospitals located in 4 districts (Ejura hospital, Nkenkaasu Hospital, Methodist Faith Healing Hospital, and Bekwai Hospital) reported hypertension admission cases constituting more than 0.1% of the district population. These 4 hospitals from 4 districts contributed 9.59% of the total admissions and 14.08% of the total deaths for 2014.

Chi-square tests of association showed no significance between the dependent variable and all independent variables except NHIS (Chi = 10.84, $p < 0.05$) as shown in Table 2.

Crude analysis of the association between the outcome of admission and predictor variables showed that gender, length of stay, and NHIS status were associated with admission

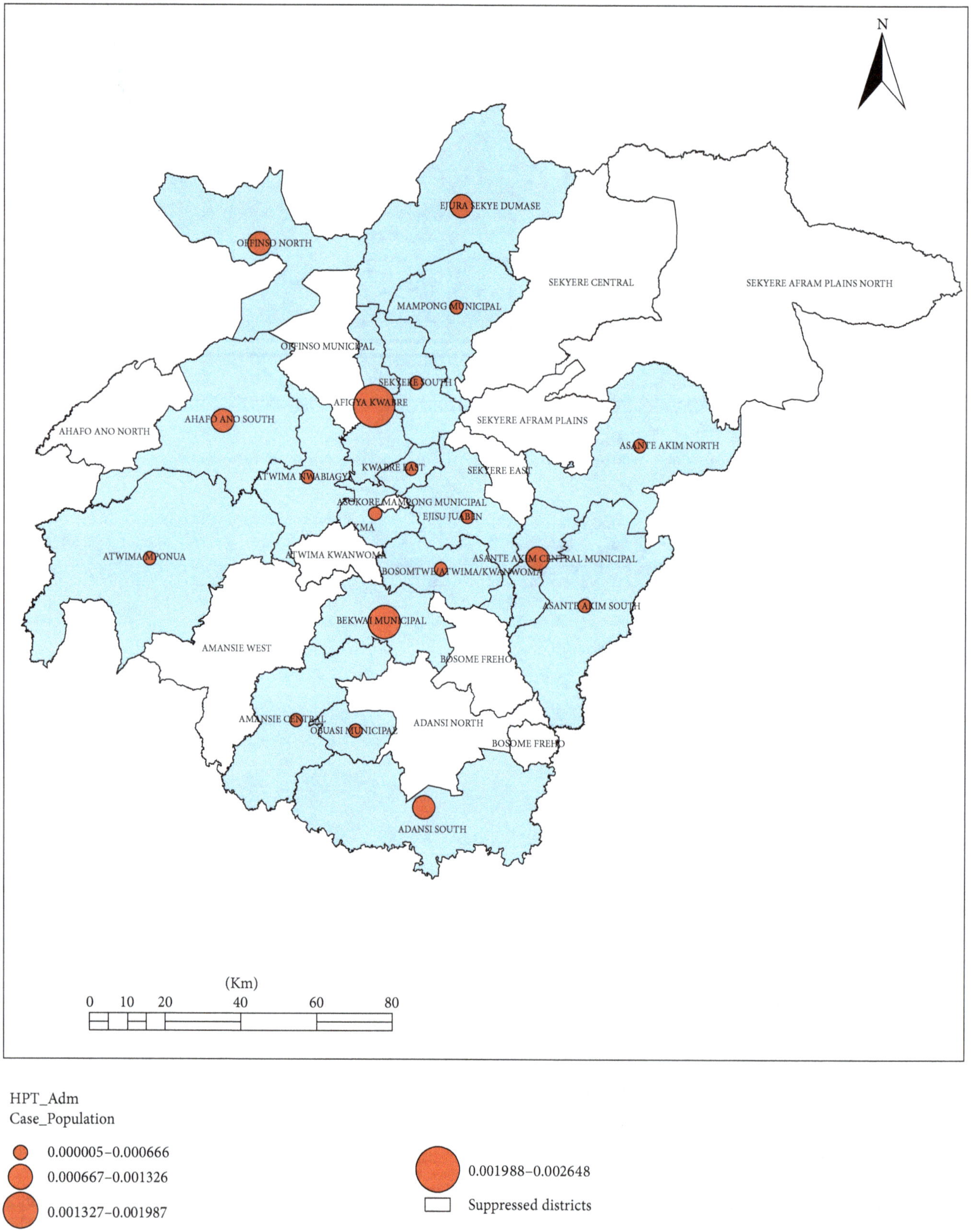


FIGURE 2: Case density of hypertension admission as reported by hospital, Ashanti, 2014.

TABLE 2: Chi-square test of association of sociodemographic characteristics of inpatient hypertensive clients and outcome of admission.

| Variables | Hypertension outcome of admission | | | | | | Total | $\chi^2$ | p – Value |
|---|---|---|---|---|---|---|---|---|---|
| | Died | | Discharged | | Referred | | | | |
| | Frequency | % | Frequency | % | Frequency | % | | | |
| Age group | | | | | | | | | |
| 25–34 | 2 | 3.9 | 86 | 5.39 | 3 | 4.5 | 91 | | |
| 35–44 | 3 | 5.8 | 218 | 13.7 | 11 | 16.4 | 232 | | |
| 45–54 | 10 | 19.2 | 355 | 22.3 | 17 | 25.4 | 382 | 8.82 | 0.304 |
| 55–64 | 8 | 15.4 | 326 | 20.4 | 14 | 20.9 | 348 | | |
| 65+ | 29 | 55.8 | 610 | 38.2 | 22 | 32.8 | 661 | | |
| *Total* | *52* | *100* | *1595* | *100* | *67* | *100* | *1714* | | |
| Sex | | | | | | | | | |
| Male | 24 | 46.2 | 506 | 31.7 | 27 | 40.3 | 557 | | |
| Female | 28 | 53.9 | 1088 | 68.3 | 40 | 59.7 | 1156 | 6.69 | 0.218 |
| *Total* | *52* | *100* | *1594* | *100* | *67* | *100* | *1621* | | |
| Educational level | | | | | | | | | |
| No formal education | 31 | 59.6 | 921 | 57.8 | 35 | 52.2 | 987 | | |
| Primary | 16 | 30.8 | 564 | 35.4 | 25 | 37.3 | 605 | | |
| Secondary | 2 | 3.9 | 66 | 4.1 | 2 | 3.0 | 70 | 7.60 | 0.414 |
| Tertiary | 3 | 5.8 | 42 | 2.6 | 5 | 7.5 | 50 | | |
| *Total* | *52* | *100* | *1593* | *100* | *67* | *100* | *1712* | | |
| NHIS status | | | | | | | | | |
| Have NHIS | 36 | 69.2 | 1350 | 85.7 | 57 | 85.1 | 1443 | | |
| Not having NHIS | 16 | 30.8 | 225 | 14.3 | 10 | 14.9 | 251 | 10.84 | 0.041* |
| *Total* | *52* | *32* | *1575* | *100* | *63* | *100* | *1694* | | |
| Occupation | | | | | | | | | |
| Unemployed | 3 | 5.8 | 113 | 7.1 | 13 | 19.4 | 129 | | |
| Formal Employment | 2 | 3.9 | 33 | 2.1 | 4 | 6.0 | 39 | | |
| Self-employed | 13 | 25.0 | 651 | 40.9 | 18 | 26.9 | 682 | | |
| Student | 0 | 0.0 | 3 | 0.2 | 0 | 0.0 | 3 | 28.09 | 0.147 |
| Unspecified | 26 | 50.0 | 583 | 36.6 | 21 | 31.3 | 630 | | |
| Others | 8 | 15.4 | 208 | 13.1 | 11 | 16.4 | 227 | | |
| *Total* | *52* | *100* | *1591* | *100* | *67* | *100* | *1710* | | |
| Length of stay | | | | | | | | | |
| 1 day | 15 | 34.88 | 477 | 31.51 | 19 | 33.93 | 511 | | |
| 2 days | 7 | 16.28 | 473 | 31.24 | 12 | 21.43 | 492 | | |
| 3 days | 5 | 11.63 | 230 | 15.19 | 9 | 16.07 | 244 | 11.92 | 0.155 |
| 4 days | 4 | 9.30 | 114 | 7.53 | 4 | 7.14 | 122 | | |
| 5+ | 12 | 27.91 | 220 | 14.53 | 12 | 21.43 | 244 | | |
| *Total* | *43* | *100* | *1514* | *100* | *56* | *100* | *1613* | | |
| Facility ownership | | | | | | | | | |
| Quasi/mission | 25 | 48.1 | 556 | 34.9 | 23 | 34.3 | | | |
| Public | 27 | 51.9 | 946 | 59.3 | 43 | 64.2 | | 8.41 | 0.706 |
| Private | 0 | 0 | 93 | 5.8 | 1 | 1.5 | | | |
| *Total* | *52* | *100* | *1595* | *100* | *67* | *100* | | | |
| District status | | | | | | | | | |
| Rural | 13 | 25.00 | 513 | 32.16 | 11 | 16.42 | 537 | | |
| Urban | 39 | 75.00 | 1082 | 67.84 | 56 | 83.58 | 1177 | 8.41 | 0.221 |
| *Total* | *52* | *100* | *1595* | *100* | *67* | *100* | *1714* | | |

*Statistically significant.

Table 3: Univariable and multivariable logistics regression analysis for the association between outcome of admission and sociodemographic characteristics of inpatient admissions of Ashanti.

| Characteristics | | | $N^* = 1552$ | |
|---|---|---|---|---|
| | Crude OR (95% CI) | $p$ value | Adjusted OR (95% CI) | $p$ value |
| Age group | | | | |
| 25–34 (reference) | 1 | | | |
| 35–44 | 0.58 | 0.475 | 0.64 (0.13–3.20) | 0.573 |
| 45–54 | 1.19 | 0.836 | 0.74 (0.05–10.40) | 0.815 |
| 55–64 | 1.05 | 0.947 | 0.44 (0.06–3.42) | 0.420 |
| 65+ | 2.04 | 0.436 | 0.54 (0.02–18.13) | 0.722 |
| Age** | 1.03 | 0.029** | 1.04 (0.99–1.10) | 0.087 |
| Sex | | | | |
| Male (reference) | 1 | | | |
| Female | 0.55 | 0.017** | 0.49 (0.29–0.82) | 0.009** |
| Educational level | | | | |
| No formal education (reference) | 1 | | | |
| Primary | 0.84 | 0.581 | 1.43 (0.80–2.56) | 0.211 |
| Secondary | 0.91 | 0.905 | 0.99 (0.13–7.86) | 0.999 |
| Tertiary | 1.97 | 0.302 | 3.42 (0.38–30.49) | 0.170 |
| Occupation | | | | |
| Unemployed (reference) | 1 | | | |
| Formal employment | 2.27 | 0.535 | Omitted | |
| Self employed | 0.82 | 0.746 | 0.83 (0.14–4.97) | 0.834 |
| Student | Omitted | | Omitted | |
| Unspecified | 1.81 | 0.324 | 2.53 (0.49–13.11) | 0.257 |
| Others | 1.53 | 0.533 | 1.15 (0.19–6.94) | 0.872 |
| NHIS status | | | | |
| Not having NHIS (reference) | 1 | | | |
| Have NHIS | 0.376 | 0.040** | 0.22 (0.11–0.45) | 0.001** |
| Length of stay on admission | | | | |
| Length of stay | 1.04 | 0.009** | 1.05 (0.99–1.10) | 0.069 |
| Facility ownership | | | | |
| Quasi/mission (reference) | 1 | | | |
| Public | 0.632 | 0.260 | 0.69 (0.29–1.61) | 0.373 |
| Private | 1 (omitted) | | | |
| District status | | | | |
| Rural (reference) | 1 | | | |
| Urban | 1.38 | 0.520 | 0.84 (0.31–2.30) | 0.726 |

$N^*$ sample size for multivariable logistic regression analysis. Age** significantly associated with the outcomes in this model when it was substituted for age category.

outcomes. After adjusting for all other variables, NHIS and sex were significant predictors of the hypertension admission outcome as shown in Table 3.

NHIS registrants were 78% less likely to die from admissions due to hypertension (AOR 0.22, 95% CI 0.11–0.45; $p = 0.001$), whilst females were 51% less likely to die from hypertension admission (AOR 0.49, 95% CI 0.29–0.82; $p = 0.009$).

In the crude analysis, for every day increase in the length of stay on admission, clients were 1.04 times more likely to die from hypertension admission. Replacing age group (categorical variable) with age (continuous variable) and using the same model, age showed a significant association with hypertension admission outcomes (OR = 1.03, 95% CI 1.00–1.05, $p = 0.029$) implying that, for every unit increase in age (years), clients were 1.04 times more likely to die from hypertension admission.

This study sought to use secondary data on hypertension admissions from the DHMIS for 2014 to determine the characteristics of inpatient hypertension cases and factors associated with admission outcomes in Ashanti Region for 2014. Females dominated the number of inpatient hypertensives in this study. This is consistent with Owusu-Sekyere and colleagues who report that there are more female hypertensives in the Kumasi metropolis than males [11]. Our finding is however not consistent with findings of Kolo and colleagues in a similar study, where females constituted 48.4% [15].

In this study, age groups were not associated with admission outcomes. However, age as a continuous variable had significant association with the outcome. Thus, for every unit increase in age (years), hypertensives on admission are 1.04 times more likely to die (OR 1.04, 95% CI 1.003–1.05 $p$ = 0.029). This is consistent with Peck et al. study which reported in 2013 that those who die of noncommunicable diseases such as hypertension are older than those who died from communicable diseases [16].

Sex and NHIS status of clients were significantly associated with admission outcomes in this study. Contrary to popular opinions, available data showed that females were 51% less likely to die from hypertension admission. This is probably because women are more conscious of their health with a better health seeking behaviour than men [15]. It can only be inferred that men's health seeking behaviour was poor. There is the need to improve upon the health seeking behaviours of men especially through information, communication, and education programs. Earlier studies by Méndez-Chacón et al. reported that the proportion in men unaware of their hypertension status is higher than that of unaware women (32% versus 20%) [17].

Majority of the deaths recorded from HPT admissions were at the age of 65 years and above with females dominating. However, Williams et al. established the tremendous burden of hypertension-related conditions in adults in sub-Saharan Africa in a similar study which also reported that majority of hypertension-related deaths occurred in the working-age males (median age of death: 61 years) [16].

Our study reports that NHIS registrants are 78% less likely to die from admissions due to hypertension (AOR 0.22, 95% CI 0.11–0.45; $p$ = 0.001). Others have reported that the blood pressure levels of clients who receive free medical care are lower than those who have to pay for the cost of care. Therefore, it is plausible that patients who have to pay for cost of care generally delay in seeking prompt care until their conditions are worsened [4]. Obviously, this is likely to lead to a poorer outcome when they are finally admitted. Although the proportion of patients with NHIS clients in this study was high (85.2%), the effects of lack of NHIS ownership on admission outcomes observed in this study bring to bear the need for a universal health care policy, which ensures that primary prevention and management of hypertension are included in the basic health care provided to all citizens.

Earlier reports from Nigeria indicate that case fatality for hypertension admissions is influenced by length of stay in the hospital, among others [15], and this study also answers in the affirmative regarding the crude analysis alone (OR 1.04, 95% CI, $p$- value = 0.009).

Our study shows that majority (59.3%) of the cases were reported by government hospitals. Out of 121 hospitals in the Ashanti Region, hospitals that reported in DHIMS by ownership were 28, 68, and 22 for mission/quasi-, private, and public facilities, respectively. However, the proportion of hospitals that reported on hypertension admission cases for the year 2014 is 35.7% of quasi-/mission, 4.4% of private, and 77.3% of public facilities. This situation contributed to the high number of cases reported by the public hospitals.

## 4. Conclusions

NHIS registrants and females were less likely to die on admission resulting from hypertension; therefore increasing NHIS access can potentially have an impact positively on hypertension admission outcomes. Also, IEC programs should pay more attention to men to help improve their health seeking behaviour, thereby improving hypertension admission outcomes.

Strategies must be adapted to resource quasi-/mission and private facilities in providing hypertension admission care to relieve the pressure on public hospitals.

## 5. Study Limitations

Due to the cross-sectional nature of this dataset, the temporal associations between NHIS status, gender, age, length of stay, and hypertension admission outcome variables may not be causal. Our study did not have any gold standard to compare the hypertension diagnosis provided in the dataset; therefore any misclassification could not have been determined. The actual cause of death could not also be validated due to the nature of the data; therefore, the death reported in this study may not be due to hypertension alone. However, generally, prescribers are all well trained and participate in compulsory continuous professional development programs coupled with regular stringent monitoring and supervisory visit from the Regional Health Administration. It could be presumed that they provide standard care to the patients. The use of routine health facility data restricted this study to the use of only variables presented in the dataset. All the public and quasi-/mission hospitals from the district levels report to the DHIMS platform, but eight out of the thirty districts in the region do not have hospitals to admit HPT cases; therefore cases from these districts could not be reported by the district. The findings of this study may not be generalizable to the whole Ashanti Region granted that even data from the only teaching hospital and biggest referral hospital (KATH) in the region was not available.

## Abbreviations

AIDS: Acquired Immune Deficiency Syndrome
AOR: Adjusted odds ratio
CI: Confidence interval
DHIMS: District Health Information Management System
ERC: Ethical Review Committee
GHS: Ghana Health Service
HIV: Human Immune Deficiency Virus
HPT: Hypertension
JHS: Junior High School
KATH: Komfo Anokye Teaching Hospital
MOH: Ministry of Health
NCD: Noncommunicable diseases
NHIS: National Health Insurance Scheme
OR: Odds ratio
OPD: Out-patient department
RHMT: Regional Health Management Team
WHO: World Health Organization.

## Ethical Approval

Ethical approval was obtained from the Ethics Review Committee (ERC) of the GHS (GHS-ERC: 24/09/15).

## Disclosure

The Ashanti Regional Director of Health Services granted permission for the use of the retrospective health facility data, provided permission for publication, and is also a co-author of this paper. The dataset consists of routine Health Service Information obtained from the database of Ghana Health Service and as such human written informed consent was not necessary. Appropriate permission was sought from the Regional Director who had oversight over the data. There was no need for consent from study participants since we relied on retrospective health facility data. The nature of the study posed no risk to individuals whose data were used because only their unique identifiers were in the dataset. Confidentiality was maintained and only the research team had access to the data. The anonymous nature of the data used does not permit the disclosure of any individual's details since the information was not connected to individual names or identity. The Global Fund and the Ghana National Malaria Control Programme had no role in the design of the study, collection, analysis, and interpretation of data and in writing the manuscript.

## Authors' Contributions

Kenneth Nuamah, Harriet Affran Bonful, Joseph Danso Yeboah, Daniel Boakye, and Ebenezer Antwi Amankwaah designed the study with inputs from Bertha Garshong, Anthony Ofosu, Margaret Gyapong, and Evelyn K. Ansah. Kenneth Nuamah, Joseph Danso Yeboah, Daniel Boakye, and Ebenezer Antwi Amankwaah extracted secondary data for analysis. Freddie Amponsah, Samuel Kwame Owusu, and Joseph Danso Yeboah generated maps for the geospatial distribution under the supervision of Anthony Ofosu. Harriet Affran Bonful, Kenneth Nuamah, Evelyn K. Ansah, Freddie Amponsah, Anthony Ofosu, Bertha Garshong, Margaret Gyapong, and Alexis Nang-Beifubah analysed and interpreted the data. Kenneth Nuamah, Harriet Affran Bonful, Joseph Danso Yeboah, Daniel Boakye, Ebenezer Antwi Amankwaah, and Evelyn K. Ansah wrote the first draft of the manuscript. Anthony Ofosu, Bertha Garshong, Margaret Gyapong, Freddie Amponsah, Adwoa Aduako Owusu, Fred Adomako-Boateng, and Alexis Nang-Beifubah contributed to the revision and finalization of the manuscript. All authors approved the final version of the manuscript. Evelyn K. Ansah and Anthony Ofosu are the guarantors.

## Acknowledgments

The authors wish to acknowledge the technical support received from Dr. Abraham Hodgson, Dr. Amanua Chinbuah, and the Research Development Division of Ghana Health Service. They also wish to acknowledge the technical support from the Policy Planning Monitoring & Evaluation Division of Ghana Health Service for the extraction and use of data from the DHIMS2 database of the Ghana Health Service. The authors wish to acknowledge the organizers of the Ghana Health Service National Research Dissemination Forum where this manuscript was earlier presented as an abstract in 2016 brochure. Finally, they wish to thank the Programme Manager and staff of the National Malaria Control Programme for facilitating access to funding this study. This study received financial support from Global Fund to Fight AIDS, Tuberculosis and Malaria through the Ghana National Malaria Control Programme.

## References

[1] W. H. Day, World Health Day 2013, A Glob. Br. Hypertens., p. 9, 2013.

[2] WHO, Global status report on noncommunicable diseases, 2010.

[3] S. S. Lim, T. Vos, and A. D. Flaxman, "A comparative risk assessment of burden of disease and injury attributable to 67 risk factors and risk factor clusters in 21 regions, 1990–2010: a systematic analysis for the Global Burden of Disease Study 2010," *The Lancet*, vol. 380, pp. 1990–2010, 2012.

[4] L. H. Opie and Y. K. Seedat, "Hypertension in Sub-Saharan African populations," *Circulation*, vol. 112, no. 23, pp. 3562–3568, 2005.

[5] P. M. Kearney, M. Whelton, K. Reynolds, P. Muntner, P. K. Whelton, and J. He, "Global burden of hypertension: analysis of worldwide data," *The Lancet*, vol. 365, no. 9455, pp. 217–223, 2005.

[6] O. S. Ogah, "Blood pressure, prevalence of hypertension and hypertension related complications in Nigerian Africans: A review," *World Journal of Cardiology*, vol. 4, no. 12, pp. 327–340, 2012.

[7] S. Sidhu and K. Kumari, "Socio-demographic variables of hypertension among adult punjabi females," *Journal of Human Ecology*, vol. 17, no. 3, pp. 211–215, 2005.

[8] J. Addo, C. Agyemang, L. Smeeth, A. de-Graft Aikins, A. K. Edusei, and O. Ogedegbe, "A review of population-based studies on hypertension in Ghana," *Ghana Medical Journal*, vol. 46, supplement, no. 2, pp. 4–11, 2012.

[9] Z. Wang, Q. Du, S. Liang et al., "Analysis of the spatial variation of hospitalization admissions for hypertension disease in shenzhen, China," *International Journal of Environmental Research and Public Health*, vol. 11, no. 1, pp. 713–733, 2014.

[10] H. Survey, "Ghana," 2014.

[11] E. Owusu-Sekyere, B. Ebenezer, and O. Linda, "Spatial Modeling of Hypertension Disease in the Kumasi Metropolitan Area of Ghana," *International Journal of Statistics and Applications*, vol. 3, no. 4, pp. 132–140, 2013.

[12] H. A. Tagoe and F. A. A. Dake, "Healthy lifestyle behaviour among Ghanaian adults in the phase of a health policy change," *Globalization and Health*, vol. 7, article no. 7, 2011.

[13] A. R. H. Directorate, "2014 Annual Report." 2014.

[14] G. Ministry of, Health, Standard Treatment Guidelines,.

[15] P. M. Kolo, Y. B. Jibrin, E. O. Sanya, M. Alkali, I. B. Peter Kio, and R. K. Moronkola, "Hypertension-related admissions and outcome in a tertiary hospital in northeast Nigeria," *International*

*Journal of Hypertension*, vol. 2012, Article ID 960546, 6 pages, 2012.

[16] R. N. Peck, E. Green, J. Mtabaji et al., "Hypertension related diseases as a common cause of hospital mortality in Tanzania: a 3-year prospective study," *Global Health Action*, vol. 9, no. 1, pp. 1806–1811, 2014.

[17] E. Méndez-Chacón, C. Santamaría-Ulloa, and L. Rosero-Bixby, "Factors associated with hypertension prevalence, unawareness and treatment among Costa Rican elderly," *BMC Public Health*, vol. 8, no. 1, article 275, 2008.

# 18

# Effects of Carvedilol on Blood Pressure, Blood Sugar and Blood Lipids in Elderly Patients with Refractory Hypertension

**Wen Zhang,[1] Guiming Deng,[1] Jia Hu,[2] Ran Yan,[3] Junliu Hu,[2] and Jianmin Fan[4]**

[1]*The First Hospital of Hunan University of Chinese Medicine, Department of Geriatrics, No. 95 Shaoshan Middle Road, Yuhua District, Changsha City, Hunan Province, China*
[2]*Hunan University of Chinese Medicine, Graduate School, Xiangzui Road, Yuelu District, Changsha City, Hunan Province, China*
[3]*Hunan University of Chinese Medicine, School of Traditional Chinese Medicine, Xiangzui Road, Yuelu District, Changsha City, Hunan Province, China*
[4]*The First Hospital of Hunan University of Chinese Medicine, Department of Cardiovascular Diseases, No. 95 Shaoshan Middle Road, Yuhua District, Changsha City, Hunan Province, China*

Correspondence should be addressed to Jianmin Fan; b20160503228@stu.ccsu.edu.cn

Academic Editor: Gang Chen

Refractory hypertension seriously affects the life safety of patients. To investigate the effect of carvedilol combined with conventional antihypertensive therapy on blood pressure, blood sugar, blood lipids, and cardiovascular and cerebrovascular complications in elderly patients with refractory hypertension, a total of 80 elderly patients with refractory hypertension who were admitted from June 2019 to September 2021 were selected as the retrospective research objects and divided into the observation group and the control group according to the random number table method, 40 cases in each group, and the control group received conventional antihypertensive therapy. On this basis, the observation group was treated with carvedilol, and the effects of blood pressure, blood sugar, blood lipids, and cardiovascular and cerebrovascular complications were analyzed in the two groups. After treatment, the systolic blood pressure, diastolic blood pressure, adrenal medulla (AM), and endothelin (ET) of the observation group were significantly lower than those of the control group, but the heart rate and NO of the observation group were significantly higher than those of the control group. After treatment, the fasting blood glucose, insulin, triacylglycerol (TG), cholesterol (CHO), and low-density lipoprotein (LDL-C) of the observation group were significantly higher than those of the control group, but the ISI and HDL-C of the observation group were significantly lower than those of the control group. After treatment, the levels of IL-1$\beta$, IL-6, TNF-$\alpha$, UAER, BUN, and SCr in the observation group were significantly lower than those in the control group. The TC of the observation group was lower than that of the control group. Combination therapy has a remarkably stable, sustained, and safe antihypertensive effect on patients with refractory hypertension.

## 1. Introduction

Refractory hypertension is defined as the application of a reasonably tolerable adequate dose of >3 antihypertensive drugs on the basis of lifestyle improvement, treatment for >1 month and still not achieving the blood pressure standard, or taking >4 antihypertensive drugs for effective blood pressure control [1–3]. The prevalence of refractory hypertension has increased gradually over a 20-year period, which may be related to the increased awareness, treatment, and management of hypertension in the United States and certainly to the increasing prevalence of aging and obesity [4]. We speculate that the prevalence of true refractory hypertension may not be high and that many patients may have pseudorefractory hypertension due to irrational medication use and poor compliance [5]. Carvedilol is a nonselective $\beta$-blocker that blocks $\beta$ receptors comprehensively and also selectively blocks $\alpha 1$ receptors, without endogenous sympathomimetic activity or peripheral $\beta$ agonism [6]. Poor control of blood pressure in refractory hypertension can easily

TABLE 1: Comparison of baseline information between the two groups of patients ($\bar{X} \pm S$).

| Group | Average age (years) | Gender (male/female) | Duration of disease (years) | Body weight (kg) |
|---|---|---|---|---|
| Comparison group (40) | 60.90 ± 1.71 | 24/26 | 3.05 ± 1.23 | 62.35 ± 2.10 |
| Observation group (40) | 61.10 ± 1.62 | 23/27 | 2.40 ± 2.03 | 60.10 ± 1.10 |
| $t$ | 0.377 | 0.731 | 0.763 | 2.107 |
| $P$ | 0.051 | 0.067 | 0.091 | 0.079 |

lead to target organ damage, leading to more serious consequences.

Carvedilol, as a third-generation $\beta$-blocker, has characteristics unmatched by other receptor blockers and is widely used in the treatment of hypertension, congestive heart failure, and coronary artery disease, with positive efficacy [7]. Some studies have shown that carvedilol can subside left ventricular hypertrophy and improve diastolic function in hypertensive patients [8]. There are few reports in the literature on the therapeutic effects of carvedilol with various antihypertensive drugs, and this paper examines the effects of carvedilol combined with conventional antihypertensive therapy on blood pressure, glucose, lipids, and cardiovascular complications in elderly patients with refractory hypertension.

## 2. Material and Methods

*2.1. Research Object.* Eighty cases of elderly patients with refractory hypertension admitted from June 2019 to September 2021 were selected for the retrospective study and were divided into 40 cases each in the observation and comparison groups according to the random number table method. Hypertension was diagnosed according to the criteria in the Chinese Guidelines for the Prevention and Treatment of Hypertension (2010 edition) [9], with an office systolic blood pressure ≥ 140 mmHg and/or diastolic blood pressure ≥ 90 mmHg, or taking antihypertensive drugs as hypertension: 140-159/90-99 mmHg as grade 1 hypertension, 160-179/100-109 mmHg as grade 2 hypertension, and ≥180/110 mmHg as grade 3 hypertension. Systolic blood pressure < 140 mmHg and diastolic blood pressure ≥ 90 mmHg were defined as pure diastolic hypertension, systolic blood pressure ≥ 140 mmHg and diastolic blood pressure < 90 mmHg were defined as pure systolic hypertension, and systolic blood pressure ≥ 140 mmHg and diastolic blood pressure ≥ 90 mmHg were defined as dual systolic-diastolic hypertension. Refractory hypertension was defined as office blood pressure ≥ 140/90 mmHg after taking ≥3 antihypertensive drugs (including a diuretic) or office blood pressure < 140/90 mmHg, but ≥4 antihypertensive drugs were required. The hypertension awareness rate was defined as the percentage of the total number of hypertensive patients who knew they had hypertension; the hypertension treatment rate was defined as the percentage of the total number of hypertensive patients who were taking antihypertensive drugs in the past two weeks; the hypertension control rate was defined as the percentage of the total number of hypertensive patients whose blood pressure was controlled to the target value (systolic blood pressure < 140 mmHg and diastolic blood pressure < 90 mmHg).

*2.2. Inclusion and Exclusion Criteria.* Inclusion criteria: (1) those with good compliance and able to cooperate with medical staff to complete our study; (2) those without congestive heart failure, acute myocarditis, acute myocardial infarction, diabetes mellitus, etc.; (3) those without history of surgery and other infectious diseases. Exclusion criteria: (1) severe diabetes mellitus with uncontrollable symptoms, infection or blood transfusion within 3 months, other chronic diseases such as malignancy, and change of treatment plan within 3 months; (2) those who do not actively cooperate with treatment, history of blood transfusion, and major trauma and surgery in the last 3 months; (3) secondary hypertension, liver and kidney dysfunction, and history of allergy to the drugs used in our study.

*2.3. Methods.* In the control group, conventional antihypertensive therapy was administered, with 80 mg/d of gelsartan (produced by Beijing Novartis Pharmaceutical Co., Ltd.) and 1 tablet/d of compound amiloride hydrochloride (produced by Jiangsu Tianhe Pharmaceutical Co., Ltd.) The first 4 weeks were the transition period of the drug, and after 4 weeks, if the blood pressure decreased to an effective level, the drug was taken for another 4 weeks at the original dose, and the blood pressure was reduced and maintained if it was stable, and the blood pressure was <120/80 mmHg and accompanied by dizziness. For those with blood pressure < 120/80 mmHg and dizziness, the compound amiloride hydrochloride could be reduced and stopped. However, the observation group was treated with carvedilol, taking 80 mg/d of gelsartan (produced by Beijing Novartis Pharmaceutical Co., Ltd.); 12.5 mg/d of carvedilol (produced by Shanghai Roche Pharmaceutical Co., Ltd.), and if tolerated, the dose was increased to 25 mg/d after two days; and 1 tablet/d of compound amiloride hydrochloride (produced by Jiangsu Tianhe Pharmaceutical Co., Ltd.). The first 4 weeks were the transition period of the drug, and after 4 weeks, if the blood pressure decreased to an effective level, then the dose was reduced again. If the blood pressure decreases effectively, the drug will be taken for another 4 weeks at the original dose; if the blood pressure is stable, the dose will be reduced and maintained; if the blood pressure is <120/80 mmHg and accompanied by dizziness, the compound amiloride hydrochloride can be reduced and stopped.

*2.4. Observation Index.* Inflammatory factors and endothelial function factors: 5 ml of fasting venous blood was drawn

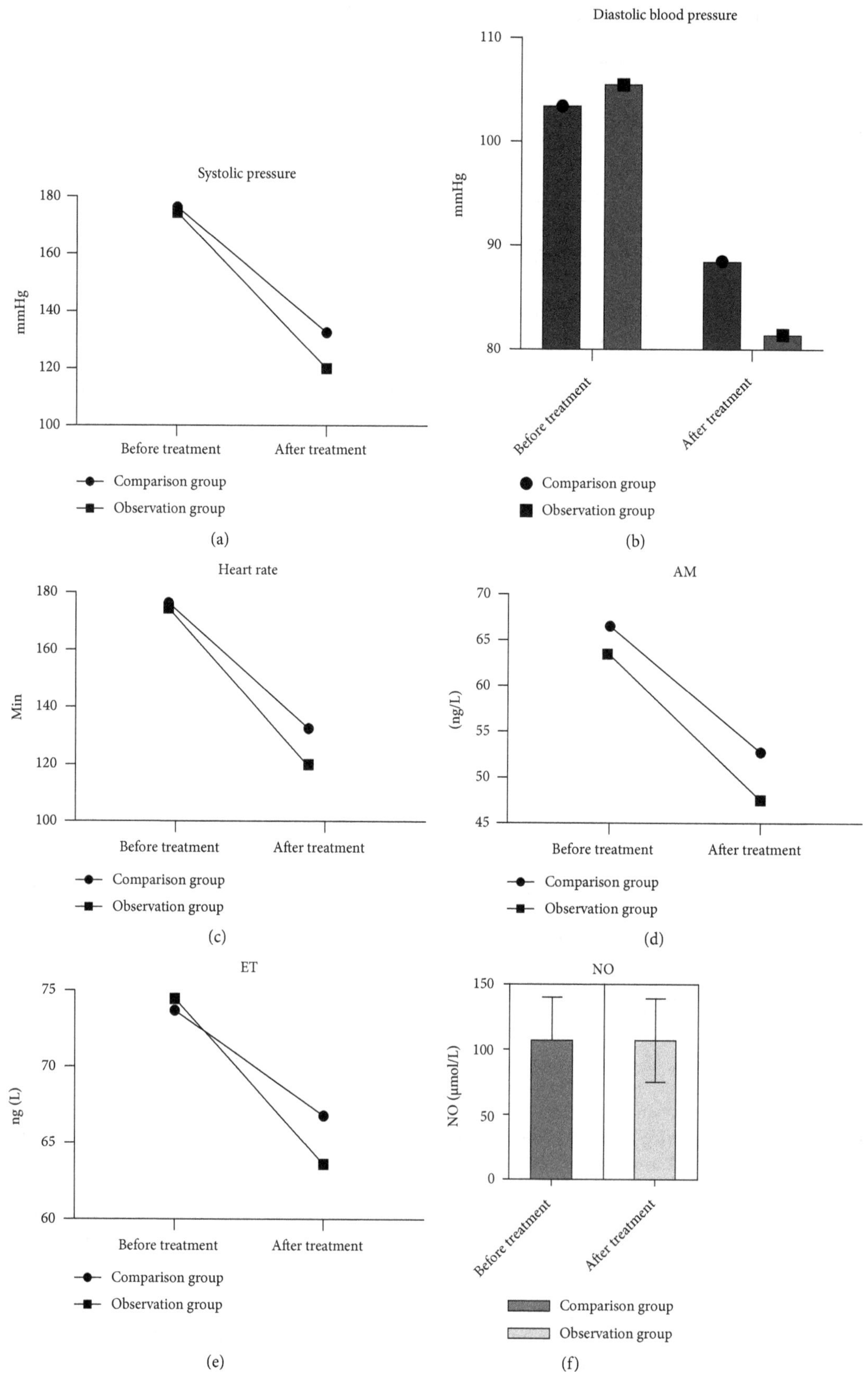


FIGURE 1: Comparison of blood pressure-related indicators. The data of blood pressure-related indicators of our study were entered into Excel software by the first and corresponding authors, and the statistical processing software was SPSS 25.0 for calculation. Using the mean ± standard deviation ($X \pm S$) representation using the independent sample $t$-test.

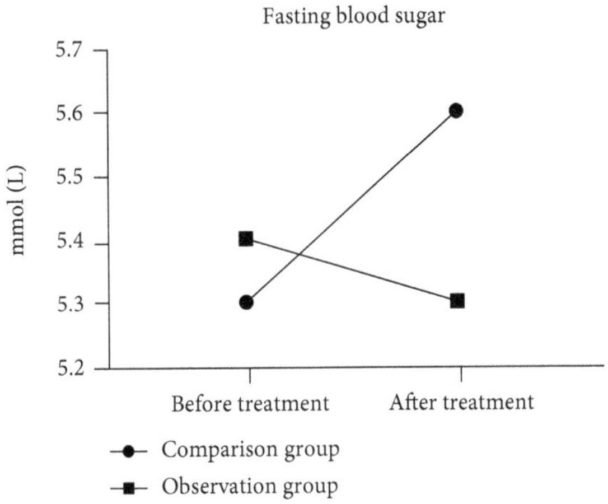


(a)

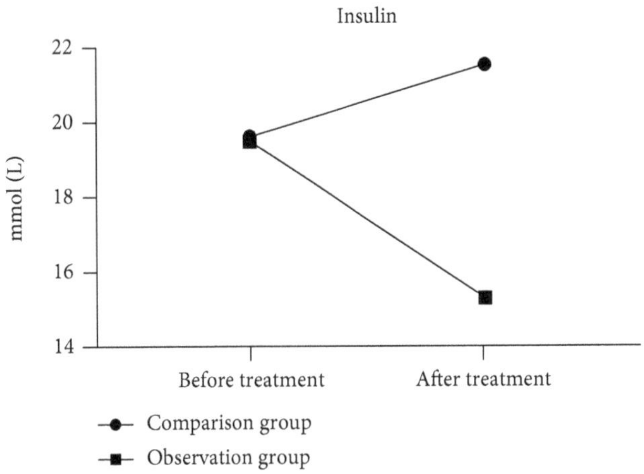


(b)

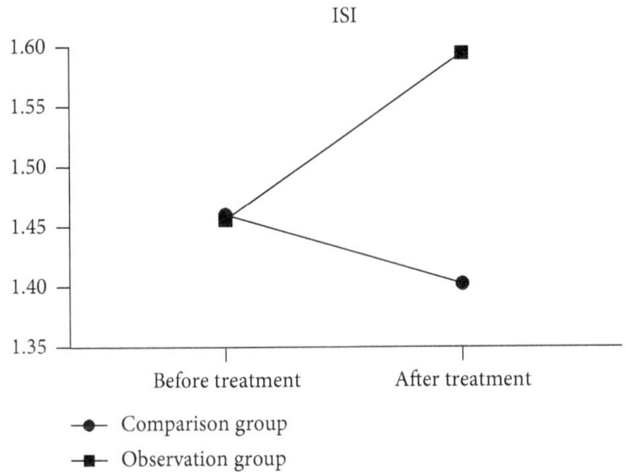


(c)

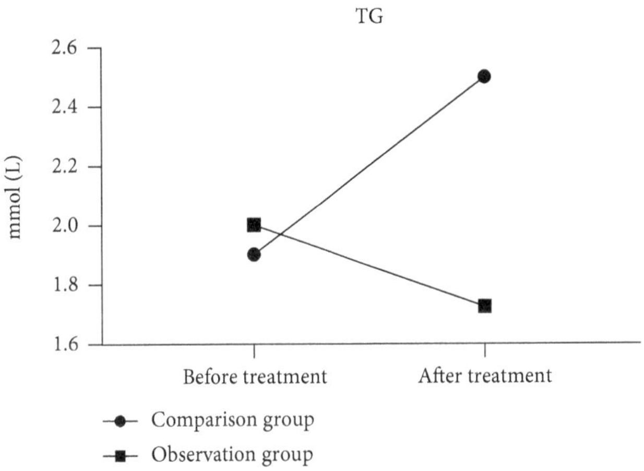


(d)

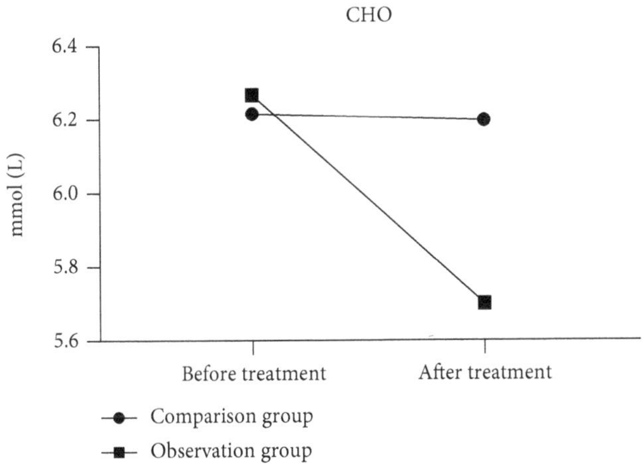


(e)

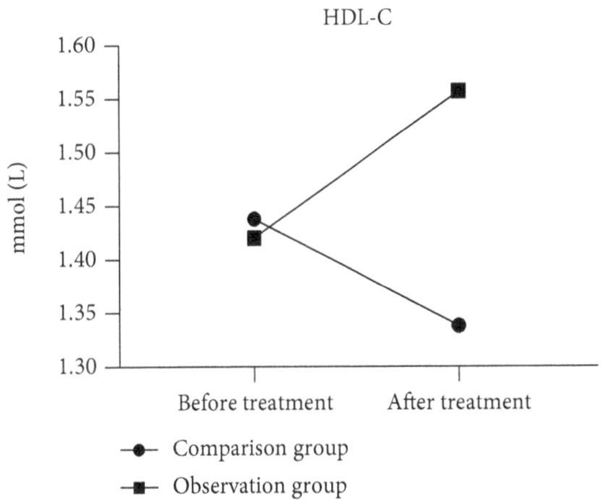


(f)

FIGURE 2: Continued.

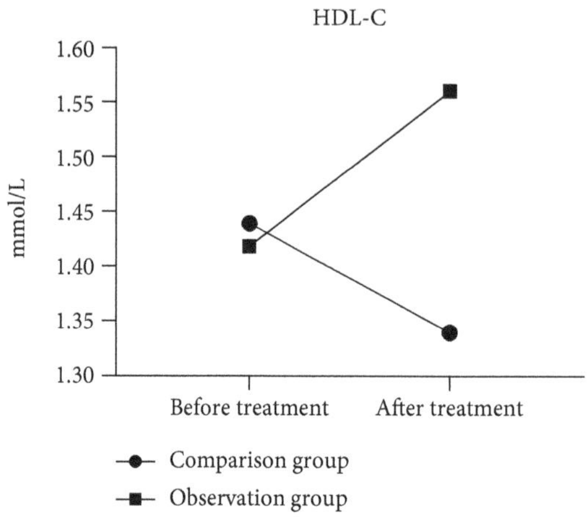


(g)

FIGURE 2: Blood lipid and blood sugar comparison. Blood lipid and blood sugar comparison data from our study were entered into Excel software by the first and corresponding authors, and statistical processing software was SPSS 25.0 for calculation. The mean ± standard deviation ($X \pm S$) was used to express the results using independent sample $t$-test.

before treatment and 1 month after treatment, respectively, and centrifuged at 3000 r/min for 5 min, and the supernatant liquid was placed in EP tubes and stored at -70°C. Serum interleukin- (IL-) 1B and IL-6 were detected in EP tubes by enzyme-linked immunosorbent assay (ELISA), and the kits were purchased from Shanghai ELISA Biotechnology Co. Plasma adrenal medulla (AM) and endothelin (ET) were detected by Beckman luminescence immunoassay, and nitric oxide (NO) was detected by nitrate reductase assay. The 24 h urinary protein excretion rate (UAER), serum creatinine (SCr), blood urea ammonia (BUN), total cholesterol (TC), and triacylglycerol (TG) were measured before and after treatment, and occasional blood pressure (OBP) and ambulatory blood pressure (ABP) were monitored. In all cases, the sitting blood pressure after 15 minutes of rest was measured three times with a mercury column sphygmomanometer on the day of treatment initiation and at the end of treatment, and the mean values were taken. Blood glucose and lipid were measured by American Beckman CX4 biochemical instrument, insulin was measured by radioimmunoassay (the kit was provided by the Reagent Research Institute of China Isotope Company), and the insulin sensitivity index (ISI) was calculated by the formula $\ln\left[1/(\text{fasting blood glucose} \times \text{fasting insulin})\right]$.

*2.5. Statistical Analysis.* All statistical data in this study were entered into Excel software by the first author and the corresponding author, respectively, and the statistical processing software was SPSS 25.0 for calculation. Repeated measures analysis of variance between groups was used to measure the measurement expressed as mean ± standard deviation ($X \pm S$) material. Count data expressed as a percentage (%) were tested by $\chi^2$. Included data that did not conform to a normal distribution were described by $M$ (QR), using the Mann–Whitney test. All statistical tests were two-sided probability tests. The statistical significance was $P < 0.05$.

## 3. Results

*3.1. Comparison of Baseline Data.* The mean age, gender, disease duration, and weight of the patients in the observation group were not significantly different from those in the comparison group, and the comparative differences were not statistically significant ($P > 0.05$). See Table 1.

*3.2. Comparison of Blood Pressure-Related Indicators.* There was no statistical significance in the blood pressure-related indexes before treatment ($P > 0.05$). After treatment, the systolic blood pressure, diastolic blood pressure, AM, and ET of the observation group were significantly lower than those of the control group, but the heart rate and NO of the observation group were significantly higher than those of the control group, and the differences were statistically significant ($P < 0.05$). See Figure 1.

*3.3. Blood Lipid and Blood Sugar Comparison.* After treatment, the fasting blood glucose, insulin, TG, CHO, and LDL-C of the observation group were significantly higher than those of the control group, but the ISI and HDL-C of the observation group were significantly lower than those of the control group, and the differences were statistically significant ($P < 0.05$). See Figure 2.

*3.4. Serum Index Comparison.* There was no significant difference in serum indexes between the two groups before treatment ($P > 0.05$). After treatment, the levels of IL-1$\beta$, IL-6, TNF-$\alpha$, UAER, BUN, and SCr in the observation group were significantly lower than those in the control group. The TC of the observation group was lower than that of the control group, and the difference was statistically significant ($P < 0.05$). See Figure 3.

## 4. Discussion

Refractory hypertension is a common clinical condition that is more difficult to treat. Carvedilol is a nonselective $\beta$-

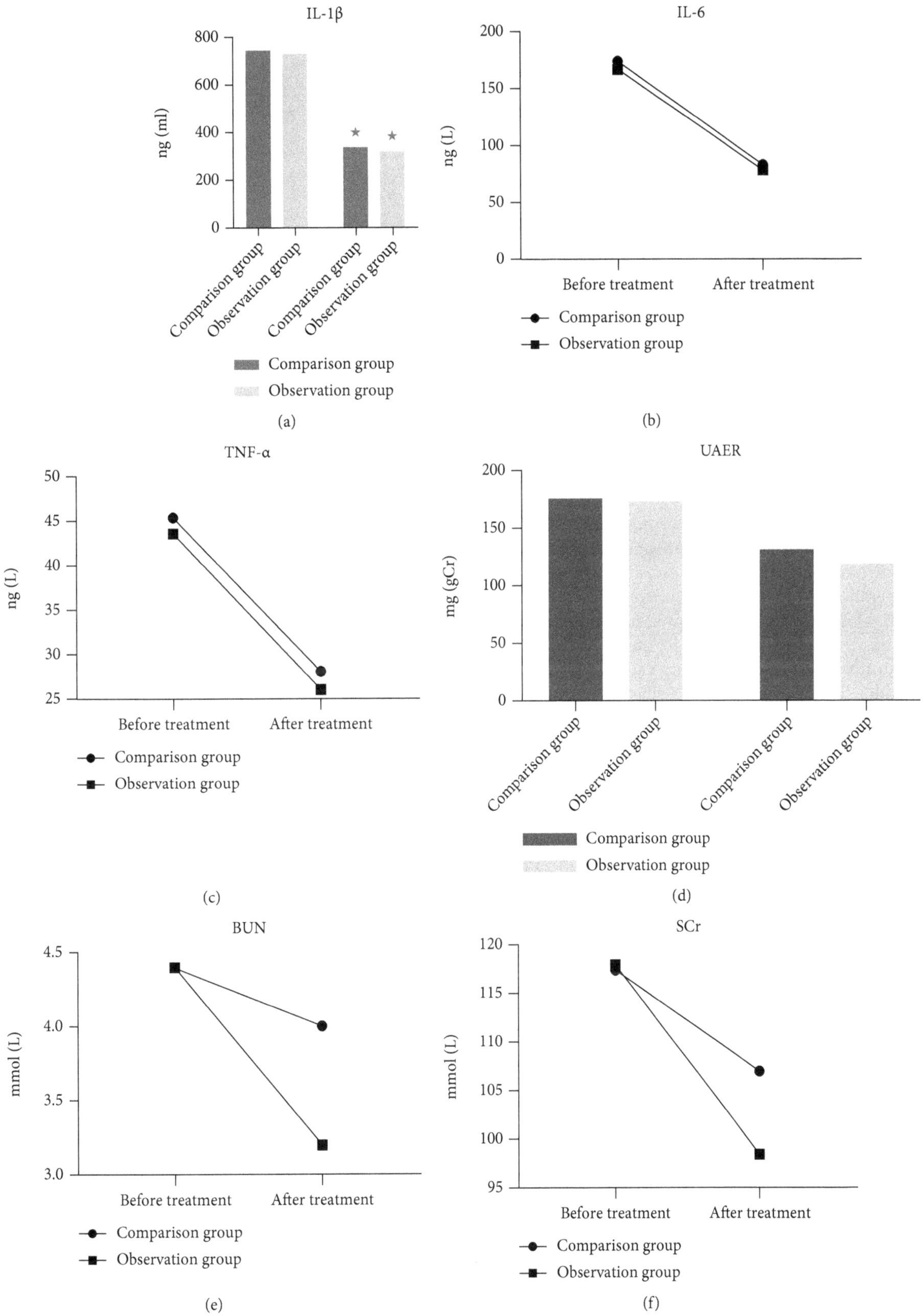


FIGURE 3: Continued.

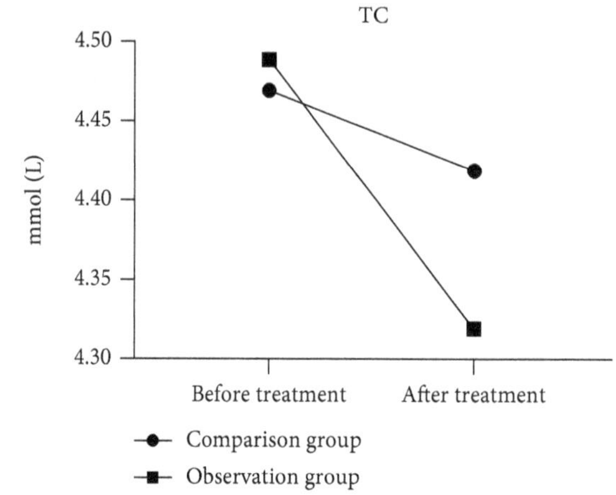


(g)

Figure 3: Serum index comparison. The comparative serum index data of our study were entered into Excel software by the first and corresponding authors, and the statistical processing software was SPSS 25.0 for calculation. Using the mean ± standard deviation ($X \pm S$) to indicate the use of independent sample $t$-test.

blocker, which can fully block $\beta$ receptors and also selectively block $\alpha 1$ receptors without endogenous sympathomimetic activity and peripheral $\beta$ agonism [10]. Carvedilol, as a third-generation $\beta$-blocker, has characteristics unmatched by other $\beta 2$-blockers and is widely used in the treatment of hypertension, congestive heart failure, and coronary artery disease with proven efficacy [11]. Some studies have shown that carvedilol can subside left ventricular hypertrophy and improve diastolic function in hypertensive patients. In contrast, spironolactone, as a potassium-preserving diuretic, has a weak diuretic and antihypertensive effect [12]. However, recent studies have found that spironolactone not only has potassium-preserving and sodium-removing effects but also has protective effects on the cardiovascular system when combined with other antihypertensive drugs as an aldosterone antagonist, which can further block RAAS to improve the antihypertensive effect [13].

Our study found that the systolic blood pressure, diastolic blood pressure, AM, and ET in the observation group were significantly lower than those in the comparison group after treatment; however, the heart rate and NO in the observation group were significantly higher than those in the comparison group, and the comparative differences were all statistically significant. IL-1$\beta$, IL-6, TNF-$\alpha$, UAER, BUN, and SCr in the observation group were significantly lower than those in the comparison group after treatment; however, TC in the observation group were lower than those in the comparison group, and the comparative differences were all statistically significant. It indicates that the combination therapy has a significantly smooth, sustained, and safe antihypertensive effect on patients with refractory hypertension. The long-term hypertensive state of patients can lead to myocardial remodeling and direct damage to vascular endothelial cells, which can even cause chronic heart failure [14]. Among them, various inflammatory cytokines and endothelial function indicators play an important regulatory role in disease progression; for example, IL-1$\beta$, IL-6, and TNF-$\alpha$ exacerbate heart failure by regulating cardiovascular function in patients [15]. Therefore, it is crucial to prevent or delay the process of heart failure in the course of antihypertension [16]. Studies have shown that carvedilol blocks B receptors while also exerting antioxidant, anti-inflammatory, and antiapoptotic effects, thereby inhibiting NF-$\kappa$B activity, suppressing the secretion of inflammatory factors by inflammatory cells, reducing the invasion of cardiomyocytes, and improving cardiac function [17]. This study showed that both can effectively improve inflammatory factor levels and endothelial function with similar effects. Studies in the literature have shown that benazepril, amlodipine, and irbesartan all improve endothelial function in patients, i.e., by increasing NO levels and decreasing AM and ET levels, thereby improving vascular endothelial function, delaying target organ damage, and reducing the risk of cardiovascular and cerebrovascular events [18]. The improvement of endothelial function can effectively respond to the improvement of blood pressure variability in patients with hypertension, thus indicating a stable antihypertensive effect [19]. Current studies confirm that the onset and development of hypertension are associated with functional and structural changes in endothelial cells, and the hypertensive state may further aggravate the functional and structural damage of vascular endothelial cells and vascular smooth muscle cells [20]. Among them, plasma ET and NO are a pair of vasoactive substances with antagonistic effects synthesized by vascular endothelial cells, which have an important role in the regulation of vascular smooth muscle function and vascular tone [21]. NO is an atomic group produced by L-arginine as a result of endothelial cell stimulation, which enters vascular smooth muscle cells to activate endoguanylate cyclase and increase intracellular CGMP content [22]. This leads to vascular smooth muscle diastole, inhibition of platelet agglutination, inhibition of endocytosis, and thus inhibition of thrombus formation, and the above effects make it useful in hypertension [23]. ET is a vasoactive peptide consisting of 21 amino acids and is the most potent long-acting vasoconstrictor known [24]. The possible mechanisms of ET involvement in the pathogenesis of EH are as follows: specific binding of ET to vascular smooth muscle on ET activates the renin-angiotensin-aldosterone system, causing a strong vasoconstrictor effect of angiotensin I. ET increases vascular responsiveness to other vasoconstrictors such as endogenous and exogenous norepinephrine substances [25]. ET promotes vascular smooth muscle cell proliferation and hypertrophy, resulting in narrowing of the lumen, thickening of the vessel wall, and increased peripheral resistance, and activation of phospholipase A2, which produces thromboxane A2, can further enhance vasoconstriction and increase blood pressure [26]. The increase in blood pressure increases the shear stress on the vessel wall and promotes the expression of ET-mRNA, and EH in turn can aggravate endothelial damage and increase endothelial dysfunction, with impaired production of diastolic substances such as nitric oxide (NO) and prostacyclin (PGL2) and increased release of thromboxane A2, along with massive secretion of ET [27].

Our study found that fasting glucose, insulin, TG, CHO, and LDL-C were significantly higher in the observation group than in the comparison group; however, ISI and HDL-C were significantly lower in the observation group than in the comparison group, and the comparative differences were all statistically significant. We know that traditional $\beta$-blockers can lead to an increase in TG and CHO levels as well as abnormalities in glucose tolerance and increased insulin resistance while exerting therapeutic effects [28]. Therefore, improving 3-blockers and improving lipid and glucose metabolism become essential. Consideration is mainly due to the fact that carvedilol is a nonselective $\beta$-blocker that selectively blocks the receptors along with the full range of B receptors [29]. At the same time, carvedilol is able to increase insulin sensitivity and improve lipid and glucose metabolism in general, which is related to the receptor blocker effect of carvedilol as well as elevating lipid oxidase activity and regulating disordered lipid and glucose metabolism [30]. Thus, carvedilol is effective in lowering blood pressure while having effects that are not found in other $\beta$-blockers, which improve insulin sensitivity [31].

This study was a case-control study, not a randomized controlled trial, and was not blinded, so there is still a certain risk of bias; the sample size included was small, there is still a need to subsequently increase the sample size and conduct multicenter clinical studies, the clinical follow-up period was short, and long-term clinical follow-up observations are still needed. In conclusion, the combination therapy had significant smooth, sustained, and safe antihypertensive effects on refractory hypertensive patients, with similar effects on endothelial function and control of various inflammatory factors and consistent recent efficacy, which is worth further promotion.

## Authors' Contributions

Deng Guiming contributed the same as Zhang Wen and shared first authorship.

## Acknowledgments

The study is supported by (1) the general project of Hunan Natural Science Foundation, project name: Study of inflammatory injury of hypertensive vascular remodeling and TCM intervention from IP3/Ca2+ signaling pathway, project no. 2021JJ30528; (2) the Academic Degree and Graduate Education Reform Project in Hunan Province, project name: Practice and exploration of cultivating clinical reasoning ability of TCM graduate students by using PBL teaching method, project no. 2019JGYB162; (3) the general project of Hunan Administration of Traditional Chinese Medicine, project name: Build the quality control system of clinical thinking ability training of TCM trainees based on PDCA cycle, project no. 2021129; and (4) the Science and Technology Innovation Platform of Science and Technology Bureau, Changsha (Cardiovascular and Cerebrovascular TCM Product Development and Key Technology Research Center).

## References

[1] A. C. Kaae, M. C. Kreissl, M. Krüger, M. Infanger, D. Grimm, and M. Wehland, "Kinase-inhibitors in iodine-refractory differentiated thyroid cancer-focus on occurrence, mechanisms, and management of treatment-related hypertension," *International Journal of Molecular Sciences*, vol. 22, no. 22, p. 12217, 2021.

[2] A. Y. Falkovskaya, V. F. Mordovin, S. E. Pekarskiy et al., "Refractory and resistant hypertension in patients with type 2 diabetes mellitus: different response to renal denervation," *Kardiologiia*, vol. 61, no. 2, pp. 54–61, 2021.

[3] C. R. L. Cardoso and G. F. Salles, "Refractory hypertension and risks of adverse cardiovascular events and mortality in patients with resistant hypertension: a prospective cohort study," *Journal of the American Heart Association*, vol. 9, no. 17, article e017634, 2020.

[4] J. Barley and C. Ellis, "Microvascular decompression: a surgical option for refractory hypertension of neurogenic etiology," *Expert Review of Cardiovascular Therapy*, vol. 11, no. 5, pp. 629–634, 2013.

[5] M. Doumas, K. P. Imprialos, M. S. Kallistratos, and A. J. Manolis, "Recent advances in understanding and managing resistant/refractory hypertension," *F1000Research*, vol. 9, 2020.

[6] M. S. Avila, S. M. Ayub-Ferreira, M. R. de Barros Wanderley et al., "Carvedilol for prevention of chemotherapy-related cardiotoxicity: the CECCY trial," *Journal of the American College of Cardiology*, vol. 71, no. 20, pp. 2281–2290, 2018.

[7] Y. Wu, Z. Li, A. Y. Xiu, D. X. Meng, S. N. Wang, and C. Q. Zhang, "Carvedilol attenuates carbon tetrachloride-induced liver fibrosis and hepatic sinusoidal capillarization in mice," *Drug Design, Development and Therapy*, vol. 13, pp. 2667–2676, 2019.

[8] A. P. Zacharias, R. Jeyaraj, L. Hobolth, F. Bendtsen, L. L. Gluud, and M. Y. Morgan, "Carvedilol versus traditional, non-selective beta-blockers for adults with cirrhosis and gastroesophageal varices," *Cochrane Database of Systematic Reviews*, vol. 10, no. 10, p. CD011510, 2018.

[9] Chinese Hypertension Prevention and Control Guidelines Revision Committee, "Chinese hypertension prevention and control guidelines 2010," *Chinese Journal of Cardiovascular Diseases*, vol. 39, no. 7, pp. 579–616, 2011.

[10] A. Y. Falkovskaya, V. F. Mordovin, S. E. Pekarskiy et al., "Refractory and resistant hypertension in patients with type 2 diabetes mellitus: differences in metabolic profile and endothelial function," *Terapevticheskii arkhiv*, vol. 93, no. 1, pp. 49–58, 2021.

[11] J. Versmissen, K. Hendriks, A. H. van den Meiracker, and M. H. Kappers, "Behandelopties voor therapieresistente hypertensive: van pseudoresistentie tot refractaire hypertensive [Treatment options for resistant hypertension: from pseudoresistant to refractory hypertension]," *Nederlands Tijdschrift voor Geneeskunde*, vol. 160, article A9937, 2015.

[12] T. Dudenbostel, M. Siddiqui, S. Oparil, and D. A. Calhoun, "Refractory hypertension: a novel phenotype of antihypertensive treatment failure," *Hypertension*, vol. 67, no. 6, pp. 1085–1092, 2016.

[13] R. Agarwal, "Refractory hypertension and kidney failure: focusing on the social determinants of health," *Hypertension*, vol. 77, no. 1, pp. 82–84, 2021.

[14] D. Meng, Z. Li, G. Wang, L. Ling, Y. Wu, and C. Zhang, "Carvedilol attenuates liver fibrosis by suppressing autophagy and promoting apoptosis in hepatic stellate cells," *Biomedicine & Pharmacotherapy*, vol. 108, pp. 1617–1627, 2018.

[15] M. Guglin, J. Krischer, R. Tamura et al., "Randomized trial of lisinopril versus carvedilol to prevent trastuzumab cardiotoxicity in patients with breast cancer," *Journal of the American College of Cardiology*, vol. 73, no. 22, pp. 2859–2868, 2019.

[16] H. R. McDowell, C. S. Chuah, D. Tripathi, A. J. Stanley, E. H. Forrest, and P. C. Hayes, "Carvedilol is associated with improved survival in patients with cirrhosis: a long-term follow-up study," *Alimentary Pharmacology & Therapeutics*, vol. 53, no. 4, pp. 531–539, 2021.

[17] T. Ajam, S. Ajam, S. Devaraj, K. Mohammed, S. Sawada, and M. Kamalesh, "Effect of carvedilol vs metoprolol succinate on mortality in heart failure with reduced ejection fraction," *American heart journal*, vol. 199, pp. 1–6, 2018.

[18] B. Kheiri, A. Abdalla, M. Osman et al., "Meta-analysis of carvedilol for the prevention of anthracycline-induced cardiotoxicity," *The American journal of cardiology*, vol. 122, no. 11, pp. 1959–1964, 2018.

[19] G. Zaatari, D. J. Fintel, H. Subacius et al., "Comparison of metoprolol versus carvedilol after acute myocardial infarction," *The American journal of cardiology*, vol. 147, pp. 1–7, 2021.

[20] T. Zhan, M. Daniyal, J. Li, and Y. Mao, "Preventive use of carvedilol for anthracycline-induced cardiotoxicity: a systematic review and meta-analysis of randomized controlled trials," *Herz*, vol. 45, no. S1, pp. 1–14, 2020.

[21] M. Krstić, L. Manić, N. Martić et al., "Binary polymeric amorphous carvedilol solid dispersions: in vitro and in vivo characterization," *European Journal of Pharmaceutical Sciences*, vol. 150, article 105343, 2020.

[22] S. Liang, M. A. Shamim, A. Shahid et al., "Prevention of skin carcinogenesis by the non-$\beta$-blocking R-carvedilol enantiomer," *Cancer Prevention Research (Philadelphia, Pa.)*, vol. 14, no. 5, pp. 527–540, 2021.

[23] R. Farhat, V. E. de Santana-Van, G. Su, L. Neely, T. Benally, and O. Chan, "Carvedilol prevents impairment of the counter-regulatory response in recurrently hypoglycaemic diabetic rats," *Endocrinology, diabetes & metabolism*, vol. 4, no. 2, article e00226, 2021.

[24] D. Banerji, R. M. Alvi, M. Afshar et al., "Carvedilol among patients with heart failure with a cocaine-use disorder," *JACC: Heart Failure*, vol. 7, no. 9, pp. 771–778, 2019.

[25] E. Martinez-Hernandez and L. A. Blatter, "Effect of carvedilol on atrial excitation-contraction coupling, Ca2+ release, and arrhythmogenicity," *American Journal of Physiology-Heart and Circulatory Physiology*, vol. 318, no. 5, pp. H1245–H1255, 2020.

[26] R. Butts, A. M. Atz, N. Baez Hernandez, D. Sutcliffe, J. Reisch, and L. Mahony, "Carvedilol does not improve exercise performance in Fontan patients: results of a crossover trial," *Pediatric Cardiology*, vol. 42, no. 4, pp. 934–941, 2021.

[27] J. Yang, K. Ge, L. Chen, and J. L. Yang, "The efficacy comparison of carvedilol plus endoscopic variceal ligation and traditional, nonselective $\beta$-blockers plus endoscopic variceal ligation in cirrhosis patients for the prevention of variceal rebleeding: a meta-analysis," *European Journal of Gastroenterology & Hepatology*, vol. 31, no. 12, pp. 1518–1526, 2019.

[28] C. T. Bussey, A. A. Babakr, R. R. Iremonger et al., "Carvedilol and metoprolol are both able to preserve myocardial function in type 2 diabetes," *Physiological Reports*, vol. 8, no. 5, article e14394, 2020.

[29] S. Ghosh and S. Verma, "Carvedilol inhibits A$\beta$25-35 fibrillation by intervening the early stage helical intermediate formation: a biophysical investigation," *International Journal of Biological Macromolecules*, vol. 188, pp. 263–271, 2021.

[30] R. M. Magadmi, M. A. Alsulaimani, A. R. Al-Rafiah, and A. Esmat, "The neuroprotective effect of carvedilol on diabetic neuropathy: an in vitro study," *Journal Diabetes Research*, vol. 2021, article 6927025, pp. 1–8, 2021.

[31] K. Amirshahrokhi and A. Zohouri, "Carvedilol prevents pancreatic $\beta$-cell damage and the development of type 1 diabetes in mice by the inhibition of proinflammatory cytokines, NF-$\kappa$B, COX-2, iNOS and oxidative stress," *Cytokine*, vol. 138, article 155394, 2021.

# 19

# Pulmonary Arterial Hypertension Specific Therapy in Patients with Combined Post- and Precapillary Pulmonary Hypertension

**Hassan Alfraidi**[1,2] **Sultan Qanash,**[1,3] **and Zoheir Bshouty**[1]

[1]*Section of Pulmonary Medicine, Department of Medicine, University of Manitoba, Winnipeg, MB, Canada*
[2]*Division of Cardiology, Department of Medicine, McGill University, Montreal, QC, Canada*
[3]*King Saud Bin Abdulaziz University for Health Sciences, King Abdulaziz Medical City, Jeddah, Saudi Arabia*

Correspondence should be addressed to Zoheir Bshouty; zbshouty@hsc.mb.ca

Academic Editor: Dimitris Georgopoulos

*Background.* Specific therapy for patients with PAH is associated with good outcomes. Little is known about the effect of this treatment in patients with Cpc-PH (PAPm ≥ 25 mmHg, PAWP > 15 mmHg, DPG ≥ 7 mmHg, and/or PVR > 3 WU). This study evaluates the outcome of treating patients with Cpc-PH using PAH specific therapy. *Methods.* The primary outcome was survival. Secondary outcomes were WHO functional class and 6-minute walk distance (6-MWD). *Results.* Twenty-six patients with Cpc-PH (half with VHD and half with HF) received PAHST. Six patients did not tolerate treatment due to pulmonary edema. No predictors for treatment intolerance were identified. In twenty patients who tolerated the treatment, the mean WHO functional class improved from 2.70 ± 0.21 at initial assessment to 2.22 ± 0.21 ($p < 0.04$) and 2.06 ± 0.21 ($p < 0.03$) at 6 and 9 months, respectively. Mean 6-MWD improved from 276.0 ± 38.50 meters at initial assessment to 343.9 ± 22.99 meters ($p < 0.04$) and 364.6 ± 34.85 meters ($p = 0.07$) at 6 and 9 months, respectively. Twelve patients died during the follow-up period. Mean survival for all patients was 1279.7 ± 193.60 days. *Conclusion.* PAHST may be beneficial in the treatment of Cpc-PH (both short and long term). Prospective randomized controlled trials of PAHST in this population are needed to assess its potential efficacy.

## 1. Background

Pulmonary Hypertension (PH) is defined as Mean Pulmonary Artery Pressure (PAPm) ≥ 25 mmHg [1]. Pulmonary Arterial Hypertension (PAH) (also termed precapillary PH) is diagnosed when, in addition, PAWP is ≤15 mmHg [1]. Postcapillary PH is defined as PH due to left ventricular dysfunction (either myocardial and/or valvular) when PAWP is >15 mmHg [2, 3]. Isolated postcapillary PH (Ipc-PH) is said to be present when Diastolic Pressure Gradient (DPG = Diastolic PAP − PAWP) is <7 mmHg and PVR ≤ 3 WU [2].

Combined postcapillary and precapillary pulmonary hypertension (Cpc-PH) is a newly recognized entity in which PAWP > 15 mmHg and DPG ≥ 7 mmHg and/or PVR > 3 WU [2–4]. This group was previously referred to as having an "out-of-proportion" elevation in PAPm [3, 4] and represents almost 30% of the PAH patients. In spite of the above, it is worth noting that criteria for what constitutes "out of proportion" are not universally accepted [3, 4]. Some experts [5] have suggested a transpulmonary pressure gradient (TPG = PAPm − PAWP) of >12 mmHg in the setting of PAWP > 15 mmHg as a diagnostic criteria. However, using a fixed TPG or DPG [6, 7] without consideration of Cardiac Output and PAWP in a quite distensible vascular bed is physiologically unsound. In the normal pulmonary circulation, previous studies have shown that the rise in PAPm as a response to a rise in left atrial pressure (LAP) is nonlinear and is highly affected by mean alveolar pressure [8–10]. Raising LAP between zero and 10 mmHg causes hardly any rise in PAPm. As LAP further increases, the rise in PAPm (in proportion to the rise in LAP) increases gradually and approaches a 1 : 1 relationship only at very high LAP (in excess of 25 mmHg) [8–11]. Furthermore, the relationship between PAPm and

LAP in the setting of PAH (and in various disease severities) is not known.

Data from the REVEAL registry has shown that PAH associated with PAWP > 19 mmHg has an increase mortality compared to PAWP < 15 mmHg [12, 13]. Despite the cardinal component of PAH (precapillary), those patients remain untreated with PAHST due to concerns extrapolated from outcomes in the management of patients with heart failure [14, 15]. PAHST is confined mainly to PAH, which mandates the absence of elevated left atrial pressure reflected by PAWP < 15 mmHg [1]. In this study, we evaluated the outcome of treating Cpc-PH with PAHST.

## 2. Methods

*2.1. Study Design.* This is a retrospective descriptive study of data obtained from the pulmonary hypertension registry (PHR) at the University of Manitoba (Health Science Centre, Winnipeg, MB). The data in the PHR is collected prospectively from a patient's initial assessment throughout every clinic visit following treatment initiation (approximately every 3 months). The PHR includes comprehensive data related to demographics, comorbidities, prior and concomitant medications, all required investigations to establish a proper diagnosis including invasive and noninvasive hemodynamic parameters, WHO functional class, and 6-minute walk distance (6-MWD). Data collection into the PHR was approved by the University of Manitoba research ethics board.

*2.2. Assessments and Definitions.* The definition of PH used in the study was based on the latest consensus [5th World Symposium of Pulmonary Hypertension, WSPH, [1]]. PH was defined as resting PAPm ≥ 25 mmHg [1]. All patients underwent right heart catheterization to confirm the diagnosis. All patients with Cpc-PH (as defined above), in addition to having TPG > 12 mmHg vascular compromise > 55% (see below), were included in the study.

We have previously developed a model of the normal pulmonary circulation, which was later adapted to simulate PAH [16]. A set of pulmonary hemodynamic data is entered into the model and through iterations, the model calculates the degree of vascular compromise (measured as percent of pulmonary arterial luminal loss at the precapillary level) that is associated with the entered data [17]. This model is applied to the hemodynamic data of all patients treated at our center. When applying model predictions to all patients in our database with PAH (PAPm ≥ 25 mmHg and PAWP ≤ 15 mmHg), vascular compromise was higher than 55%. This is why a vascular compromise threshold > 55% was used in addition to the criteria of Cpc-PH described above.

PH severity was assessed using WHO functional class and 6-MWD. WHO functional class and 6-MWD were assessed at baseline and at least every 3 months thereafter for one year. After one year, WHO functional class and 6-MWD were assessed every 3–6 months until being lost to follow-up or death. The 6-MWD was performed by trained and certified pulmonary function laboratory technicians according to the American Thoracic Society (ATS) guidelines [18]. Predicted distance for each individual was calculated using reference equations published by Enright and Sherrill in 1998 [19]. The primary end point was survival. Secondary end points included WHO functional class and 6-MWD 6 and 9 months following treatment initiation.

*2.3. Treatment Protocol.* All patients were initiated on monotherapy with either an endothelin receptor antagonist (ERA) or a phosphodiesterase-5 (PDE-5) inhibitor. Intolerance to a medication prompted a switch to another medication either within the same group or within another group dependent on the cause of the intolerance. The treatment protocol used in the PH clinic is a stepwise approach based on the goal-oriented treatment of PAH [20] as described by Hoeper et al. (and in conjunction with 5th WSPH). Patients who reported inadequate improvement in symptoms or did not achieve 380 meters within 3 to 6 months of monotherapy were stepped up to combination therapy. A drop in 6-MWD of greater than 50 meters was considered clinically significant when assessing individual patients. NYHA classification for dyspnea was recorded, although patients' lack of subjective improvement in symptoms was considered the more relevant clinical response.

*2.4. Statistical Analysis.* The statistical package used was Statistica. Analysis of variance for repeated measures (ANOVAR) with Tukey's test for specific comparisons was used to compare 6-MWD at 6 and 9 months after treatment initiation to baseline. Friedman ANOVA followed by Wilcoxon signed-rank tests with Bonferroni correction were used to compare WHO functional class at 6 and 9 months after treatment initiation to baseline. Unpaired $t$-test was used to compare parametric demographics (chi-square was used for nonparametric data), baseline hemodynamics, and functional capacity between patients who did and those who did not tolerate PAHST. Cox proportional hazards regression was used to identify predictors of survival.

## 3. Results

*3.1. Study Population.* Between July 2001 and December 2015, twenty-six patients with Cpc-PH underwent initial assessment. Six patients developed pulmonary edema within the first 3 months of treatment that was deemed due to PAHST and were excluded from the short- and long-term outcome analysis. Of the twenty patients who tolerated PAHST, half had a valvular heart disease (VHD) while the other half suffered from heart failure (HF). At our center, patients with VHD are considered for PAHST only if they have persistent PAH or Cpc-PH following valve repair and/or replacement with no evidence of significant residual stenosis and/or regurgitation (of either aortic or mitral valve). In the other ten patients who were diagnosed with HF, six had diastolic dysfunction (DD) with preserved CO and four had systolic dysfunction (SD). Of the six patients who did not tolerate PAHST, four had VHD and two had HF (one DD and one SD). Of the twenty patients who tolerated treatment, 13 (65%) were females and 7 (35%) were males. The mean age (±SE) for all patients was 64.7 ± 2.93 years (females

TABLE 1: Descriptive statistics of patients enrolled in the study.

| Variable | Patients who tolerated PAHST* | | | Patients who did not tolerate PAHST* | | |
|---|---|---|---|---|---|---|
| | Number of patients | Mean | SE | Number of patients | Mean | SE |
| Age | 20 | 64.6 | 2.93 | 6 | 67.4 | 4.61 |
| CCI | 20 | 3.80 | 0.36 | 6 | 4.0 | 0.37 |
| PAPm | 20 | 51.3 | 2.71 | 6 | 48.8 | 3.45 |
| PAWP | 20 | 23.6 | 0.84 | 6 | 27.0 | 2.80 |
| TPG | 20 | 27.7 | 2.53 | 6 | 21.8 | 2.27 |
| PVR | 19 | 6.5 | 0.78 | 6 | 7.14 | 2.47 |
| DPG | 20 | 8.3 | 1.65 | 6 | 4.2 | 2.06 |
| CO | 19 | 4.46 | 0.21 | 6 | 3.68 | 0.25 |
| Vascular compromise | 19 | 71.2 | 1.20 | 6 | 71.4 | 2.47 |
| WHO-baseline | 20 | 2.70 | 0.21 | 6 | 3.00 | 0.37 |
| WHO-3 months | 18 | 2.33 | 0.23 | | | |
| WHO-6 months | 18 | 2.22 | 0.21 | | | |
| WHO-9 months | 16 | 2.06 | 0.21 | | | |
| 6-MWD-baseline | 23 | 276.0 | 38.50 | 6 | 268.0 | 50.52 |
| 6-MWD-3 months | 17 | 360.5 | 29.01 | | | |
| 6-MWD-6 months | 17 | 343.9 | 22.99 | | | |
| 6-MWD-9 months | 15 | 364.6 | 34.85 | | | |
| 6-MWD (% pre)-baseline | 23 | 56.4 | 6.83 | 6 | 58.3 | 8.99 |
| 6-MWD (% pre)-3 months | 17 | 72.6 | 3.82 | | | |
| 6-MWD (% pre)-6 months | 17 | 72.8 | 3.58 | | | |
| 6-MWD (% pre)-9 months | 15 | 74.1 | 4.26 | | | |
| Survival (in days) | 20 | 1350.8 | 173.44 | | | |

*PAHST = Pulmonary Arterial Hypertension Specific Therapy, CCI = Charlson Comorbidities Index, PAPm = Mean Pulmonary Artery Pressure (mmHg), PAWP = Pulmonary Arterial Wedge Pressure (mmHg), CO = Cardiac Output (L/min), TPG = Transpulmonary Gradient (mmHg), DPG = Diastolic Pressure Gradient (mmHg), PVR = Pulmonary Venous Resistance (WU), WHO = World Health Organization functional class, 6-MWD = 6-minute walk distance (meters), and SE = standard error.

63.0 ± 2.65 and males 67.8 ± 7.01). Basic demographics, invasive hemodynamic data, baseline, 3-month, 6-month, and 9-month WHO, and 6-MWD are shown in Table 1. Data are shown as mean and standard error (SE).

*3.2. Treatment.* Out of the twenty patients who tolerated treatment, fifteen patients were treated with Bosentan monotherapy, two patients were on Sildenafil monotherapy, and three patients were treated with a combination of both. None of these patients required a change in treatment during the observation period. The six patients who did not tolerate treatment all received Bosentan. All discontinuations were due to pulmonary edema and none because of liver function abnormalities. All patients who tolerated treatment received treatment for at least 6 months and eighteen patients were treated for at least 9 months.

*3.3. Right Heart Catheterization (RHC) Data.* All patients underwent RHC. Mean (±SE) pulmonary artery pressure was 51.3 ± 2.71 mmHg, mean PAWP was 23.6 ± 0.84 mmHg, mean TPG was 27.7 ± 2.53 mmHg, mean DPG was 8.3 ± 1.65 mmHg, and mean PVR was 6.5 ± 0.78 WU. Based on model predictions, mean vascular compromise was 71.2 ± 1.20%. The rest of the hemodynamic data is shown in Table 1.

*3.4. WHO Functional Class.* Mean (±SE) WHO functional class for all patients at initial assessment was 2.70 ± 0.21. Mean WHO functional class at 6 and 9 months after treatment initiation was 2.22 ± 0.21 ($p < 0.04$, compared to baseline) and 2.06 ± 0.21 ($p < 0.03$), respectively (Figure 1).

*3.5. 6-MWD.* Mean (±SE) 6-MWD for all patients at initial assessment was 276.0±38.50 meters (56.4±6.84% predicted). Mean 6-MWD distances at 6 and 9 months after treatment initiation were 343.9 ± 22.99 meters (72.8 ± 3.58% predicted) ($p < 0.04$, compared to baseline) and 364.6 ± 34.85 meters (74.1 ± 4.26% predicted) ($p = 0.073$, compared to baseline), respectively (Figure 2).

*3.6. Survival.* Out of twenty patients, 12 patients died during the follow-up period (6 years). Mean (±SE) survival for all patients was 1279.7 ± 193.6 days (1383.2 ± 250.4 days for females and 1087.4 ± 311.0 days for males). Kaplan Meier survival curve showed slightly lower survival for patients

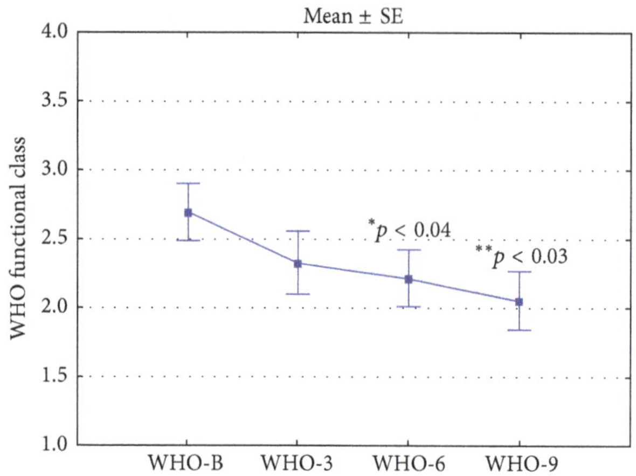


FIGURE 1: WHO functional class at baseline, 3 months, 6 months, and 9 months after initiation of PAHST.

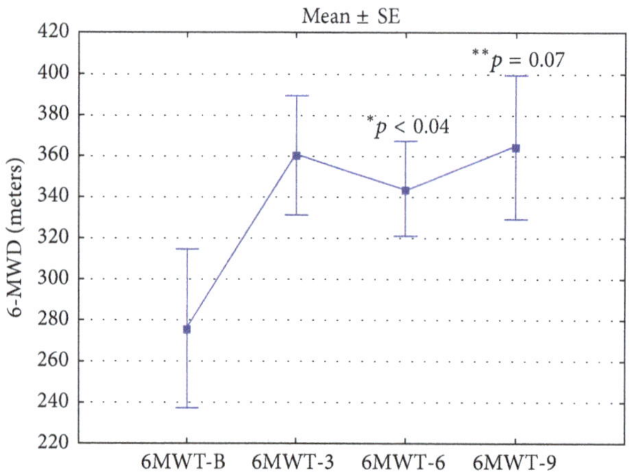


FIGURE 2: 6-minute walk test distance (6-MWT) at baseline, 3 months, 6 months, and 9 months after initiation of PAHST.

with Cpc-PH when compared to patients with pure PAH. A survival rate of 80%, 75%, and 53% at one, two, and three years (Figure 3) was noted, respectively. During the same period of observation, one, two, and three years survival rates in patients with pure PAH in our registry were 89%, 79%, and 67%, respectively. No predictors of survival could be identified among the parameters shown in Table 1.

## 4. Discussion

In the absence of mitral stenosis, PAWP and LVEDP are both considered accurate surrogates for left atrial pressure [21, 22]. Chronic elevations in left arterial pressure are associated with more than pressure related effects on the pulmonary circulation [23]. Vascular remodeling [24] and endothelial dysfunction [25], resembling PAH, have been described. Combined precapillary and postcapillary PH is a newly recognized entity which has specific hemodynamic parameters that include a PAWP > 15 mmHg, DPG ≥ 7 mmHg, and/or PVR > 3 WU [2–4, 7]. These patients tend to be obese, have more comorbidities, and perform less in 6-MWD [12, 13]. Data from the REVEAL registry has shown that patients with PAH associated with PAWP > 19 mmHg have a higher mortality rate over 2 years when compared to patients with PAWP < 15 mmHg [13].

In the present study, we combined the criteria of Cpc-PH, TPG > 12 mmHg, and we used model predictions of vascular compromise > 55% to ensure that the observed PAPm is out of proportion to the associated rise in PAWP. Calculated mean vascular compromise in both groups (those who tolerated and those who did not tolerate treatment) was higher (71.2 and 71.4%, resp.) than patients with pure PAH (55%) in our database suggesting that these patients had significant precapillary vasculopathy.

Several trials were performed to test the efficacy of PAHST on the treatment of heart failure [13–15]. In these studies, increased mortality and safety concerns have outweighed the beneficial effects on hemodynamics, exercise tolerance, and quality of life [14, 26, 27]. The effect of PAHST on Cpc-PH has been studied with variable outcomes [28–31]. The REVEAL registry has included patients with PAWP 15–18 mmHg. Compared to isolated PAH, PAH with

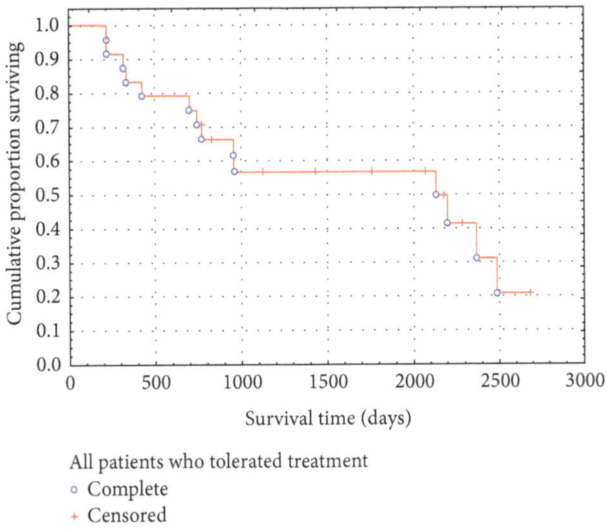


FIGURE 3: Survival rate of the study population receiving PAHST up to 6 years.

PAWP > 19 mmHg is associated with increased mortality [13]. A recent trial in patients with PH and DPG > 20 mmHg who were treated with PAHST had promising results [32].

In the present study, twenty of twenty-six patients with Cpc-PH tolerated PAHST. In those patients, we noted some improvement in WHO functional class and 6-MWD at 6 and 9 months after treatment initiation (Figures 1 and 2).

Pulmonary Arterial Hypertension Specific Therapy has resulted in increased survival at one, two, and three years in patients with PAH (93%, 75% and 66%, resp.) [33]. It is comforting to see that our survival rates in patients with PAH (89%, 79% and 67%, resp.) are comparable to the published survival rates. In our observational study, patients with Cpc-PH who received and tolerated PAHST had slightly lower survival rates of 80%, 75%, and 53%, respectively (Figure 3).

All six patients who did not tolerate PAHST had their treatment discontinued because of developing pulmonary edema and none of these patients sustained end-organ damage or died due to this treatment trial. We could not identify, among the monitored factors, predictors that would identify patients who are more likely to tolerate PAHST.

This study has many limitations including its retrospective design, small sample size, and lack of a control group. The lack of a control group is a legitimate concern as we have no way of predicting whether not treating these patients would have resulted in similar or even better outcomes, although the sustained improvement in WHO functional class and 6-MWD led us to believe that we have not caused harm. It may be considered a pilot study or case series that is alerting us to a group of patients with Cpc-PH, some of whom may benefit from PAHST. Randomized controlled trials, on a much larger scale, are needed to answer the question of benefit and survival in this group of patients. These studies may also help identify predictors of good outcome that would lead to a better selection of patients who are likely to benefit from PAHST.

## 5. Conclusion

Pulmonary Arterial Hypertension Specific Therapy may be beneficial in the treatment of combined post- and precapillary pulmonary hypertension (both short and long term). Prospective randomized controlled trials of PAHST in this population are needed to assess its potential efficacy.

## Data Access

The data is available in electronic form (Excel sheets) and in the PAH Database (PHMS) at the Division of Pulmonary Medicine, Department of Medicine, University of Manitoba.

## Ethical Approval

The database and data derivation from the database were approved by the ethics board at University of Manitoba.

## Disclosure

Dr. Hassan Alfraidi is the principle author. The study includes no identifiable information.

## Authors' Contributions

Dr. Hassan Alfraidi contributed in writing the proposal, collecting data, and writing the manuscript. Dr. Sultan Qanash contributed in reviewing the proposal and manuscript. Dr. Zoheir Bshouty contributed in reviewing proposal, data, and manuscript, editing manuscript, revisions, and final review prior to final submission following reviewer's comments.

## Acknowledgments

The authors would like to thank the pulmonary hypertension clinic nurse.

## References


[1] M. M. Hoeper, H. J. Bogaard, and R. Condliffe, "Definitions and diagnosis of pulmonary hypertension," *Journal of the American College of Cardiology*, vol. 62, no. 25, pp. D42–D50, 2013.

[2] N. Galiè, M. Humbert, JL. Vachiery, S. Gibbs, I. Lang et al., "2015 ECS/ERS Guidelines for the diagnosis and treatment of pulmonary hypertension," *European Heart Journal*, vol. 37, no. 1, pp. 67–119, 2015.

[3] M. Guazzi and B. A. Borlaug, "Pulmonary hypertension due to left heart disease," *Circulation*, vol. 126, no. 8, pp. 975–990, 2012.

[4] J.-L. Vachiéry, Y. Adir, J. A. Barberà et al., "Pulmonary hypertension due to left heart diseases," *Journal of the American College of Cardiology*, vol. 62, no. 25, pp. D100–D108, 2013.

[5] R. Naeije, J.-L. Vachiery, P. Yerly, and R. Vanderpool, "The transpulmonary pressure gradient for the diagnosis of pulmonary vascular disease," *European Respiratory Journal*, vol. 41, no. 1, pp. 217–223, 2013.

[6] C. Gerges, M. Gerges, M. B. Lang et al., "Diastolic pulmonary vascular pressure gradient: A predictor of prognosis in "out-of-proportion" pulmonary hypertension," *CHEST*, vol. 143, no. 3, pp. 758–766, 2013.

[7] E. Tampakakis, P. J. Leary, V. N. Selby et al., "The diastolic pulmonary gradient does not predict survival in patients with pulmonary hypertension due to left heart disease," *JACC: Heart Failure*, vol. 3, no. 1, pp. 9–16, 2015.

[8] H. P. Chaliki, D. G. Hurrell, R. A. Nishimura, R. A. Reinke, and C. P. Appleton, "Pulmonary venous pressure: Relationship to pulmonary artery, pulmonary wedge, and left atrial pressure in normal, lightly sedated dogs," *Catheterization and Cardiovascular Interventions*, vol. 56, no. 3, pp. 432–438, 2002.

[9] R. K. Albert and W. J. E. Lamm, "Left atrial pressure can be accurately transmitted to the pulmonary artery despite Zone 1 conditions," *American Journal of Respiratory and Critical Care Medicine*, vol. 167, no. 7, pp. 1016–1020, 2003.

[10] N. Saouti, N. Westerhof, P. E. Postmus, and A. Vonk-Noordegraaf, "The arterial load in pulmonary hypertension," *European Respiratory Review*, vol. 19, no. 117, pp. 197–203, 2010.

[11] R. Ilsar, B. P. Bailey, T. A. Dobbins, and D. S. Celermajer, "The Relationship Between Pulmonary Artery and Pulmonary Capillary Wedge Pressure for the Diagnosis of Pulmonary Vascular Disease," *Heart, Lung and Circulation*, vol. 19, no. 1, pp. 38–42, 2010.

[12] D. B. Badesch, G. E. Raskob, C. G. Elliott et al., "Pulmonary arterial hypertension: baseline characteristics from the REVEAL registry," *CHEST*, vol. 137, no. 2, pp. 376–387, 2010.

[13] A. E. Frost, H. W. Farber, R. J. Barst, D. P. Miller, C. G. Elliott, and M. D. McGoon, "Demographics and outcomes of patients diagnosed with pulmonary hypertension with pulmonary capillary wedge pressures 16 to 18 mm Hg: Insights from the REVEAL registry," *CHEST*, vol. 143, no. 1, pp. 185–195, 2013.

[14] R. M. Califf, K. F. Adams, W. J. McKenna, and et al, "A randomized controlled trial of epoprostenol therapy for severe congestive heart failure: the Flolan International Randomized Survival Trial (FIRST)," *American Heart Journal*, vol. 134, no. 1, pp. 44–54, 1997.

[15] M. Packer, J. McMurray, B. M. Massie et al., "Clinical effects of endothelin receptor antagonism with bosentan in patients with severe chronic heart failure: Results of a pilot study," *Journal of Cardiac Failure*, vol. 11, no. 1, pp. 12–20, 2005.

[16] Z. Bshouty and M. Younes, "Distensibility and pressure-flow relationship of the pulmonary circulation. II. Multibranched model," *Journal of Applied Physiology*, vol. 68, no. 4, pp. 1514–1527, 1990.

[17] Z. Bshouty, "Vascular compromise and hemodynamics in pulmonary arterial hypertension: Model predictions," *Canadian Respiratory Journal*, vol. 19, no. 3, pp. e15–e17, 2012.

[18] "ATS statement: guidelines for the six-minute walk test," *American Journal of Respiratory and Critical Care Medicine*, vol. 166, no. 1, pp. 111–117, 2002.

[19] P. L. Enright and D. L. Sherrill, "Reference equations for the six-minute walk in healthy adults," *American Journal of Respiratory and Critical Care Medicine*, vol. 158, no. 5, part 1, pp. 1384–1387, 1998.

[20] M. M. Hoeper, I. Markevych, E. Spiekerkoetter, T. Welte, and J. Niedermeyer, "Goal-oriented treatment and combination therapy for pulmonary arterial hypertension," *European Respiratory Journal*, vol. 26, no. 5, pp. 858–863, 2005.

[21] E. D. Flores, R. A. Lange, and L. D. Hillis, "Relation of mean pulmonary arterial wedge pressure and left ventricular end-diastolic pressure," *American Journal of Cardiology*, vol. 66, no. 20, pp. 1532-1533, 1990.

[22] R. K. F. De Oliveira, E. V. M. Ferreira, R. P. Ramos et al., "Usefulness of pulmonary capillary wedge pressure as a correlate of left ventricular filling pressures in pulmonary arterial hypertension," *The Journal of Heart and Lung Transplantation*, vol. 33, no. 2, pp. 157–162, 2014.

[23] N. R. Dayeh, J. Ledoux, and J. Dupuis, "Lung Capillary Stress Failure and Arteriolar Remodelling in Pulmonary Hypertension Associated with Left Heart Disease (Group 2 PH)," *Progress in Cardiovascular Diseases*, vol. 59, no. 1, pp. 11–21, 2016.

[24] J. B. West and O. Mathieu-Costello, "Vulnerability of pulmonary capillaries in heart disease," *Circulation*, vol. 92, no. 3, pp. 622–631, 1995.

[25] M. Farrero, I. Blanco, M. Batlle et al., "Pulmonary hypertension is related to peripheral endothelial dysfunction in heart failure with preserved ejection fraction," *Circulation: Heart Failure*, vol. 7, no. 5, pp. 791–798, 2014.

[26] G. D. Lewis, R. Shah, K. Shahzad et al., "Sildenafil improves exercise capacity and quality of life in patients with systolic heart failure and secondary pulmonary hypertension," *Circulation*, vol. 116, no. 14, pp. 1555–1562, 2007.

[27] P. Botha, G. Parry, J. H. Dark, and G. A. MacGowan, "Acute Hemodynamic Effects of Intravenous Sildenafil Citrate in Congestive Heart Failure: Comparison of Phosphodiesterase Type-3 and -5 Inhibition," *The Journal of Heart and Lung Transplantation*, vol. 28, no. 7, pp. 676–682, 2009.

[28] D. Bonderman, S. Ghio, S. B. Felix et al., "Riociguat for patients with pulmonary hypertension caused by systolic left ventricular dysfunction: A phase IIb double-blind, randomized, placebo-controlled, dose-ranging hemodynamic study," *Circulation*, vol. 128, no. 5, pp. 502–511, 2013.

[29] R. Jiang, L. Wang, C.-T. Zhu et al., "Comparative effectiveness of sildenafil for pulmonary hypertension due to left heart disease with HFrEF," *Hypertension Research*, vol. 38, no. 12, pp. 829–839, 2015.

[30] E. S. Hoendermis, L. C. Y. Liu, Y. M. Hummel et al., "Effects of sildenafil on invasive haemodynamics and exercise capacity

in heart failure patients with preserved ejection fraction and pulmonary hypertension: A randomized controlled trial," *European Heart Journal*, vol. 36, no. 38, pp. 2565–2573, 2015.

[31] E. Kaluski, G. Cotter, M. Leitman et al., "Clinical and hemodynamic effects of bosentan dose optimization in symptomatic heart failure patients with severe systolic dysfunction, associated with secondary pulmonary hypertension - A multi-center randomized study," *Cardiology*, vol. 109, no. 4, pp. 273–280, 2008.

[32] C. Gerges, M. Gerges, N. Skoro-Sajer et al., "Hemodynamic thresholds for precapillary pulmonary hypertension," *CHEST*, vol. 149, no. 4, pp. 1061–1073, 2016.

[33] T. Thenappan, S. J. Shah, S. Rich, L. Tian, S. L. Archer, and M. Gomberg-Maitland, "Survival in pulmonary arterial hypertension: A reappraisal of the NIH risk stratification equation," *European Respiratory Journal*, vol. 35, no. 5, pp. 1079–1087, 2010.

# 20

# Circulating Sestrin Levels are Increased in Hypertension Patients

**Cao Fang,[1] Zicong Yang,[2] Lei Shi,[2] Tao Zeng,[2] Ying Shi,[2] Ling Liu,[2] Hongtao Liu,[3] and Yingzhong Lin[2]**

[1]*Xishui County People's Hospital Affiliated to Hubei University of Science and Technology, Hubei 530021, China*
[2]*Department of Cardiology, The People's Hospital of Guangxi Zhuang Autonomous Region, Nanning 530021, China*
[3]*Department of Cardiovascular Medicine, Shenzhen Longhua District Central Hospital, Longhua Central Hospital Affiliated to Guangdong Medical University, Shenzhen, Guangdong Province, 518110, China*

Correspondence should be addressed to Hongtao Liu; liuhongtaosz@163.com and Yingzhong Lin; yingzhonglin@126.com

Academic Editor: Benoit Dugue

*Background.* Sestrins (Sesns), a group of oxidative stress-related proteins, have been reported to be involved in various cardiovascular diseases, including aortic dissection and chronic heart failure. This study is aimed at investigating the level of circulating Sesn1, Sesn2, and Sesn3 in hypertension patients. *Methods.* Plasma levels of Sesn1, Sesn2, and Sesn3 in 400 hypertensive patients and 100 normotensive subjects were detected using enzyme-linked immunosorbent assay (ELISA) kits. The hypertension patients were divided into groups with grade I ($n = 140$), grade II ($n = 180$), and grade III ($n = 80$) hypertension. *Results.* Compared with the normotensive subjects, Sesn1, Sesn2, and Sesn3 levels were increased in patients with hypertension, with a gradual increase between the groups with grade I, grade II, and grade III hypertension. Elevated Sesn1, Sesn2, and Sesn3 levels were positively correlated with both the systolic blood pressure (SBP) and diastolic blood pressure (DBP). Moreover, Sesn1, Sesn2, and Sesn3 levels were elevated in patients with dipper hypertension and further increased in patients with nondipper hypertension. In addition, smokers, as well as patients with higher levels of angiotensin II (Ang II) and carotid atherosclerotic plaque (CAP), exhibited increased Sesn1, Sesn2, and Sesn3 levels when compared with patients without these clinical characteristics. Furthermore, plasma levels of Sesn1, Sesn2, and Sesn3 were negatively correlated with the presence of CAP. *Conclusions.* Circulating Sesn levels are increased in patients with hypertension and may be a target for the prevention and treatment of clinical hypertension.

## 1. Introduction

Hypertension is the most common risk factor of cardiovascular disease, leading to significantly higher morbidity and mortality than other risk factors. Numerous previous studies have used the immune effects and inflammatory response of blood vessels to strengthen the pathogenesis of hypertension [1, 2]. In recent years, more and more studies have proved that oxidative stress was closely related to the progression of hypertension [3–5].

Sestrin (Sesn) family members, including Sesn1, Sesn2, and Sesn3 in mammals, are proteins that regulate oxidative stress both *in vivo* and *in vitro* [6, 7]. Sesn is widely present in a variety of tissues and organs, and its expression is majorly regulated by oxidative stress levels and, to a lesser extent, by inflammatory responses, aging, and other pathophysiological effects [8–10]. A number of studies have confirmed that Sesns are involved in the development and progression of various diseases, by regulating oxidative stress. Moreover, some studies have reported that Sesns can also regulate inflammation, apoptosis, aging, and autophagy [9–13].

Sesn1, Sesn2, and Sesn3 were also shown to play a critical role in cardiovascular diseases [14]. Elevated plasma Sesn1, Sesn2, and Sesn3 levels were observed in patients with coronary artery disease (CAD). Furthermore, they were positively correlated with malondialdehyde (MDA) levels and negatively correlated with superoxide dismutase (SOD) levels [15]. Knockdown of Sesn1 significantly alleviated phenylephrine-(PE-) induced cardiac hypertrophy by regulating the AMPK/mTORC1/autophagy axis, while Sesn1 overexpression

Table 1: Clinical characteristics in each group.

| Characteristics | Control | Hypertension | | | |
|---|---|---|---|---|---|
| | | Total | Grade I | Grade II | Grade III |
| Age (years) | 48.2 ± 9.4 | 47.8 ± 9.9 | 48.8 ± 10.3 | 47.1 ± 9.4 | 47.6 ± 9.6 |
| Male (*n*, %) | 66 (66.0) | 287 (71.8) | 102 (72.9) | 126 (70.0) | 59 (73.4) |
| Smoking (*n*, %) | 33 (33.0) | 145 (36.3) | 47 (33.6) | 62 (34.4) | 36 (45.0) |
| History (years) | — | 10.1 ± 7.4 | 11.4 ± 8.6 | $9.4 \pm 7.7^{\$}$ | $9.5 \pm 7.1^{\$}$ |
| SBP (mmHg) | 111 ± 11 | $165 \pm 18^{*}$ | $147 \pm 12^{*,\#}$ | $169 \pm 15^{*,\$}$ | $189 \pm 20^{*,\#,\$,\&}$ |
| DBP (mmHg) | 74 ± 8 | $95 \pm 10^{*}$ | $86 \pm 9^{*,\#}$ | $98 \pm 10^{*,\$}$ | $104 \pm 11^{*,\#,\$,\&}$ |
| HR (HR) | 68 ± 6 | 70 ± 9 | 71 ± 9 | 68 ± 8 | 72 ± 10 |
| BMI (kg/m$^2$) | 24.5 ± 3.1 | 24.5 ± 3.2 | 24.3 ± 2.9 | 24.7 ± 3.1 | 25.3 ± 3.5 |
| TC (mmol/L) | 4.5 ± 0.8 | 4.4 ± 0.9 | 4.6 ± 1.0 | 4.3 ± 0.8 | 4.5 ± 0.9 |
| TG (mmol/L) | 1.8 ± 1.1 | 1.8 ± 1.2 | 2.0 ± 1.3 | 1.7 ± 1.2 | 1.9 ± 0.9 |
| HDL-C (mmol/L) | 1.3 ± 0.3 | $1.1 \pm 0.3^{*}$ | $1.1 \pm 0.3^{*}$ | 1.2 ± 0.3 | $1.0 \pm 0.3^{*,\&}$ |
| LDL-C (mmol/L) | 2.6 ± 0.7 | 2.7 ± 0.8 | 2.8 ± 0.8 | 2.5 ± 0.7 | 2.9 ± 0.9 |
| Glu (mmol/L) | 5.4 ± 0.6 | 5.5 ± 0.8 | 5.7 ± 0.8 | 5.3 ± 0.9 | 5.5 ± 0.8 |
| HbAlc (%) | 4.7 ± 0.8 | 4.5 ± 0.8 | 4.4 ± 0.6 | 4.6 ± 0.8 | 4.5 ± 0.9 |
| CRRA (μmol/L) | 71 ± 11 | $93 \pm 20^{*}$ | $81 \pm 15^{*,\#}$ | $94 \pm 19^{*,\$}$ | $111 \pm 24^{*,\#,\$,\&}$ |
| CRP (mg/L) | 0.9 ± 0.6 | $6.6 \pm 3.6^{*}$ | $3.9 \pm 1.6^{*,\#}$ | $7.5 \pm 3.8^{*,\#,\$}$ | $9.3 \pm 4.4^{*,\#,\$,\&}$ |
| Hcy (pg/mL) | 10.6 ± 3.4 | $15.3 \pm 5.8^{*}$ | $11.7 \pm 4.6^{*,\#}$ | $15.9 \pm 5.2^{*,\$}$ | $20.2 \pm 7.3^{*,\#,\$,\&}$ |
| Ang II (pg/mL) | 34.9 ± 14.1 | $57.5 \pm 24.1^{*}$ | $45.5 \pm 19.5^{*,\#}$ | $59.9 \pm 24.4^{*,\$}$ | $72.9 \pm 29.1^{*,\#,\$,\&}$ |
| CAP | — | 200 (50.0) | $52 (37.1)^{\#}$ | $93 (51.7)^{\$}$ | $55 (68.8)^{\#,\$,\&}$ |
| Medical treatments (*n*, %) | | | | | |
| ACEI/ARB | — | 244 (61.0) | $70 (50.0)^{\#}$ | 111 (61.1) | $63 (78.8)^{\#}$ |
| β-Blocker | — | 179 (44.8) | 52 (37.1) | 83 (46.1) | 44 (55.0) |
| CCB | — | 338 (84.5) | $109 (77.9)^{\#}$ | 159 (88.3) | 70 (87.5) |
| Diuretics | — | 244 (41.3) | $30 (21.4)^{\#}$ | $74 (41.1)^{\$}$ | $61 (76.3)^{\#,\$,\&}$ |

History: the duration of hypertension; SBP: systolic blood pressure; DBP: diastolic blood pressure; HR: heart rate; BMI: body mass index; TC: total cholesterol; TG: total triglycerides; HDL-C: high-density lipoprotein cholesterol; LDL-C: low-density lipoprotein cholesterol; Glu: fasting glucose; HbA1c: hemoglobin a1c; CRP: C-reactive protein; CREA: creatinine; Hcy: homocysteine; Ang II: angiotensin II; CAP: carotid atherosclerotic plaque; ACEI: angiotensin-converting enzyme inhibitor; ARB: angiotensin receptor blocker; CCB: calcium channel blocker. $^{*}p < 0\ 05$ vs. the control group, $^{\#}p < 0\ 05$ vs. the total group, $^{\$}p < 0\ 05$ vs. the grade I group, and $^{\&}p < 0\ 05$ vs. the grade II group.

led to the opposite effect [16]. Expression of circulating Sesn2 was shown to be increased in aortic dissection and chronic heart failure (CHF) patients. Moreover, CHF patients with elevated Sesn2 levels exhibited poor outcomes and more cardiac events [17, 18]. Knockout of Sesn2 enlarged the area of myocardial infarction after ischemia-reperfusion and aggravated myocardial injury after radiation [19, 20]. In addition, Sesn2 protected against age-related intolerance to postmyocardial infarction and phenylephrine- (PE-) induced cardiomyocyte hypertrophy [21, 22]. However, the current expression levels of circulating Sesns in patients with hypertension are still unknown. Therefore, this study is aimed at examining plasma Sesn1, Sesn2, and Sesn3 levels in hypertension patients.

## 2. Methods

*2.1. Study Populations.* In the present study, 100 normotensive and 400 primary hypertension patients were enrolled. The patients diagnosed with diseases, including secondary hypertension, chronic heart failure, chronic renal failure, stroke, valvular heart disease, collagen disease, advanced liver disease, malignant disease, septicemia, or other diseases that may affect Sesn expression, were excluded from this study. According to the value of systolic blood pressure (SBP) and/or diastolic blood pressure (DBP), the hypertension patients were divided into three groups, namely, grade I hypertension ($n = 140$), grade II hypertension ($n = 180$), and grade III hypertension ($n = 80$). All subjects underwent ambulatory blood pressure monitoring to determine the type of hypertension and were further divided into two groups, namely, the scoop-shaped hypertension group ($n = 240$) and nonscoop-shaped hypertension group ($n = 160$). In addition, all subjects received a carotid ultrasound to determine the presence of carotid atherosclerotic plaque (CAP). The blood samples were collected from the People's Hospital of Guangxi Zhuang Autonomous Region from March 2016 to May 2018. All patients signed informed consent forms, and the study was approved by the Ethics Committee of the People's Hospital of Guangxi Zhuang Autonomous Region.

*2.2. Blood Sample Collection.* Blood samples were collected from each subject at 6-7 A.M. on the day following admission. All the samples were collected in sodium heparin vacutainers and quickly taken to the laboratory. The samples were then centrifuged as at $4000 \times g$ for 20 min to obtain the plasma, which was subsequently frozen and preserved in liquid nitrogen until use. The blood samples were collected by nurses with more than 8 years of experience, and the time from blood samples collection to plasma storage was no longer than 45 min.

*2.3. Detection of Plasma Sesn1, Sesn2, and Sesn3 Levels.* The Sesn1, Sesn2, and Sesn3 enzyme-linked immunosorbent assay (ELISA) kits were purchased from Cloud-Clone Corp. (USA). The performance of these ELISA kits was tested. The lower detection limit of Sesn1 was approximately 10.5 ng/mL, the intra-assay and interassay coefficients of variation were <5% and <7%, respectively, the recovery range was between 90.5 and 115.2%, and the sensitivity was approximately 1.0 ng/mL. The lower detection limit of Sesn2 was approximately 0.5 ng/mL, the intra-assay and interassay coefficients of variation were <4% and <8%, respectively, the recovery range was between 93.4 and 110.5%, and the sensitivity was approximately 0.2 ng/mL. For Sesn3, the lower detection limit was approximately 3.2 ng/mL, the intra-assay and interassay coefficients of variation were <4.5% and <9.5%, respectively, the recovery range was between 92.5 and 116.6%, and the sensitivity was approximately 0.5 ng/mL.

Plasma samples were taken from liquid nitrogen and defrosted at 4°C. The plasma levels of Sesn1, Sesn2, and Sesn3 were detected using the respective ELISA kits, according to the manufacturer's instructions. All tests were performed in duplicate.

*2.4. Statistical Analysis.* Data regarding the enumeration variables were expressed as the mean ± standard deviation (SD). Student's *t*-test was performed to compare the difference between the two groups, and one-way ANOVA, followed by the LSD test, was performed for multiple comparisons between more than two groups. The categorical variables are presented as counts (percentages) and compared with the chi-square test. The correlations between Sesn2 levels and blood pressure (including SBP and DBP) were calculated using Spearman's correlation analysis. The simple linear regression analysis and subsequent multiple linear regression analysis were performed to investigate the role of Sesns in the presence of CAP. All the data were analyzed using the SPSS 23.0 software, and $p < 0.05$ was considered statistically significant.

## 3. Results

*3.1. The Differences in the Clinical Characteristics of Each Group.* Compared with the control group, hypertension patients exhibited higher SBP, DBP, high-density lipoprotein cholesterol (HDL-C), creatinine (CREA), C-reactive protein (CRP), homocysteine (Hcy), and angiotensin II (Ang II). No other differences in clinical characteristics were identified between the two groups, including age, male gender, smoking, the duration of hypertension (history), heart rate (HR), body mass index (BMI), total cholesterol (TC), total triglycerides (TG), low-density lipoprotein cholesterol (LDL-C), fasting glucose (Glu), and hemoglobin a1c (HbA1c). In addition, the SBP, DBP, CREA, CRP, Hcy, Ang II, and CAP percentages were shown to gradually increase between the grade I, grade II, and grade III groups. The history in the grade II and grade III groups was higher than that in the grade I group, while the level of high-density lipoprotein cholesterol (HDL-C) in the grade III group was lower than that of the other two groups. The clinical characteristics of each group are listed in Table 1.

In addition, the dipper group and nondipper group exhibited higher SBP, DBP, CREA, CRP, Hcy, and Ang II when compared to the control group. Moreover, SBP and CRP were higher in the dipper group when compared with the nondipper group, while DBP, HR, CREA, and CAP percentages exhibited the opposite trend. The clinical characteristics of the dipper and nondipper groups are listed in Table 2.

Table 2: Clinical characteristics in the dipper group and nondipper group.

| Characteristics | Control | Hypertension | |
|---|---|---|---|
| | | Dipper | Nondipper |
| Age (years) | 48.2 ± 9.4 | 48.0 ± 10.1 | 47.5 ± 8.9 |
| Male (*n*, %) | 66 (66.0) | 167 (69.6) | 120 (75.0) |
| Smoking (*n*, %) | 33 (33.0) | 78 (32.5) | 77 (48.1)$^{*,\#}$ |
| History (years) | — | 9.9 ± 7.5 | 10.5 ± 8.8 |
| SBP (mmHg) | 111 ± 11 | 167 ± 15$^*$ | 163 ± 11$^{*,\#}$ |
| DBP (mmHg) | 74 ± 8 | 94 ± 9$^*$ | 96 ± 10$^*$ |
| HR (HR) | 68 ± 6 | 71 ± 9$^*$ | 68 ± 8$^\#$ |
| BMI (kg/m$^2$) | 24.5 ± 3.1 | 24.5 ± 2.8 | 25.0 ± 3.4 |
| TC (mmol/L) | 4.5 ± 0.8 | 4.4 ± 0.8 | 4.5 ± 0.9 |
| TG (mmol/L) | 1.8 ± 1.1 | 1.8 ± 1.1 | 1.9 ± 1.2 |
| HDL-C (mmol/L) | 1.3 ± 0.3 | 1.1 ± 0.3$^*$ | 1.2 ± 0.4 |
| LDL-C (mmol/L) | 2.6 ± 0.7 | 2.6 ± 0.7 | 2.8 ± 0.9 |
| Glu (mmol/L) | 5.4 ± 0.6 | 5.4 ± 0.7 | 5.6 ± 0.9 |
| HbAlc (%) | 4.7 ± 0.8 | 4.5 ± 0.7 | 4.5 ± 0.9 |
| CRRA (μmol/L) | 71 ± 11 | 90 ± 18$^*$ | 97 ± 23$^{*,\#}$ |
| CRP (mg/L) | 0.9 ± 0.6 | 7.4 ± 4.6$^*$ | 5.4 ± 2.9$^{*,\#}$ |
| Hcy (pg/mL) | 10.6 ± 3.4 | 15.1 ± 5.7$^*$ | 15.6 ± 6.4$^*$ |
| Ang II (pg/mL) | 34.9 ± 14.1 | 57.1 ± 24.7$^*$ | 58.1 ± 26.2$^*$ |
| CAP | — | 109 (45.4) | 91 (56.9)$^*$ |
| Medical treatments (*n*, %) | | | |
| ACEI/ARB | — | 146 (60.8) | 98 (61.2) |
| β-Blocker | — | 101 (40.1) | 78 (48.8) |
| CCB | — | 200 (83.3) | 138 (86.3) |
| Diuretics | — | 141 (58.8) | 101 (63.1) |

$^*p < 0.05$ vs. the control group; $^\#p < 0.05$ vs. the dipper group.

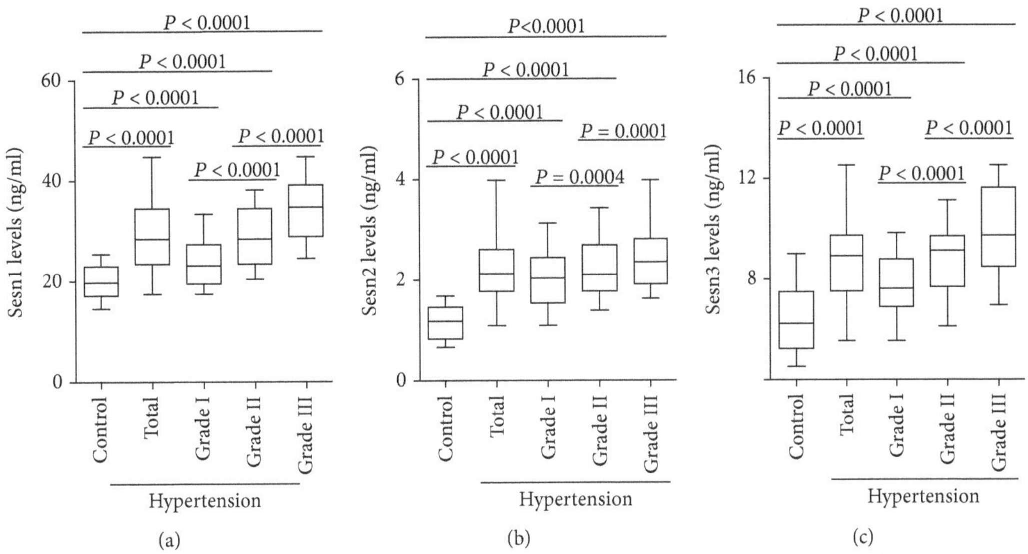


FIGURE 1: Circulating Sesn levels in normotensive subjects (control) and hypertension patients. (a) Plasma Sesn1 levels in the control group ($n = 100$), total hypertension group ($n = 400$), grade I group ($n = 140$), grade II group ($n = 180$), and grade III group ($n = 80$) were measured using ELISA kits. (b) Plasma Sesn2 levels were detected in each group. (c) Plasma levels of Sesn3 were determined in the four groups.

*3.2. Plasma Sesn1, Sesn2, and Sesn3 Levels Were Increased in Hypertension Patients.* Plasma Sesn1 levels were significantly increased in hypertension patients when compared with the control group and gradually increased between the grade I, grade II, and grade III groups (Figure 1(a)). Plasma Sesn2 and Sesn3 exhibited similar trends to Sesn1 (Figures 1(b) and 1(c)). Furthermore, plasma Sesn1, Sesn2, and Sesn3 levels were positively correlated to both SBP and DBP in hypertension patients. The $r$ values and $p$ values are listed in Table 3.

*3.3. Nondipper Hypertension Patients Exhibited Higher Sesn1, Sesn2, and Sesn3 Levels.* According to the results of the ambulatory blood pressure monitoring, the hypertension patients were divided into the dipper and nondipper groups. The ELISA results revealed that plasma Sesn1, Sesn2, and Sesn3 levels gradually increased between the dipper and nondipper groups (Figures 2(a)–2(c)).

*3.4. Effects of Clinical Characteristics on Plasma Sesn1, Sesn2, and Sesn3 Levels.* Subjects were divided into two groups based on the median of several characteristics, such as HDL-C, CREA, CRP, Hcy, Ang II, smoking status, CAP, and medication use. The results showed that smokers and patients with CAP and higher Ang II (≥Median) exhibited higher plasma Sesn1, Sesn2, and Sesn3 levels. HDL-C, CREA, CRP, Hcy, and use of ACEI/ARB, $\beta$-blockers, CCB, and diuretics did not affect Sesn expression. Sesn1, Sesn2, and Sesn3 levels in each group are listed in Table 4.

*3.5. Sesn1, Sesn2, and Sesn3 Were Negatively Correlated with CAP Occurrence.* To determine the effects of Sesns on CAP occurrence, Sesn1, Sesn2, and Sesn3 levels, as well as smoking status, SBP, DBP, LDL-C, Glu, CRP, Hcy, and Ang II were used to perform simple linear regression analysis. The results revealed that Sesn1, Sesn2, Sesn3, smoking, SBP, DBP, CRP, Hcy, and Ang II showed a trend. These variables were further used to perform a multivariate linear regression analysis. The results showed that Sesn1, Sesn2, and Sesn3, respectively, were independently associated with the presence of CAP. The $\beta$ value, 95% CI of $\beta$, and $p$ values are listed in Table 5.

TABLE 3: Correlation between blood pressure and the Sesn levels.

| Characteristic | SBP | | DBP | |
|---|---|---|---|---|
| | $r$ value | $p$ value | $r$ value | $p$ value |
| Sesn1 | 0.3262 | <0.0001 | 0.4198 | <0.0001 |
| Sesn2 | 0.4511 | <0.0001 | 0.3309 | <0.0001 |
| Sesn3 | 0.2987 | <0.0001 | 0.4419 | <0.0001 |

## 4. Discussion

In the present study, the plasma levels of the antioxidant proteins Sesn1, Sesn2, and Sesn3 in hypertension patients were detected. The results of our study revealed that Sesn1, Sesn2, and Sesn3 levels were significantly increased in hypertension patients when compared with the normotensive subjects. A further analysis showed a positive correlation between plasma Sesn levels and blood pressure values, including SBP and DBP. In addition, we identified a variety of variables, including smoking status, Ang II, and CAP, which could promote Sesn expression. Furthermore, the results of the multiple linear regression analysis suggested that Sesn1, Sesn2, and Sesn3 levels were negatively correlated with the presence of CAP. Our study is the first to show the increased expression of Sesns in hypertension patients, which may have a protective effect against the development of CAP.

Elevated Sesn levels have been widely reported in a variety of diseases. In a previous study, circulating Sesn1, Sesn2, and Sesn3 were reported to be increased in patients with coronary artery diseases, while the amplitude of the increase in

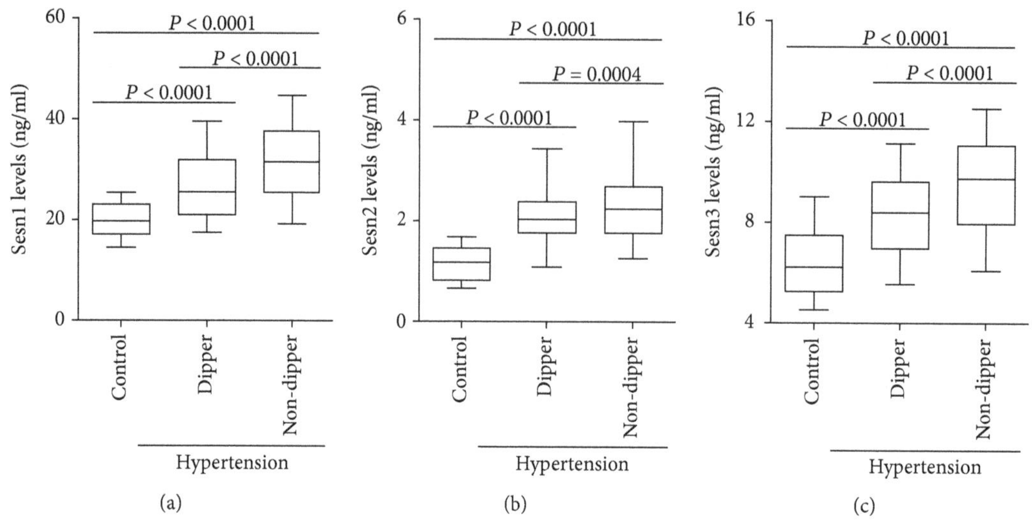


FIGURE 2: Plasma Sesn levels in dipper hypertension and nondipper hypertension patients. The plasma (a) Sesn1, (b) Sesn2, and (c) Sesn3 levels in the control group ($n = 100$), dipper hypertension group ($n = 240$) and nondipper hypertension group ($n = 160$) were analyzed by ELISA.

TABLE 4: Sesn levels according to characteristics in hypertensive patients.

| Characteristics | Factors | Sesn1 (ng/mL) | Sesn2 (ng/mL) | Sesn3 (ng/mL) |
|---|---|---|---|---|
| Smoking | Yes | 30.6 ± 7.9 | 2.49 ± 0.81* | 9.44 ± 2.8* |
| | No | 27.4 ± 5.1 | 2.0 ± 0.51 | 8.1 ± 1.6 |
| HDL-C | ≥Median | 29.1 ± 6.8 | 2.19 ± 0.68 | 8.8 ± 1.7 |
| | <Median | 28.9 ± 7.4 | 2.30 ± 0.64 | 8.7 ± 1.6 |
| CREA | ≥Median | 28.8 ± 5.7 | 2.24 ± 0.69 | 8.8 ± 1.9 |
| | <Median | 29.2 ± 7.6 | 2.25 ± 0.59 | 8.8 ± 1.6 |
| CRP | ≥Median | 30.1 ± 6.7 | 2.39 ± 0.77 | 9.0 ± 2.0 |
| | <Median | 26.9 ± 6.1 | 2.10 ± 0.49 | 8.6 ± 1.5 |
| Hcy | ≥Median | 28.8 ± 5.9 | 2.20 ± 0.62 | 8.7 ± 1.4 |
| | <Median | 29.2 ± 6.5 | 2.29 ± 0.68 | 8.8 ± 1.9 |
| Ang II | ≥Median | 36.6 ± 7.2* | 2.88 ± 0.79* | 10.7 ± 2.4* |
| | <Median | 21.4 ± 5.9 | 1.95 ± 0.54 | 6.8 ± 1.4 |
| CAP | Yes | 32.8 ± 6.9* | 2.69 ± 0.75* | 9.8 ± 2.1* |
| | No | 25.1 ± 6.8 | 1.80 ± 0.66 | 7.7 ± 1.3 |
| ACEI/ARB | Yes | 29.1 ± 5.9 | 2.21 ± 0.49 | 8.7 ± 1.2 |
| | No | 28.8 ± 7.1 | 2.28 ± 0.76 | 8.8 ± 1.5 |
| $\beta$-Blocker | Yes | 28.6 ± 7.3 | 2.19 ± 0.66 | 8.6 ± 1.1 |
| | No | 29.3 ± 7.7 | 2.30 ± 0.74 | 8.9 ± 1.8 |
| CCB | Yes | 29.1 ± 7.9 | 2.24 ± 0.61 | 8.8 ± 1.6 |
| | No | 28.8 ± 7.1 | 2.24 ± 0.77 | 8.8 ± 2.0 |
| Diuretics | Yes | 28.9 ± 5.5 | 2.27 ± 0.55 | 8.7 ± 1.5 |
| | No | 29.1 ± 7.9 | 2.22 ± 0.81 | 8.8 ± 2.4 |

*$p < 0.05$.

TABLE 5: Association between plasma Sesns and the presence of CAP was assessed by simple linear regression analysis and subsequent multiple linear regression analysis.

| Variables | Simple linear | | | Multiple linear | | |
|---|---|---|---|---|---|---|
| | $\beta$ | 95% CI | $p$ value | $\beta$ | 95% CI | $p$ value |
| Sesn1 | -0.415 | -0.636 to -0.194 | <0.001 | -0.218 | -0.304 to -0.132 | 0.011 |
| Sesn2 | -0.556 | -0.794 to -0.318 | <0.001 | -0.301 | -0.408 to -0.194 | <0.001 |
| Sesn3 | -0.487 | -0.715 to -0.259 | <0.001 | -0.247 | -0.342 to -0.152 | 0.009 |
| Smoking | 0.339 | 0.154 to 0.524 | 0.002 | 0.144 | 0.086 to 0.201 | 0.039 |
| SBP | 0.357 | 0.167 to 0.547 | 0.009 | 0.157 | 0.094 to 0.220 | 0.068 |
| DBP | 0.289 | 0.115 to 0.463 | 0.011 | 0.112 | 0.052 to 0.172 | 0.104 |
| LDL-C | 0.109 | 0.062 to 0.156 | 0.198 | | | |
| Glu | 0.212 | 0.104 to 0.320 | 0.239 | | | |
| CRP | 0.117 | 0.071 to 0.163 | 0.019 | 0.046 | -0.017 to 0.109 | 0.042 |
| Hcy | 0.098 | 0.047 to 0.149 | 0.026 | 0.087 | 0.022 to 0.152 | 0.672 |
| Ang II | 0.614 | 0.383 to 0.845 | <0.001 | 0.356 | 0.455 to 0.257 | <0.001 |

Sesn levels was closely related to the degree of stenosis and oxidative stress in CAD patients [15]. In another study of human aortic dissection, plasma Sesn2 levels were found to be positively correlated with MDA levels and negatively correlated with SOD levels [16]. Considering that oxidative stress is the most important factor that affects Sesn expression, we suspected that the level of increase in Sesn expression may reflect the severity of the oxidative stress. Indeed, treatment with Ang II and oxidized low-density lipoprotein, which were shown to induce intense oxidative stress, increased Sesn2 mRNA levels in macrophages in a dose-dependent manner [17, 23, 24]. These findings further support our hypothesis that there is a strong association between oxidative stress levels and Sesn expression and that they can influence each other.

In this study, we found that plasma Sesn levels were increased in patients with hypertension and were positively correlated with the value of blood pressure. These results suggest that there are different degrees of oxidative stress imbalance among hypertensive patients. Moreover, intense oxidative stress may be one of the key players in the pathogenesis of hypertension. As such, it may be useful to pay attention to the dynamic changes in both blood pressure and oxidative stress.

In healthy subjects, blood pressure variability over a 24 h period presents as a double peak and a valley; namely, the highest blood pressure appears in the morning and afternoon, while the lowest blood pressure appears at night. This is due to a drop in sympathetic nerve excitability in the evenings and is called the dipper blood pressure. In some patients with hypertension, this blood pressure trend is disrupted and the blood pressure at night is higher than that in the morning, which is called nondipper hypertension. Since nondipper hypertension is not easy to detect and the damage to target organs is significantly higher than that of dipper hypertension, nondipper hypertension is more harmful to patients [25, 26]. There is evidence that sympathetic excitation promotes the release of large amounts of peroxidation-related substances [27]. In our study, we found a significant increase in Sesn levels in nondipper hypertension patients, which represents excessive oxidative stress. One possible reason is that sympathetic hyperactivity may mediate the formation of nondipper hypertension by enhancing oxidative stress and that reducing the oxidative stress levels may be beneficial to the treatment of nondipper hypertension and the reduction of target organ injury mediated by this condition.

Previously, we revealed that Sesns are involved in the regulation of hypertension, mainly via its antioxidant effects. In an early study, Yang et al. reported that silencing Sesn2 aggravated oxidative stress and elevated the blood pressure in dopamine D2 receptor (D2R) knockout-induced hypertension mice [28]. In a recent study, Xiao et al. found that Sesn2 promoted the expression of the nuclear factor erythroid-2-related factor-2 (Nrf2), which then alleviated Ang II-induced smooth muscle cells apoptosis [17]. While we found that Sesn levels increase in the oxidative stress environment of hypertension, the conclusion of the studies mentioned above seems to contradict our results. One possible explanation is that Sesn levels increase in response to oxidative stress and that Sesns act as antioxidants that protects organs and tissues from damage.

Smoking, angiotensin, atherosclerosis, and a variety of antihypertensive drugs are closely related to oxidative stress [29–31]. To determine whether these factors affect Sesn expression, the hypertension patients were divided into 2 groups. The results showed that patients with higher Ang II, smoking, and CAP exhibited higher plasma Sesn1, Sesn2, and Sesn3 levels, while other factors and the use of antihypertensive drugs did not affect Sesn expression. To investigate the role of Sesns in the occurrence of CAP, multivariate linear regression analysis was performed. The results revealed that Sesn1, Sesn2, and Sesn3 were independently associated with the presence of CAP. These results suggest that Sesns may be useful in preventing and delaying the development and progression of atherosclerosis. However, this hypothesis requires further confirmation in animal models.

In conclusion, we found that plasma Sesn1, Sesn2, and Sesn3 levels were increased in hypertension patients and positively correlated to the blood pressure values. Nondipper hypertension patients exhibited higher plasma Sesn1, Sesn2, and Sesn3 levels when compared to dipper hypertension patients. Moreover, Sesns may be involved in hypertension or CAP through the regulation of oxidative stress. As such, Sesns may be a novel target for the treatment and prevention of hypertension and CAP. However, there were some limitations in the present study. The oxidative stress markers such as SOD and MDA levels were not quantified in the patients included in the study, and the correlation between SOD, MDA, and Sesns was not analyzed. Moreover, while there is a strong relationship between inflammatory response and oxidative stress, Sesn expression and oxidative stress levels can affect each other. However, we did not explore the potential link between them.

## Authors' Contributions

Cao Fang and Zicong Yang contributed equally to this work.

## References

[1] A. Agita and M. T. Alsagaff, "Inflammation, immunity, and hypertension," *Acta Medica Indonesiana*, vol. 49, no. 2, pp. 158–165, 2017.

[2] E. L. Schiffrin, "Immune mechanisms in hypertension and vascular injury," *Clinical Science*, vol. 126, no. 4, pp. 267–274, 2014.

[3] P. Pignatelli, D. Menichelli, D. Pastori, and F. Violi, "Oxidative stress and cardiovascular disease: new insights," *Kardiologia Polska*, vol. 76, no. 4, pp. 713–722, 2018.

[4] D. La Russa, E. Brunelli, and D. Pellegrino, "Oxidative imbalance and kidney damage in spontaneously hypertensive rats: activation of extrinsic apoptotic pathways," *Clinical Science*, vol. 131, no. 13, pp. 1419–1428, 2017.

[5] E. Brunelli, D. La Russa, and D. Pellegrino, "Impaired oxidative status is strongly associated with cardiovascular risk factors," *Oxidative Medicine and Cellular Longevity*, vol. 2017, Article ID 6480145, 11 pages, 2017.

[6] N. Sinha and P. K. Dabla, "Oxidative stress and antioxidants in hypertension-a current review," *Current Hypertension Reviews*, vol. 11, no. 2, pp. 132–142, 2015.

[7] M. Cordani, M. Sánchez-Álvarez, R. Strippoli, A. V. Bazhin, and M. Donadelli, "Sestrins at the interface of ROS control and autophagy regulation in health and disease," *Oxidative Medicine and Cellular Longevity*, vol. 2019, Article ID 1283075, 11 pages, 2019.

[8] S. D. Chen, J. L. Yang, T. K. Lin, and D. I. Yang, "Emerging roles of sestrins in neurodegenerative diseases: counteracting oxidative stress and beyond," *Journal of Clinical Medicine*, vol. 8, no. 7, p. 1001, 2019.

[9] M. Wang, Y. Xu, J. Liu et al., "Recent insights into the biological functions of sestrins in health and disease," *Cellular Physiology and Biochemistry*, vol. 43, no. 5, pp. 1731–1741, 2018.

[10] A. A. Dalina, I. E. Kovaleva, and A. V. Budanov, "Sestrins are gatekeepers in the way from stress to aging and disease," *Molekuliarnaia Biologiia*, vol. 52, no. 6, pp. 948–962, 2018.

[11] J. H. Yang, K. M. Kim, M. G. Kim et al., "Role of sestrin2 in the regulation of proinflammatory signaling in macrophages," *Free Radical Biology & Medicine*, vol. 78, pp. 156–167, 2015.

[12] A. L. B. C. Morsch, E. Wisniewski, T. F. Luciano et al., "Cigarette smoke exposure induces ROS-mediated autophagy by regulating sestrin, AMPK, and mTOR level in mice," *Redox Report*, vol. 24, no. 1, pp. 27–33, 2019.

[13] S. Rafia and S. Saran, "Sestrin-like protein from dictyostelium discoideum is involved in autophagy under starvation stress," *Microbiological Research*, vol. 220, pp. 61–71, 2019.

[14] H. H. Liao, J. Y. Ruan, H. J. Liu, Y. Liu, H. Feng, and Q. Z. Tang, "Sestrin family may play important roles in the regulation of cardiac pathophysiology," *International Journal of Cardiology*, vol. 202, pp. 183-184, 2016.

[15] J. Ye, M. Wang, Y. Xu et al., "Sestrins increase in patients with coronary artery disease and associate with the severity of coronary stenosis," *Clinica Chimica Acta*, vol. 472, pp. 51–57, 2017.

[16] R. Xue, J. Zeng, Y. Chen et al., "Sestrin 1 ameliorates cardiac hypertrophy via autophagy activation," *Journal of Cellular and Molecular Medicine*, vol. 21, no. 6, pp. 1193–1205, 2017.

[17] T. Xiao, L. Zhang, Y. Huang et al., "Sestrin2 increases in aortas and plasma from aortic dissection patients and alleviates angiotensin II-induced smooth muscle cell apoptosis via the Nrf2 pathway," *Life Sciences*, vol. 218, pp. 132–138, 2019.

[18] H. Wang, N. Li, X. Shao et al., "Increased plasma sestrin2 concentrations in patients with chronic heart failure and predicted the occurrence of major adverse cardiac events: a 36-month follow-up cohort study," *Clinica Chimica Acta*, vol. 495, pp. 338–344, 2019.

[19] A. Morrison, L. Chen, J. Wang et al., "Sestrin2 promotes LKB1-mediated AMPK activation in the ischemic heart," *The FASEB Journal*, vol. 29, no. 2, pp. 408–417, 2014.

[20] Y. C. Zeng, F. Chi, R. Xing et al., "Sestrin2 protects the myocardium against radiation-induced damage," *Radiation and Environmental Biophysics*, vol. 55, no. 2, pp. 195–202, 2016.

[21] N. Quan, L. Wang, X. Chen et al., "Sestrin2 prevents age-related intolerance to post myocardial infarction via AMPK/PGC-1$\alpha$ pathway," *Journal of Molecular and Cellular Cardiology*, vol. 115, pp. 170–178, 2018.

[22] B. Dong, R. Xue, Y. Sun, Y. Dong, and C. Liu, "Sestrin 2 attenuates neonatal rat cardiomyocyte hypertrophy induced by phenylephrine via inhibiting ERK1/2," *Molecular and Cellular Biochemistry*, vol. 433, no. 1-2, pp. 113–123, 2017.

[23] L. Yi, F. Li, Y. Yong et al., "Upregulation of sestrin-2 expression protects against endothelial toxicity of angiotensin II," *Cell Biology and Toxicology*, vol. 30, no. 3, pp. 147–156, 2014.

[24] H. J. Hu, Z. Y. Shi, X. L. Lin, S. M. Chen, Q. Y. Wang, and S. Y. Tang, "Upregulation of Sestrin2 expression protects against macrophage apoptosis induced by oxidized low-density lipoprotein," *DNA and Cell Biology*, vol. 34, no. 4, pp. 296–302, 2015.

[25] Y. Chen, J. H. Liu, Z. Zhen et al., "Assessment of left ventricular function and peripheral vascular arterial stiffness in patients with dipper and non-dipper hypertension," *Journal of Investigative Medicine*, vol. 66, no. 2, pp. 319–324, 2018.

[26] E. Aksit, E. Gursul, F. Aydin, M. Samsa, and F. Ozcelik, "Non-dipper hypertension is associated with slow coronary flow among hypertensives with normal coronary angiogram," *Cardiovascular Journal of Africa*, vol. 28, no. 1, pp. 14–18, 2017.

[27] R. S. Moheimani, M. Bhetraratana, F. Yin et al., "Increased cardiac sympathetic activity and oxidative stress in habitual electronic cigarette users: implications for cardiovascular risk," *JAMA Cardiology*, vol. 2, no. 3, pp. 278–284, 2017.

[28] Y. Yang, S. Cuevas, S. Yang et al., "Sestrin2 decreases renal oxidative stress, lowers blood pressure, and mediates dopamine D2 receptor-induced inhibition of reactive oxygen species production," *Hypertension*, vol. 64, no. 4, pp. 825–832, 2014.

[29] L. Zuo, F. He, G. G. Sergakis et al., "Interrelated role of cigarette smoking, oxidative stress, and immune response in COPD and corresponding treatments," *American Journal of Physiology-Lung Cellular and Molecular Physiology*, vol. 307, no. 3, pp. L205–L218, 2014.

[30] H. N. Siti, Y. Kamisah, and J. Kamsiah, "The role of oxidative stress, antioxidants and vascular inflammation in cardiovascular disease (a review)," *Vascular Pharmacology*, vol. 71, pp. 40–56, 2015.

[31] G. Zhou, X. Liu, A. K. Cheung, and Y. Huang, "Efficacy of aliskiren, compared with angiotensin II blockade, in slowing the progression of diabetic nephropathy in db/db mice: should the combination therapy be a focus?," *American Journal of Translational Research*, vol. 7, no. 5, pp. 825–840, 2015.

# Permissions

All chapters in this book were first published by Hindawi Publishing Corporation; hereby published with permission under the Creative Commons Attribution License or equivalent. Every chapter published in this book has been scrutinized by our experts. Their significance has been extensively debated. The topics covered herein carry significant findings which will fuel the growth of the discipline. They may even be implemented as practical applications or may be referred to as a beginning point for another development.

The contributors of this book come from diverse backgrounds, making this book a truly international effort. This book will bring forth new frontiers with its revolutionizing research information and detailed analysis of the nascent developments around the world.

We would like to thank all the contributing authors for lending their expertise to make the book truly unique. They have played a crucial role in the development of this book. Without their invaluable contributions this book wouldn't have been possible. They have made vital efforts to compile up to date information on the varied aspects of this subject to make this book a valuable addition to the collection of many professionals and students.

This book was conceptualized with the vision of imparting up-to-date information and advanced data in this field. To ensure the same, a matchless editorial board was set up. Every individual on the board went through rigorous rounds of assessment to prove their worth. After which they invested a large part of their time researching and compiling the most relevant data for our readers.

The editorial board has been involved in producing this book since its inception. They have spent rigorous hours researching and exploring the diverse topics which have resulted in the successful publishing of this book. They have passed on their knowledge of decades through this book. To expedite this challenging task, the publisher supported the team at every step. A small team of assistant editors was also appointed to further simplify the editing procedure and attain best results for the readers.

Apart from the editorial board, the designing team has also invested a significant amount of their time in understanding the subject and creating the most relevant covers. They scrutinized every image to scout for the most suitable representation of the subject and create an appropriate cover for the book.

The publishing team has been an ardent support to the editorial, designing and production team. Their endless efforts to recruit the best for this project, has resulted in the accomplishment of this book. They are a veteran in the field of academics and their pool of knowledge is as vast as their experience in printing. Their expertise and guidance has proved useful at every step. Their uncompromising quality standards have made this book an exceptional effort. Their encouragement from time to time has been an inspiration for everyone.

The publisher and the editorial board hope that this book will prove to be a valuable piece of knowledge for researchers, students, practitioners and scholars across the globe.

# List of Contributors

**Talha Ahmed**
Department of Medicine, University of Maryland Midtown Campus, USA

**Gautam V. Ramani**
Department of Medicine, University of Maryland, USA

**Mehrdad Ghoreishi and Bartley P. Griffith**
Department of Surgery, University of Maryland, USA

**Ayesha Safdar**
Army Medical College, Pakistan

**Chuanchen Zhang and Shuhua Li**
Department of Radiology, Liaocheng People's Hospital, Shandong University, 67 Dongchang West Road, Liaocheng District, Shandong 252000, China

**Xiaoyong Huang**
Department of Radiology, Anzhen Hospital, Capital Medical University, 2 Anzhen Road, Chaoyang District, Beijing 100029, China

**Hengchen Yao**
Department of Cardiology, Liaocheng People's Hospital, Shandong University, 67 Dongchang West Road, Liaocheng District, Shandong 252000, China

**Bin Zhang**
Department of Surgery, Liaocheng People's Hospital, Shandong University, 67 Dongchang West Road, Liaocheng District, Shandong 252000, China

**Narangoda Liyanage Ajantha Shyamali**
University of Sri Jayewardenepura, Gangodawila, Nugegoda, Sri Lanka

**Chandrike Ponnamperuma**
National Hospital of Sri Lanka, Colombo 10, Sri Lanka

**Mahmood Mubasher, Amir Hanafi, Tausif Syed, Abir Zinal, Ibrahim Y. Abubeker, Mohan Rao and Ryan Hoefen**
Rochester Regional Health-Unity Hospital, Rochester, NY, USA

**Mouhand F. H. Mohamed and Mohammed Danjuma**
Internal Medicine Department, Hamad General Hospital, Hamad Medical, Corporation, Doha, Qatar

**Raunak Rao, Spoorthy Kulkarni and Ian B. Wilkinson**
Division of Experimental Medicine and Immunotherapeutics, University of Cambridge, Cambridge, UK

**Kanyanatt Boonyatarp**
Department of Internal Medicine, Lampang Hospital, Lampang, Tailand

**Kanoksri Samintharapanya**
Division of Neurology, Department of Internal Medicine, Lampang Hospital, Lampang, Tailand

**Thanawat Vongchaiudomchoke**
Division of Nephrology, Department of Internal Medicine, Lampang Hospital, Lampang, Tailand

**Nuttaya Wachiraphansakul**
Division of Endocrinology and Metabolism, Department of Internal Medicine, Lampang Hospital, Lampang, Tailand

**Elizabeth Walter-Nicolet and Delphine Mitanchez**
Service de Néonatologie, Hôpital Armand Trousseau, AP-HP, Faculté de Médecine, Université Pierre et Marie Curie, 75012 Paris, France

**Magali Leblanc**
Service de Réanimation Néonatale, Hôpital Universitaire D'Angers, 49033 Angers, France

**Marianne Leruez-Ville**
Laboratoire de Virologie, Hôpital Necker-Enfants Malades, AP-HP, Faculté de Médecine, Université Paris-Descartes, 75015 Paris, France

**Philippe Hubert**
Service de Réanimation Polyvalente Pédiatrique et Néonatale, Hôpital Necker-Enfants Malades, AP-HP, Faculté de Médecine, Université Paris-Descartes, 75015 Paris, France

**Barreto Ana Terra Fonseca and Barreto Lucas Vinícius da Fonseca**
Departamento de Medicina, Universidade Federal de Sergipe (UFS), São Cristóvão, SE, Brazil

**Cavalcante Felipe Naze Rodrigues**
Departamento de Medicina, Universidade Tiradentes, Aracaju, SE, Brazil

**Oliveira Joselina Luzia Menezes**
Departamento de Medicina, Universidade Federal de Sergipe (UFS), São Cristóvão, SE, Brazil
Centro de Ensino e Pesquisa da Fundação Lucas, Aracaju, SE, Brazil
Núcleo de Pós-Graduação em Medicina da UFS, São Cristóvão, SE, Brazil

**Almeida-Santos Marcos Antônio**
Departamento de Medicina, Universidade Tiradentes, Aracaju, SE, Brazil
Centro de Ensino e Pesquisa da Fundação Lucas, Aracaju, SE, Brazil

**Garcez Juliane Dantas Seabra**
Departamento de Medicina, Universidade Federal de Sergipe (UFS), São Cristóvão, SE, Brazil
Centro de Ensino e Pesquisa da Fundação Lucas, Aracaju, SE, Brazil

**Barreto-Filho José Augusto Soares**
Departamento de Medicina, Universidade Federal de Sergipe (UFS), São Cristóvão, SE, Brazil
Centro de Ensino e Pesquisa da Fundação Lucas, Aracaju, SE, Brazil
Núcleo de Pós-Graduação em Medicina da UFS, São Cristóvão, SE, Brazil

**Sousa Antônio Carlos Sobral**
Departamento de Medicina, Universidade Federal de Sergipe (UFS), São Cristóvão, SE, Brazil
Centro de Ensino e Pesquisa da Fundação Lucas, Aracaju, SE, Brazil
Núcleo de Pós-Graduação em Medicina da UFS, São Cristóvão, SE, Brazil
The American College of Cardiology, New York, NY, USA

**Bryan Yong**
Clinical School, University of Melbourne, Parkville, Victoria, Australia

**David A. Power**
Department of Nephrology, Austin Health, Studley Road, Heidelberg 3084, Victoria, Australia

**Saurabh Gupta and Jose Melendez**
University of Connecticut Health Center, Farmington, CT 06030, USA

**Apurv Khanna**
SUNY Upstate Medical University, Syracuse, NY 13210, USA

**Yueming Shao, Tingting Qin, Ruihua Zhang, Yu Zhang and Xiaoyu Wen**
Department of Hepatology, First Hospital of Jilin University, Xinmin Street, No. 71, Changchun, Jilin Province 130021, China

**Xin Yin**
Center for Infectious Diseases, West China Hospital of Sichuan University, Chengdu, Sichuan Province 610041, China

**Jozef Bulas, Mária Potolárová, Ján Murín and Martin Haprnda**
1st Department of Internal Medicine, Comenius University, Faculty of Medicine, Mickiewiczova 13, 813 69 Bratislava, Slovakia

**Katarína Kozlíková**
Institute of Medical Physics, Biophysics, Informatics and Telemedicine, Comenius University, Faculty of Medicine, Sasinkova 2, 813 72 Bratislava, Slovakia

**Ján Luha**
Institute of Medical Biology, Genetics and Clinical Genetics, Comenius University, Faculty of Medicine, Sasinkova 4, 813 72 Bratislava, Slovakia

**Chi Zhang, Jun Li, Jian Zhou, Qiaoling Zheng, Ruicong Dong, Enhong Xing and Zhijie Dou**
Affiliated Hospital, Chengde Medical College, Chengde 067000, China

**Mark Hamer**
Psychobiology Group, Department of Epidemiology and Public Health, University College London, 1-19 Torrington Place, London WC1E 6BT, UK

**Nancy Frasure-Smith and François Lespérance,**
Department of Psychiatry and School of Nursing, McGill University CHUM Research Center, QC, Canada
Montreal Heart Institute Research Center, University of Montreal, Montreal, QC, Canada H3C 3J7

**Brian H Harvey**
Unit for Drug Research and Development, Division of Pharmacology, School of Pharmacy, North-West University, Potchefstroom 2520, South Africa

**Nico T Malan and Leoné Malan**
Hypertension in Africa Research Team (HART), School for Physiology, Nutrition, and Consumer Sciences, North-West University, Potchefstroom 2520, South Africa

**Geofrey Musinguzi**
Department of Disease Control and Environmental Health, School of Public Health, Makerere University, Kampala, Uganda
Primary and Interdisciplinary Care, University of Antwerp, Antwerp, Belgium

**Sibyl Anthierens and Hilde Bastiaens**
Primary and Interdisciplinary Care, University of Antwerp, Antwerp, Belgium

**Fred Nuwaha and Rhoda K. Wanyenze**
Department of Disease Control and Environmental Health, School of Public Health, Makerere University, Kampala, Uganda

**Jean-Pierre Van Geertruyden**
International Health, University of Antwerp, Antwerp, Belgium

**Kirubel Zemedkun Gebreselassie**
Epidemiology and Global Health, Department of Public Health and Clinical Medicine, Umeå University, 901 85 Umeå, Sweden

**Mojgan Padyab**
Centre for Population Studies, Ageing and Living Conditions Programme, Umeå University, Umeå, Sweden

**Kenneth Nuamah, Ebenezer Antwi Amankwaah, Daniel Boakye, Samuel Kwame Owusu, Fred Adomako-Boateng and Alexis Nang-Beifubah**
Ashanti Regional Health Directorate, Kumasi, Ghana

**Harriet Affran Bonful**
Department of Epidemiology and Disease Control, School of Public Health, University of Ghana, Legon, Accra, Ghana

**Joseph Danso Yeboah**
Sekyere Central District Health Directorate, Nsuta, Ashanti, Ghana

**Adwoa Aduako Owusu**
Suntreso Government Hospital, Kumasi, Ghana

**Freddie Amponsah and Anthony Ofosu**
Policy Planning Monitoring and Evaluation Division, Ghana Health Service, PMB Ministries, Accra, Ghana

**Margaret Gyapong and Evelyn K. Ansah**
Research Development Division, Ghana Health Service, Accra, Ghana
Institute of Health Research, University of Health & Allied Science, PMB 31, Ho, Ghana

**Bertha Garshong**
Research Development Division, Ghana Health Service, Accra, Ghana

**Wen Zhang and Guiming Deng**
The First Hospital of Hunan University of Chinese Medicine, Department of Geriatrics, No. 95 Shaoshan Middle Road, Yuhua District, Changsha City, Hunan Province, China

**Jia Hu and Junliu Hu**
Hunan University of Chinese Medicine, Graduate School, Xiangzui Road, Yuelu District, Changsha City, Hunan Province, China

**Ran Yan**
Hunan University of Chinese Medicine, School of Traditional Chinese Medicine, Xiangzui Road, Yuelu District, Changsha City, Hunan Province, China

**Jianmin Fan**
The First Hospital of Hunan University of Chinese Medicine, Department of Cardiovascular Diseases, No. 95 Shaoshan Middle Road, Yuhua District, Changsha City, Hunan Province, China

**Hassan Alfraidi**
Section of Pulmonary Medicine, Department of Medicine, University of Manitoba, Winnipeg, MB, Canada
Division of Cardiology, Department of Medicine, McGill University, Montreal, QC, Canada

**Sultan Qanash**
Section of Pulmonary Medicine, Department of Medicine, University of Manitoba, Winnipeg, MB, Canada
King Saud Bin Abdulaziz University for Health Sciences, King Abdulaziz Medical City, Jeddah, Saudi Arabia

**Zoheir Bshouty**
Section of Pulmonary Medicine, Department of Medicine, University of Manitoba, Winnipeg, MB, Canada

**Cao Fang**
Xishui County People's Hospital Affiliated to Hubei University of Science and Technology, Hubei 530021, China

**Zicong Yang, Lei Shi, Tao Zeng, Ying Shi, Ling Liu and Yingzhong Lin**
Department of Cardiology, The People's Hospital of Guangxi Zhuang Autonomous Region, Nanning 530021, China

**Hongtao Liu**
Department of Cardiovascular Medicine, Shenzhen Longhua District Central Hospital, Longhua Central Hospital Affiliated to Guangdong Medical University, Shenzhen, Guangdong Province, 518110, China

# Index

www.ingramcontent.com/pod-product-compliance
Lightning Source LLC
LaVergne TN
LVHW082237200926
848484LV00008B/2365
*9798887406046*